Forensic Learning Series

Forensic Pathology of
Child Death Assessment

For Autopsy Results & Diagnoses

Forensic Learning Series

STM **Learning,** Inc.

Leading Publisher of Scientific, Technical, and Medical Educational Resources

Saint Louis

www.stmlearning.com

Forensic Pathology of
Child Death Assessment

For Autopsy Results & Diagnoses

Forensic Learning Series

Mary E. Case, MD
Professor Emerita of Pathology
St. Louis University School of Medicine
Chief Medical Examiner
St. Louis, St. Charles, Jefferson, and Franklin Counties
St. Louis, Missouri

STM **Learning,** Inc.

Leading Publisher of Scientific, Technical, and Medical Educational Resources
Saint Louis
www.stmlearning.com

Publishers: Glenn E. Whaley and Marianne V. Whaley
Acquisitions Editors: Glenn E. Whaley and Samantha Koester
Graphic Design Director: Glenn E. Whaley
Graphic Designer: Connie H. C. Wang
Color Prepress Specialist: Kevin Tucker
Managing Editor: Holly Henry
Developmental Editor/Curriculum Developer: Olivia Sigmund
Copy Editor: Samantha Koester

Printed in the United States of America.

Publisher:
STM Learning, Inc.
Saint Louis, Missouri 63033
Phone: (314) 434-2424
http://www.stmlearning.com orders@stmlearning.com

Library of Congress Control Number: 2021923417
ISBN 9781953119056 (Print) | ISBN 9781953119063 (eBook)

Foreword

Around 2000 children die in the United States each year from some form of child maltreatment. Within this text, Dr. Mary Case provides a rich and well-organized approach to better understanding what has happened to these children. The forensic pathologist, along with the child death investigation team, is in a vital position to unravel the truth.

Key clusters of injuries help to define abuse in the absence of admission by the perpetrator. In the legal arena, lawyers, judges, and juries want to know what the evidence is and how they can be sure. By systematically showing injuries at all levels and types, it becomes clear how abusive trauma occurs and what happens to the child when it does.

One of the major advantages of this assessment book is the inclusion of detailed case studies, which vividly illustrate key points in the pathological evaluation of suspected child abuse. They help to cement concepts about trauma around the narrative of what has happened to the child. Additionally, this text provides detailed pictures that are rarely seen elsewhere. For students and educators, such high-quality photographs bring to light what words alone cannot.

By providing evidence-based research on various topics, case studies detailing specific instances of child death, images for analysis, and an assessment section designed to ensure the understanding of content, this book engrains in the reader a deeper understanding of forensic pathology and causes of child death as a whole.

Forensic Pathology of Child Death Assessment will be a key resource for those seeking to understand the details of abusive trauma and to make such important diagnoses.

Randell Alexander, MD, PhD
Professor and Chief
Division of Child Protection and Forensic Pediatrics
University of Florida
Jacksonville, Florida

Our Mission

To become the world leader in publishing and information services on child abuse, maltreatment, diseases, and domestic violence. We seek to heighten awareness of these issues and provide relevant information to professionals and consumers.

Preface

My vision for this assessment book was to document the findings of my many years of experience as a forensic pathologist, neuropathologist, and medical examiner and to create a way for members of the child fatality review team, especially forensic pathologists, medical examiners, and coroners, to learn from my experiences and research.

I began handling medical examiner cases in February of 1975 in St. Louis County, Missouri, but I did not see a child abuse fatality in St. Louis County until 1981. From there, the number of abusive fatalities gradually increased over the following years. In 1977, I began working as a medical examiner in the St. Louis City Medical Examiner's Office, which had just transitioned from a coroner's office to a medical examiner's system. When I began managing medical examiner cases in the City of St. Louis, I was struck by the large number of fatal child abuse cases we encountered in our work. I am both a forensic pathologist and a neuropathologist, so my experience with child abuse fatalities has been greatly influenced by my neuropathology background.

In 2014, Elizabeth Kermgard was a medical student at St. Louis University where I was a professor of pathology and is now a pediatric resident. She abstracted much of the data on the cases included in this text which include child deaths from 1999 to 2017 in the St. Louis metropolitan area (ie, St. Louis County and the adjacent counties of St. Charles, Jefferson, and Franklin with a total population of 1.75 million) and the City of St. Louis from 1986 to 1994. Access to the case data from St. Louis City was generously provided by Dr. Michael Graham, Chief Medical Examiner of St. Louis City.

One of the main objectives of this assessment book is to guide the reader through what the medical examiner finds when an autopsy is done by well-trained forensic pathologists. The intent is to document every mark on the child's body, thus every case in this text was performed by a forensic pathologist that I had a role in training and to whom I stressed that a child's autopsy should include documentation of each and every mark on the body. Documentation of each detail is of extreme importance as the mechanisms of accidental death, natural death, and homicide death are considerably different.

A majority of the cases in this book were ruled deaths by homicide, a conclusion that requires medical, social, and investigative histories from birth to the time of the fatal incident. While there was extensive circumstantial and historical information that factored into the determination of the cause and manner of death in each of these cases, only brief histories have been provided in the context of this book for the sake of brevity.

Since 1991, the state of Missouri has had a child fatality review system that is county based and includes members of the medical examiner's office, child and social services, juvenile court, prosecution, police agencies, public health, and a variety of other agencies who might have knowledge of a particular case. Members meet monthly in order to share any new information because it is critical that all members of the child fatality review team have full access to all findings in order to coordinate a successful investigation.

This text and accompanying assessment are written for health professionals, including medical examiners, coroners, and forensic pathologists, and others involved in the investigation of child death, such as social workers, law enforcement, and legal professionals. While the images in this text are often graphic, their intent is to educate and inform, not to shock. The children in this book are gone, but they are not forgotten. Their stories and autopsies will hopefully help us better understand, diagnose, and prevent future child deaths.

Mary E. Case, MD

Reviews

The investigations of sudden unexpected death in children are some of the most challenging for the forensic pathologist. These deaths are even more challenging when they involve neuropathological injury. This book, whose lead author is both a forensic pathologist and neuropathologist, is organized by body region, which offers an extremely practical approach for the forensic pathologist. An entire chapter, as it should be, is devoted to the neuropathology of pediatric head trauma. Detailed discussions of injuries and mechanisms of injury are intermixed with referenced studies which put our understanding of these injuries in proper context and elevate this work beyond the typical descriptive forensic pathology text. It is an academic, well-referenced work that also includes over 150 color images and numerous case studies. Not only will forensic pathologists and fellows find this valuable, but given the well-written, concise discussions and descriptions, the non-medical pediatric death investigator will also find it understandable and beneficial.

Forensic Pathology of Child Death Assessment *is a condensed and restructured version of Dr. Case's original work in an assessment format that includes an assessment section, allowing readers to test their newly gained knowledge. This assessment contains an extra quality educational tool for forensic pathologists, medical examiners, coroners, and others who investigate or teach about these deaths.*

James R. Gill, MD
Chief Medical Examiner
State of Connecticut
Office of the Chief Medical Examiner

Forensic Pathology of Child Death Assessment *demystifies jurisdiction issues and protocol questions that surround pediatric autopsies. An abundance of high resolution color photos adds to the quality of the case discussions and highlights the impact of findings recovered throughout the evaluation of a child's death–from scene investigation findings to hospital documentation and finally post mortem radiographs and the in situ appearance of trauma to the central nervous system, soft tissues, organs, and young bones. This is an impressive and thorough text that will benefit readers across multiple disciplines. Child fatality review team partners working in health care services, law enforcement, social services, and the legal system will be able to practically apply the information presented in this book to better serve child victims.*

Marcella Donaruma, MD, FAAP
Associate Professor of Pediatrics
Baylor College of Medicine
Section of Public Health Pediatrics
Texas Children's Hospital
Houston, TX

As usual, Dr. Mary Case has produced an essential work on the investigation of child death. The writing is brilliantly clear, and the detail is very helpful. I would strongly recommend this book for fellows in child abuse pediatrics who are studying for their board examinations. It would also be helpful for emergency department and pediatric intensive care unit providers to review to understand their roles in documenting and protecting evidence of possible child death. I give this book an A+ for usefulness and thoroughness.

Carole Jenny, MD, MBA, FAAP
Professor Emerita
University of Washington School of Medicine

In her book Forensic Pathology of Child Death Assessment, *Dr. Mary Case offers the reader a comprehensive review of child deaths that is not only a reference for forensic pathologists but can also be useful for forensic autopsy technicians, death investigators, professional nurses, and physician assistants. Dr. Case explores the role of the forensic pathologist and medical examiner/coroner, the medicolegal system's responsibilities, and the components of a forensic autopsy, and she includes photographs that largely depict the information given within the text. Dr. Case explains the deaths and categories of deaths that jurisdiction is taken regarding organ and tissue procurement, and why there is an acute need for children's tissues and organs, and she summarizes the decision-making process of the medical examiner/coroner. She presents case studies with ample photographs that support the importance of being familiar with documentation and bodily injuries when making decisions. This book, with its extensive descriptions, photographs, and discussions, will provide a practical approach to assist in making determinations and decisions when faced with a fatal child maltreatment case.*

Annette A. Cannon, PhD, MA, RN, MSN, D-ABMDI
Jefferson County Coroner
Jefferson County Government
Golden, Colorado

Contents in Brief

Contents in Detail

Forensic Pathology of
Child Death Assessment

For Autopsy Results & Diagnoses

Forensic Learning Series

STM **Learning,** Inc.

Leading Publisher of Scientific, Technical, and Medical Educational Resources
Saint Louis
www.stmlearning.com

Section I

Definitions

Objectives:

After reviewing this section, the reader will be able to:

1. *Clearly identify and define key terms related to forensic pathology.*
2. *Accurately apply terms when analyzing cases of child fatality.*

Instructions:

The following terms are found throughout the text. This section should serve as a convenient reference for readers as they move through the chapters.

— ***Abrasion:*** The wearing away of the upper layer of skin as a result of applied friction force.

— ***Accident:*** A manner of death; an unnatural death resulting from an inadvertent chance happening.

— ***Adrenal glands:*** A small gland located on top of the kidney; sometimes referred to as "suprarenal" gland.

— ***Anoxia:*** An absence or deficiency of oxygen reaching the tissues; severe hypoxia.

— ***Apnea:*** A temporary cessation of breathing.

— ***Ascites:*** The accumulation of fluid in the peritoneal cavity, causing abdominal swelling.

— ***Aspiration:*** The action of drawing a breath and inhaling foreign substances (eg, food particles, objects, or fluid).

— ***Asphyxia:*** The failure of cells to receive or use oxygen.

— ***Autopsy:*** A postmortem assessment or examination of a body to determine the cause of death.

— ***Beta-amyloid precursor protein (BAPP):*** An immunohistochemical stain that is helpful in viewing damaged axons. BAPP staining can demonstrate damage to axons within 2 hours of injury.

— ***Bilateral:*** Affecting both the right and left sides of the body.

— ***Blunt abdominal trauma:*** Forceful impact made to the central abdominal area, typically inflicting injury to the celiac and mesenteric arteries.

— ***Blunt force trauma:*** Physical injury caused by forceful impact with a blunt object (ie, one that does not possess any sharp edges and therefore is nonpenetrating).

— ***Brain contusion:*** A type of traumatic brain injury (TBI) that causes localized bruising of the brain, typically occurring alongside a severe head injury.

— ***Brain death:*** Irreversible cessation of all functions of the entire brain, including the brainstem.

— ***Brain swelling:*** Recognizable by the flattening of the gyral surfaces and narrowing of the sulci, along with the appearance of the brain filling the cranial cavity when the brain is removed. Brain weight is also a good indicator of swelling if the weight is 10% to 15% greater than the expected value.

— ***Bridging vein:*** Arises from the cortical surface of the brain and passes to the dural sinus. Bridging vein failure (and the subsequent bleeding) is the source of subdural bleeding, which begins within the interhemispheric sulcus and spreads out over the cerebral convexities.

— ***Bronchopneumonia:*** A form of pneumonia that affects both the alveoli in the lungs and the bronchi.

— ***Cardiopulmonary resuscitation (CPR):*** A life-saving emergency procedure that involves applying external chest compression in an effort to make the heart pump and restore breathing.

— ***Cause of death:*** The disease or injury that creates the physiologic disturbance that leads to death (eg, a gunshot wound to the chest).

— ***Cecum:*** A small pouch that forms the first portion of the large intestine; connects the small intestine to the colon of the large intestine.

— ***Central nervous system (CNS):*** Comprised of the brain and spinal cord, it is the complex of nerve tissues that controls the activities of the body.

— ***Chemical asphyxia:*** The failure of cells to receive or use oxygen due to the inhaling of a chemical.

— ***Child death review team:*** Varies state to state, but typically consists of a panel of individuals such as the medical examiner, prosecuting attorney, family services employee, law enforcement member, pediatrician, and any other individual who might have information about a particular child's death.

— ***Child protective services (CPS):*** A branch of the state's social services department that is responsible for the assessment, investigation, and intervention regarding cases of child abuse and neglect, including sexual abuse.

— ***Chronic subdural hematoma:*** A liquefied hematoma with a membrane that consists of fibroblastic proliferation and neovascularization.

— ***Closed head trauma:*** An injury to the head that does not pierce the skull (ie, a nonpenetrating head injury). In infants, closed head trauma often results in diffuse brain atrophy.

— ***Computed tomography (CT) scan:*** A common diagnostic imaging procedure that uses x-rays to generate images of the anatomy.

— ***Conjunctiva:*** The clear, thin membrane that covers part of the front surface of the eye and the inner surface of the eyelids. It is comprised of 2 segments: the bulbar conjunctiva and the palpebral conjunctiva.

— ***Contact burns:*** A burn that is the result of contact with a hot object for several seconds; typically have patterns that are recognizable (eg, curling irons, heat grids, cigarettes, irons, heater grates).

— ***Contrecoup contusion:*** An injury that occurs on the opposite side of which the blow or impact was made (eg, the brain hitting the right side of the skull after a blow to the left).

— ***Contusion:*** Also called a ***bruise***; a region of injured soft tissue in which blood vessels have been ruptured as a result of blunt trauma.

— ***Coroner:*** An elected public officer who is typically not required to have specific medical qualifications and whose principal duty is to inquire into the cause of any death in which there is suspicion of unnatural causes.

— ***Craniocerebral trauma:*** Also called ***traumatic brain injury (TBI);*** an injury to the brain from external blunt force (eg, car accident, severe beating, large fall).

— ***Craniotomy:*** A type of surgery in which part of the skull is temporarily removed to expose the brain for repair.

— ***Crepitance:*** Identifiable by an internal crackling sound; occurs when air abnormally infiltrates an area of the body (eg, breathing through an inflamed lung).

— ***Crushing head injury:*** Relatively rare injury that occurs when a heavy weight crushes the stationary head (eg, head being run over by a motor vehicle wheel, a heavy object falling onto the child's head).

— ***Death investigation:*** An investigation that begins when a death is reported to the medicolegal death investigator; the depth of the investigation depends on the complexity of the case and may include a detailed scene investigation. This investigation is separate from the police investigation.

— ***Department of family services (DFS):*** A government-sponsored department that ensures the safety and well-being of children and their families by assisting and supporting caregivers.

— ***Diffuse axonal injury:*** A form of TBI in which the brain's connecting nerve fibers tear; happens when the brain is injured from shifting and rotating inside the skull.

— ***Distended:*** Swollen from internal pressure (eg, an enlarged abdomen).

— ***Distraction injury:*** A rare, abusive injury of the cervical cord; typically results from severe shaking while grasping the head.

— ***Drowning:*** A death as a result of submersion in and inhalation of water. Drowning in all cases, at all ages, is a diagnosis of exclusion. A homicidal drowning in a child is difficult to distinguish from an accidental drowning; however, most homicidal drownings occur alone in the bathtub at an odd time.

— ***Duodenum:*** The first part of the small intestine, leading from the stomach to the jejunum. The location of the duodenum provides some degree of protection against blunt trauma so that, when injury does occur, it is the result of significant force applied to the abdomen.

— ***Dura:*** The toughest, outermost membrane that envelops the brain and spinal cord; made up of fibroblasts and large amounts of extracellular collagen.

— ***Dynamic injury:*** A type of head injury that occurs when force is rapidly loaded onto the head in less than 200 milliseconds; caused by impulse loading or impact loading.

— ***Ecchymosis:*** A discoloration of the skin resulting from ruptured blood vessels.

— ***Edema:*** The swelling of soft tissues as a result of excess fluid accumulation (eg, cerebral edema).

— ***Electrocution:*** A death or injury as a result of electric shock; typically an accident.

— ***Emergency medical services (EMS):*** Emergency services that provide urgent pre-hospital treatment and stabilization for serious illness and injuries as well as transportation to definitive care.

— ***Endocrine system:*** A series of glands that produce and secrete hormones that the body uses for a wide range of functions (eg, respiration, metabolism, and reproduction).

— ***Epidural hemorrhage:*** A traumatic accumulation of blood between the inner table of the skull and the stripped-off dura membrane; results from traumatic head injury.

— ***Erythrocyte:*** A red blood cell that contains hemoglobin, which transports oxygen and carbon monoxide to and from the tissues of the body.

— ***External examination:*** A forensic autopsy of the body in the condition in which it arrived to the morgue. Each anatomic part of the body—face, scalp, neck, chest, abdomen, back, genitalia, buttocks, and extremities—is examined and described regarding the presence of identifying marks, scars, fresh injury, healing injury, and healed injuries.

— ***Failure to thrive:*** Refers to children whose current weight or rate of weight gain and/or height is much lower than that of other children of similar age and sex.

— ***Focal head injury:*** A brain injury that is concentrated in one area of the brain (eg, short fall); this does not mean that only one brain system is affected, however.

— ***Forensic autopsy:*** An autopsy that fulfills the needs of the medical examiner through procedures that are not typically used by other hospital pathologists (eg, the removal of bones, digits, eyes, or inner ears; extensive dissection of soft tissue; other special dissections).

— ***Forensic pathologist:*** Works in the office of the medical examiner; performs autopsies and carries out record reviews to determine cause and manner of death of individuals whose death may have some impact on the well-being of others.

— ***Gyri:*** Ridges or folds between 2 clefts on the cerebral surface in the brain; typically appears flat and mushy after injury.

— ***Head trauma:*** Refers to any injury to the scalp, skull, or brain. As many as 80% of lethal cases of child physical abuse are a result of head trauma.

— ***Hematoma:*** A localized swelling that is filled with blood from a break in the wall of a blood vessel.

— ***Hematomyelia:*** A hemorrhage into the spinal cord, of which trauma is the leading cause.

— ***Hematoxylin-eosin (HE) staining:*** A laboratory method that uses 2 different dyes (hematoxylin and eosin) in order to more clearly identify the parts of a cell. Hematoxylin stains the ribosomes, chromatin within the nucleus, and other structures a deep purple color. Eosin stains the cytoplasm, cell wall, collagen, connective tissue, and other structures that surround and support the cell an orange-pink-red color.

— ***Hemorrhage:*** Bleeding or an abnormal flow of blood; could be external (ie, outside the body) or internal (ie, inside the body).

— ***Histology:*** The study of tissues and cells under a microscope.

— ***Histologic examination:*** Examining tissues and cells under a microscope in order to discover any differential diagnoses that could be attributed to the child's death; also used to evaluate and estimate the age of injuries in child abuse cases.

— ***Hollow viscus injury:*** A blunt force injury to the gastrointestinal system; more common in inflicted abdominal trauma than in accidental trauma, and it most commonly occurs in the proximal small bowel.

— ***Homicide:*** A manner of death; the deliberate and unlawful killing of one person by another.

— ***Hyperpigmentation:*** A common, usually harmless condition in which patches of skin become darker in color than the normal surrounding skin; an excess of melanin deposits in the skin.

— ***Hypopigmentation:*** A condition in which patches of skin appear lighter than the normal surrounding skin; an absence of melanin.

— ***Hypoxic encephalopathy:*** Injury to the cells in the brain and spinal cord as result of inadequate oxygen. Any child found to have hypoxic encephalopathy of undetermined etiology must be thoroughly examined and evaluated for possible asphyxia events.

— ***Ileum:*** The third and last portion of the small intestine; situated between the jejunum and the cecum.

— ***Impact loading:*** Imparts inertial movement of the brain within the cranial cavity causing the brain to move and displace away from the skull (eg, torn bridging veins, traumatic axonal injury).

— ***Impulse loading:*** Caused by an action to the body that causes the head to move (eg, shaking).

— ***Internal examination:*** The viewing, describing, and photographically documenting of injuries to the soft tissue of the anterior surface of the body.

— ***Jejunum:*** The middle portion of the small intestine; situated between the duodenum and the ileum.

— ***Laceration:*** Also called a ***cut***; a tear to skin or flesh.

— ***Leptomeninges:*** The innermost layers of tissue covering the brain and spinal cord. There are 2 layers: the arachnoid mater and pia mater.

— ***Lethal neglect:*** The death of a child as a result of caregivers failing to supply essential requirements that children cannot supply for themselves (eg, food, a safe environment, and medical care).

— ***Ligament of treitz:*** Also called the ***suspensory ligament***; a broad, flat band of smooth muscle and fibrous tissue attached to the right crus of the diaphragm and the duodenum at its junction with the jejunum.

— ***Ligature strangulation:*** Strangulation by means of a constricting cord or band (eg, jump rope, electrical cord, belt).

— ***Magnetic resonance imaging (MRI):*** A non-invasive imaging technology that produces a 3-dimensional detailed anatomical image.

— ***Malnutrition:*** Any condition in which the body does not receive enough nutrients for proper function. In many child abuse cases, malnutrition is a result of the caregiver failing to feed the child(ren).

— ***Manner of death:*** Describes how the cause of death occurred. Manners of death include natural, accident, suicide, homicide, and undetermined.

— ***Marantic endocarditis:*** Lesions on otherwise undamaged heart valves without a bacterial infection; lesions may be microscopic or large enough to visualize.

— ***Mastoid:*** The rounded protrusion of bone just behind the ear.

— ***Mechanical asphyxia:*** Physical force or abnormality that interferes with the uptake and/or delivery of oxygen (eg, strangulation at the hands of another).

— ***Mechanism of death:*** The pathophysiologic derangements that result in death (eg, exsanguination, renal failure, respiratory failure, cardiac arrest).

— ***Medical child abuse (MCA):*** Previously called ***Munchausen syndrome by proxy***. A child receiving unnecessary and harmful or potentially harmful medical care at the instigation of the caretaker. It is a factitious disorder in which a parent, usually the mother, either feigns a disorder in a child or creates an illness by some harmful practice, such as dosing the child with adult blood pressure medication or injecting fecal material into the child. This results in medical investigation with extensive testing and diagnostic procedures in an attempt to determine the source of the problem.

— ***Medical examiner:*** An appointed public officer who is typically required to have specific medical training (ie, pathology) and is qualified to conduct medical examinations and autopsies; has similar duties to a coroner.

— ***Medicolegal death investigator:*** Death investigations begin with a report to these persons. Their duties include taking telephone reports of deaths, responding to death scenes and carrying out death scene investigations, obtaining a thorough history from the victim (eg, development, social, and family history), ordering medical records and police reports, and arranging the transportation of bodies to the medical examiner's office.

— ***Medicolegal system:*** An interdependent system that relies on both medicine and law.

— ***Mesentery:*** A fold of the peritoneum that attaches the intestines and other organs to the posterior wall of the abdomen.

— ***Metabolic acidosis:*** A condition in which the fluids of the body contain too much acid.

— ***Microscopic examination:*** An examination of tissue or bone that is too small to be viewed with the naked eye; thus, the examination is done under a microscope.

— ***Neuropathology:*** The study of diseases or injuries to the central nervous system, typically using microscopic examination techniques.

— ***Optic nerve sheath hemorrhage:*** Commonly associated with the retinal hemorrhages that accompany abusive head trauma in young children. Blood in the optic nerve sheath may also be seen in other causes of intracranial hemorrhage not associated with abusive injury.

— ***Ora serrata:*** Located in the eye, it is the serrated junction between the ciliary body and the retina. It marks the transition from the non-photosensitive area of the retina to the photosensitive area.

— ***Pattern injury:*** An imprint left on the skin that is in the pattern of the object that caused injury (eg, belt buckle).

— ***Petechial hemorrhages:*** Also called ***petechiae***, small, pin-point size red/purple marks left on the skin as a result of asphyxia. Petechial hemorrhages are typically found in cases of manual strangulation or smothering.

— ***Parietal peritoneum:*** The section of the peritoneum that lines the abdominal walls.

— ***Periosteal reaction:*** A radiographic finding that indicates irritation to the periosteum.

— ***Peritoneal cavity:*** A potential space that is situated between the parietal peritoneum and the visceral peritoneum; typically only a thin film containing peritoneal fluid, but it is called a "potential" space because excess fluid may accumulate.

— ***Poisoning:*** Occurs as a result of the inhalation, injection, or absorption of a toxic substance. Children may be poisoned by a variety of substances, including medications, alcohol, drugs, and even salt or water.

— ***Purulent peritonitis:*** An inflammation of the peritoneum located in the abdomen.

— ***Radiographs:*** A photograph that is created using a form of radiation; either an x-ray or a gamma ray photograph. In most medical examiner offices, all children under 3 will have radiographs taken, as well as older children in specific cases.

— ***Renal failure:*** A type of mechanism of death; happens when the kidneys cease to function properly, meaning that they are unable to remove waste and excess water from the blood stream and cannot regulate body chemicals.

— ***Retinal hemorrhage:*** Bleeding in the retina of the eye.

— ***Retinoschisis:*** The splitting of the layers of the retina. The condition results from vitreous traction on the retina during acceleration-deceleration motions of the head transmitted to the eye. It is highly associated with acceleration-deceleration abusive head injury.

— ***Scalding burns:*** Produced by holding someone under hot water or submerging someone in a tub or sink of hot water.

— ***Scaphoid:*** Refers to the shape of a body part (ie, concave, boat-shaped, hollow).

— ***Scene:*** The location where the incident surrounding the death or injury occurred.

— ***Scene investigation:*** An investigation with the purpose of assessing the scene, the circumstances, and the body if it is still in place; or, if the body has been transported for care, an assessment of the site where the child was found.

— ***Scene recreation:*** A recreation of the scene in which a child was found or a demonstration of how the child was injured using a scene recreation doll; allows the investigator to photographically document a complex scene.

— ***Sepsis:*** The body's extreme response to an infection; occurs when an existing infection triggers a chain reaction throughout the body. In cases of suspected infection, swabs, blood, or cerebrospinal fluid may be obtained postmortem and sent for culture to a microbiology laboratory.

— ***Shaken baby syndrome:*** A severe brain injury caused by forcefully shaking a young child; used to describe situations in which infants present with subdural or subarachnoid hemorrhages, retinal hemorrhages, and little or no extreme marks of trauma to the head. Evidence of shaking includes 2 or more of the following: (1) fingermarks and/or rib fractures, (2) subdural and/or subarachnoid hemorrhage, and (3) a history of vigorous shaking.

— ***Small bowel:*** Also called ***small intestine***; most commonly injured organ in inflicted abdominal trauma.

— ***Smothering:*** Caused by occluding the nose and mouth; can be easily done to children and infants without always leaving evidence.

— ***Static injury:*** Occurs over longer periods of time, usually longer than 200 milliseconds; causes crushing head injury.

— ***Strangulation:*** A type of asphyxial death that can be manual or ligature; the compression of the neck structure to cease the circulation of blood and oxygen. Strangulation in infants and young children is difficult to recognize due to a typical lack of any external markings on the neck, lack of petechial hemorrhages, or lack of internal injury to the muscles, hyoid, or larynx.

— ***Stress cardiomyopathy:*** Lesions in the heart believed to be related to catecholamine release from stress, causing damage to the heart.

— ***Subarachnoid hemorrhage:*** Bleeding into the space between the brain its surrounding membrane (ie, the subarachnoid space). This can be caused by head trauma and is life-threatening, especially if the injury goes untreated.

— ***Subdural hemorrhage:*** Also called ***subdural hematoma***; bleeding that often occurs outside of the brain tissue due to ruptured blood vessels, often from head trauma. Subdural hemorrhage is present in 90% to 95% of cases of fatal inflicted head injury at autopsy and can be imaged in 40% to 55% of living children with such head injuries.

— ***Subgaleal hemorrhage:*** A large collection of blood in the soft tissue space between the galea aponeurotica and the skull's periosteum. When a subgaleal hemorrhage is considered "massive," it may lead to profound hypovolemic shock.

— ***Subtle lethal abusive injury:*** In contrast to overt forms of child maltreatment, subtle lethal child abuse injuries are sustained through drownings, poisonings, asphyxia, and neglect of medical care, safety, or nutrition. In cases of subtle lethal deaths, deciding the manner of death can be a difficult choice.

— ***Sudden infant death syndrome (SIDS):*** Also called ***sudden unexpected infant death (SUID)*** or sleep-related infant death; describes the sudden and unexpected death of an infant less than 1 year of age, typically while sleeping. There is currently no known cause.

— ***Suffocation:*** A type of asphyxial death that includes entrapment, smothering, choking, mechanical asphyxia, and/or suffocating gases; the death results from oxygen deprivation.

— ***Suicide:*** A manner of death; death as a result of causing lethal harm to oneself with the intent of dying.

— ***Thermal injury:*** Occurs when there is excessive heat applied to the skin (eg, burns from an oven, iron, hot liquid, or flames) or from indirect heat (eg, radiation).

— ***Thoracic cavity:*** The cavity composing the thorax; located under the diaphragm and enclosed by the sternum, ribs (including the heart and lungs), and thoracic vertebrae.

— ***Thoracic injury:*** Injury to the thorax or thoracic cavity.

— ***Thorax:*** The section of the body between the neck and the abdomen; contains the thoracic cavity.

— ***Toxicology:*** During the autopsy, specimens are taken of blood, urine, vitreous fluid, gastric contents, bile, liver, brain, and sometimes other organs to test for the presence of alcohol, drugs, medications, poisons, or gases (eg, carbon monoxide).

— ***Traumatic diffuse axonal injury (tDAI):*** A type of TBI; occurs when the brain's long, connective nerve fibers (ie, axons) are sheared as a result of the brain shifting and rotating inside the skull during an injury. Typically causes injury to multiple spots on the brain.

— ***Traumatic compression fracture:*** An injury to the spine caused by weakening of the bone.

— ***Uncal herniation:*** A type of brain herniation; occurs as a result of excessive intracranial pressure that forces portions of the brain to displace downward, causing severe injury to brainstem functions.

— ***Undetermined:*** A manner of death; unnatural deaths in which there is not enough evidence to support any other particular manner of death (eg, homicide, suicide, or accident).

— ***Visceral peritoneum:*** The section of the peritoneum that lines the abdominal viscera, including the intestines.

— ***Wedging:*** To force into a narrow space, leading to entrapment.

Section II

Introduction

Chapter 1

Fatal Child Maltreatment, Medical Examiners, and Forensic Autopsy

Objectives

After reviewing this chapter, the reader will be able to:

1. *Analyze and describe the role of the forensic pathologist, medical examiner, and coroner.*
2. *Evaluate and describe the medicolegal system's responsibilities in relation to death and scene investigations.*
3. *Categorize and describe the components of a forensic autopsy, including the distinctions between an external and internal examination, toxicology, and other laboratory studies.*

Introduction

Forensic pathology is a medical specialty that functions within the role of the medical examiner. The medical examiner is part of the medicolegal death investigation system, which is created by a state statute. The forensic pathologist works within the office of the medical examiner. Forensic pathologists perform autopsies and carry out record reviews to determine the cause and manner of death of individuals whose death may have some impact on the well-being of others. While these vary by state, the types of deaths that fall into the jurisdiction of the medical examiner are deaths that:

— Occur suddenly or unexpectedly

— Are by possibly unnatural causes

— Are from accidents, homicides, or suicides

— May be related to dangers in the workplace or a public place

— Occur outside of hospitals or the care of a physician

— Fall into certain categories of interest (eg, children, individuals in custody of the law or in the care of others, or at home unattended by a physician or other care provider)

Currently in the United States, all states have specific medical examiner or coroner laws for the investigation of children's deaths. Child death laws generally require that a death investigation be carried out by the medical or coroner system unless a child in a particular age group died from a known natural disease. These laws also specify that certain categories of children *must* have autopsies and may further indicate which physicians will conduct them. In most medical examiner systems, these children are autopsied by forensic pathologists.

It is important to note that the forensic approach to an autopsy is significantly different from a hospital autopsy. Hospital autopsies are performed to determine why the patient has died and to evaluate the treatment modalities and the accuracy of diagnostic procedures. Forensic autopsies are performed on a select group of individuals when there is concern for a possible unnatural death or harm to society. State statutes usually allow medical examiners to autopsy those who fall into their jurisdiction without family permission or consent.

Death Investigation

The death investigation begins when a death is reported to the medicolegal death investigator, who works closely with forensic pathologists. Every medical examiner system has protocols for hospitals, police departments, funeral homes, hospice agencies, nursing homes, and other professionals who might interact with a dead body. When conducting a death investigation, the following duties fall to the medicolegal system[1]:

— Taking telephone reports of deaths

— Responding to certain death scenes and carrying out death scene investigations

— Determining the cause and manner of death

— Identifying the deceased, if unknown

— Determining the time of death

— Collecting all necessary evidence (eg, toxicology specimens, DNA materials, hair, fibers, etc.)

— Documenting injuries or lack of injuries

— Determining how the injuries occurred

— Documenting any natural disease present

— Determining or excluding other contributory or causative factors to the death

— Ordering medical records and police reports

— Arranging the transportation of bodies coming into the medical examiner office

— Providing expert testimony if the case goes to trial

This medicolegal death investigation is separate from the police investigation, which also generates information needed by the forensic pathologist in order to fully evaluate a case.

The ***cause of death*** is the disease or injury that creates the physiologic disturbance that leads to death (eg, a gunshot wound to the chest). The ***manner of death*** describes how the cause of death occurred. Manners of death include: natural, accident, suicide, homicide, and undetermined. In certain cases, even after all information from the autopsy, toxicology report, histologic examination, and accessory investigation is gathered, the pathologist is still unable ascertain a manner of death, which is then considered to be undetermined.

Many people, including nonforensic physicians, confuse cause of death with mechanism of death. The ***mechanism of death*** refers to the actual pathophysiologic derangements that result in death (eg, a gunshot wound to the chest might cause death through the mechanism of exsanguination). Mechanisms of death include:

exsanguinations, renal failure, respiratory failure, and cardiac arrest. Additionally, determining the mechanism of death can be immensely helpful in child maltreatment cases. The most effective way to study the mechanisms of death is to study collections of case histories with known similar injuries and observing the appearance and progression of these cases, thus making it easier to understand how the clinical presentation of an injured child would look (eg, a liver laceration in a young child causes exsanguination, comparable to liver lacerations seen in adults who have been in a vehicular accident).

Death Investigation of a Child

To properly evaluate the death of a child, a number of records need to be reviewed. These records are aimed at creating a comprehensive report meant to aid the child fatality review process. They include:

— All medical records, beginning from birth and extending to time of death (includes: birth records, pediatrician visits, emergency medical service records, emergency department records, and hospital records)

— Growth charts (especially helpful when suspected nutritional neglect is present)

— Information gathered from family service agencies, Child Protective Services, and the juvenile court system

— Police department records

— Insurance examinations (helpful in finding missing details of a child's life)

— School records

— A detailed history of the child's developmental, medical, and social history

— Significant family medical and social history including family size, structure, ages, and any recent changes or sources of stress such as criminal background, drug use, divorce, or death

— Statements made by the parents or caretakers, siblings, or any others with knowledge of the circumstances surrounding a child's death (note the reaction of all individuals who were caring for the child when the death occurred [eg, do the individuals appear appropriate in their emotional state, is there any evidence of intoxication or mental disturbance?])

The child fatality review process is one of the most efficient methods of accessing all of the information needed by the forensic pathologist before decisions are made about the cause and manner of a child's death; it allows for all of the knowledge of involved agencies to be shared with those conducting the death investigation. The child death review process varies from state to state but generally involves a panel of individuals such as the medical examiner, prosecuting attorney, family services specialists, police, juvenile court personnel, pediatricians, and any others who might have information about a particular death.

Scene Investigation

The ***scene*** refers to the location where the incident surrounding the death or injury occurred. The purpose of the scene investigation is to assess the scene, the circumstances, and the body if it is still in place, or, if the body has been transported for care, the site where the child was found. Information of interest at the scene investigation is detailed in **Table 1-1**.

The details of the scene listed in **Table 1-1** should be documented by photography and written descriptions so that the information can be reviewed by the pathologist before the autopsy.

Table 1-1. Information of Interest at the Scene of the Crime

Site or Objects of Investigation	Information of Interest
Home or incident site	— Geographic location — Urban — Suburban — Rural — How the home compares with other homes in the same area — Dwelling appearance — State of repair — Cleanliness — Furnishings — Dangerous conditions — Infestations — Temperature — Weather — Clothing — Available food — Siblings — Behavior of everyone — Drug paraphernalia — Electric and plumbing
Bedding/ sleeping surface	— Toys, objects near body — Presence of purges, exudates — Type of bedding, sheets, blankets, pillows — Others present in bed/sleeping surface
Physical evidence	— Stains — Blood — Medications — Formula — Bottles
Body	— Terminal position — Initial position if different from terminal position — Moved or altered position — Pattern of lividity — Presence of rigor — Body temperature — Odor — Hygiene

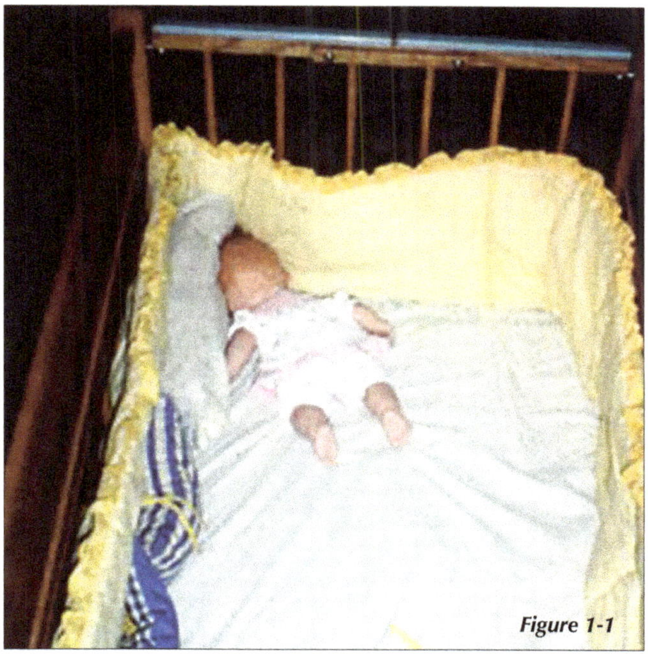

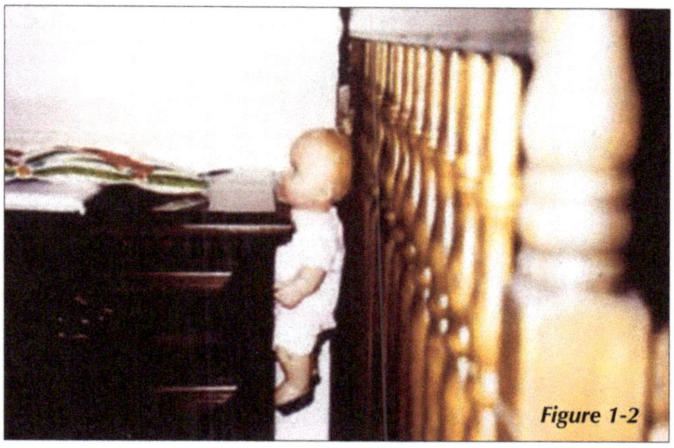

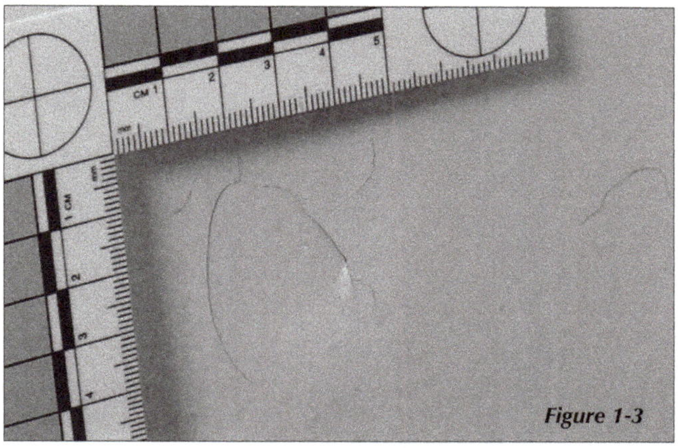

Figure 1-1. *Scene recreation doll used to recreate unsafe sleeping conditions.*

Figure 1-2. *Scene recreation doll illustrating a 10-month-old boy who fell out of bed and became caught between the dresser and crib, causing asphyxia.*

Figure 1-3. *Hole indented in the wall where a 5-year-old girl's head was slammed.*

Scene recreation involves having the individual who found the child demonstrate the position in which the child was found or how the child was injured using a scene recreation doll. In specific types of deaths (eg, an infant found dead or unresponsive in bed potentially due to sudden infant death syndrome [SIDS], sudden unexpected infant death [SUID], or a sleep-related death), recreation dolls and scenarios may be useful, especially because most people are not sufficiently verbal or detail oriented enough to accurately describe the circumstances.

Using a scene recreation doll allows the investigator to photographically document a complex scene (**Figure 1-1**). Many asphyxial deaths are best understood by studying scene recreations. Children can easily fall into positions that interfere with breathing or chest excursion (**Figure 1-2**). Sometimes children fall into areas that entrap them, and the scene might have findings that are directly related to injuries on the child, such as an indented wall where a child's head was impacted (**Figure 1-3**). Detailed scene recreations are imperative in determining whether the injuries found on a child could in fact be sustained by the caretaker's described scenario.

Forensic Autopsy

The purpose of the forensic autopsy is to fulfill the needs of the medical examiner system, as noted previously.[1] Although the forensic autopsy will note and document all findings in the body, the forensic pathologist or medical examiner will use a number of autopsy procedures that are unfamiliar or strange to hospital pathologists. Those procedures include:

— Removal of bones for documentation of injury and aging injury

— Removal of digits, fingers, or hands for identification

— Extensive dissection of soft tissue

— Skeletonization of the face or body for examination of wounds

— Removal of eyes and inner ears

— Retention of the body after autopsy for later reexamination

— Removal of the entire rib cage or spine

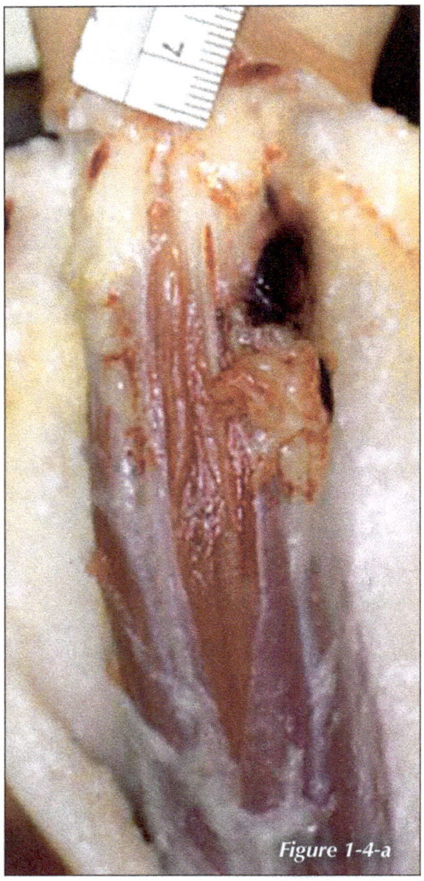

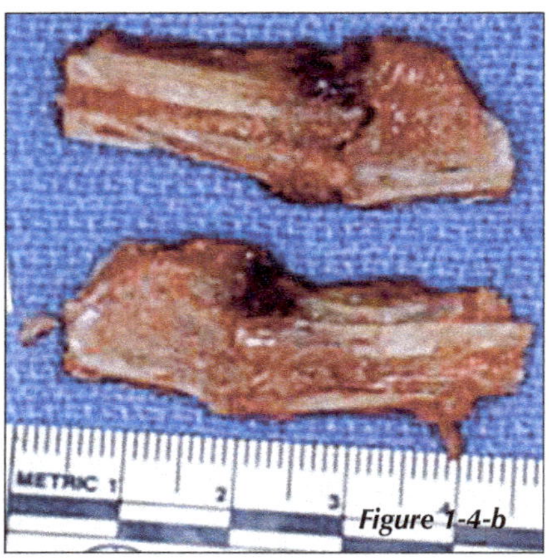

Figure 1-4-a. *Fracture of radius with surrounding soft tissue hemorrhage.*

Figure 1-4-b. *Radius removed and incised to submit for microscope sections for aging of fracture.*

In addition, special dissections may be used to investigate specific areas of injures (eg, posterior neck, palms of the hands or soles of the feet, genitalia).

Before the autopsy, radiographs are taken in appropriate cases: *all* children under 3 years of age and older children involved in select cases. Images should be taken of all areas of the body, using as many views as necessary to see the child's entire anatomy. In most cases, the following views are suggested:

— Anterior/posterior skull and lateral skull

— Anterior/posterior torso to include chest, abdomen, and pelvis with adequate penetration to view posterior ribs

— Anterior/posterior views of upper and lower extremities

— Anterior/posterior joints

— Lateral view of entire spine

When any bony injury is found or is questionable, the soft tissue surrounding the injured bone is dissected to look for hemorrhage and to take samples of the tissue for microscopic examination. Microscopic slides of the soft tissue are used to determine the age of the injury by measuring the state of the progression of the inflammatory response to the injury (**Figure 1-4-a** and **b**). A relatively new technique used in cases of obvious abusive injury is to expose all the long bones during the autopsy by dissecting away the soft tissue, even if no injury is visible on the radiograph. This technique is aimed at discovering a subtle bony injury. Hemorrhaging in the periosteum, pointing to an underlying bony injury, may also be found by this technique.

External Examination

The forensic autopsy begins with a detailed examination of the body in the condition in which it arrived to the morgue. The clothing on the body is examined for evidence and documented. Measurements of height, weight and, in young children, the dimensions of the head, chest, and abdomen, are noted. The forensic pathologist then proceeds systematically through a detailed external examination of the body, which is of paramount importance.

The external examination may take several hours in order to complete the necessary descriptive and photographic documentation. Each anatomic part of the body – face, scalp, neck, chest, abdomen, back, genitalia, buttocks, and extremities – is examined and described regarding the presence of identifying marks, scars, fresh injury, healing injury, and healed injury. Injuries are then individually characterized as an abrasion, contusion, incised wound, burn, or penetrating injury (eg, gunshot or stab wound). Each injury is described by size, color, and shape. Sections of tissues from the injuries are taken for microscopic examination to determine the age of the injury (**Figure 1-5**). If patterned injuries are noted, these are documented photographically and the

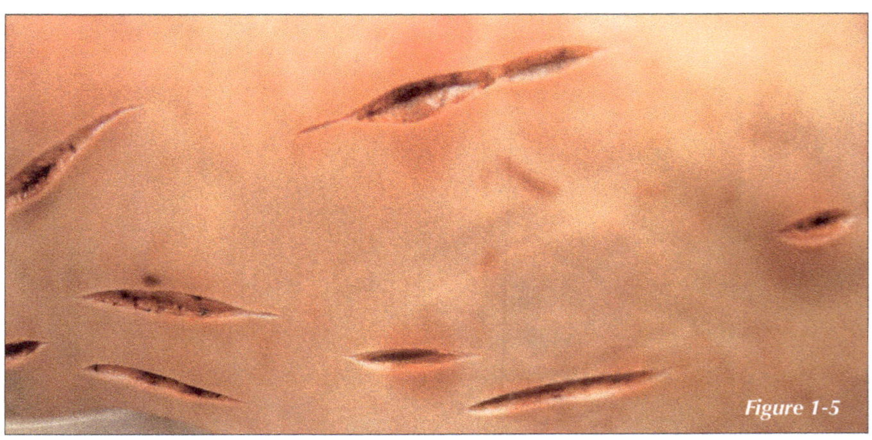

Figure 1-5. *Many contusions on back incised for photography and to take sections to submit for microscopic examination for aging of contusions.*

type of pattern suggested is described (eg, loop mark). If bite marks are present, the injury is swabbed for possible DNA collection. Additionally, the degree and distribution of livor and rigor are described and photographed.

The external examination of a child includes the state of nutrition, hygiene, hair growth, unusual soiling with urine or feces, and any congenital abnormalities. Evidence of dehydration is noted (eg, sunken fontanel or eyes, poor skin turgor, and dry mucosal membranes).

The child's mouth is also closely inspected for injury of the teeth, lips, gums, and frenula. These must be distinguished from injuries that were related to intubation and resuscitation efforts. Inflicted injuries of the mouth are often associated with other abusive injuries (**Figure 1-6-a** and **b**).

The child's genitalia are examined for any evidence of injury, and if assault is suspected, swabs are taken from the oral cavity, vagina, rectum, and penis for DNA. The injuries are also examined by taking microscopic sections in order to establish the age of injury. Injuries to the female genitalia are fairly easy to recognize if there are gross tears or contusion; however, there may be injuries to the genitalia, in both males and females, that are not sexually inflicted but rather caused by blunt trauma (**Figure 1-7**). Additionally, it is important to note that in young children the mucosal surfaces surrounding the anus often roll up or sluff off after death, and this change should not be mistaken for injury. Obvious tears in the rectum, though, are usually evident by associated hemorrhages and can be further studied by removing the rectum internally (**Figure 1-8**).

Internal Examination

The internal examination begins as the skin and soft tissue of the anterior body are reflected to expose the rib cage and peritoneal cavity, thus making injuries in the soft tissue of the anterior surface able to be viewed, described, and documented pho-

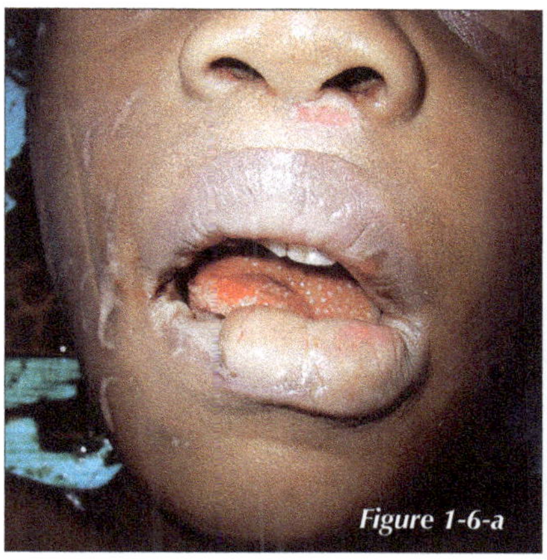

Figure 1-6-a. Mouth of a 5-year-old girl showing healed avulsion of right lower lip and fractured upper right central incisor.

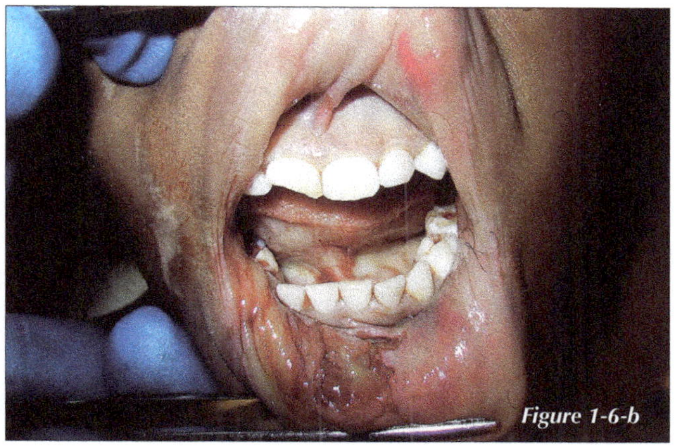

Figure 1-6-b. Inner mucosal surface of mouth showing laceration of right lower lip.

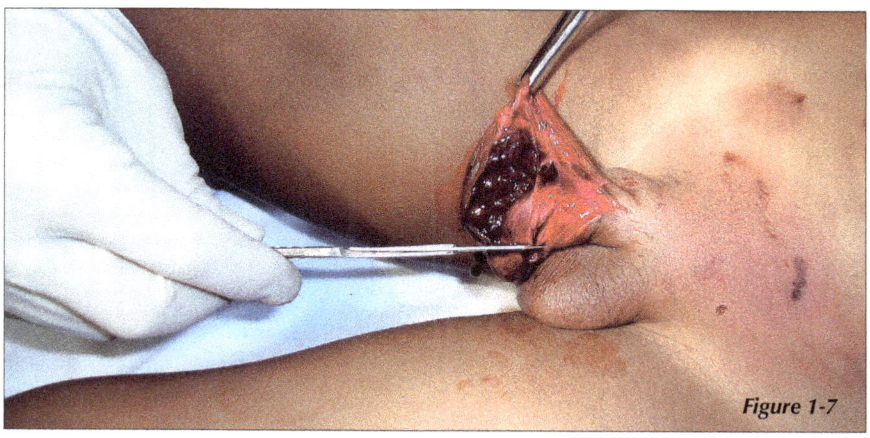

Figure 1-7. A 17-month-old boy with blunt trauma to penis with incision of foreskin to demonstrate hematoma in foreskin and to take sections for microscopic examination.

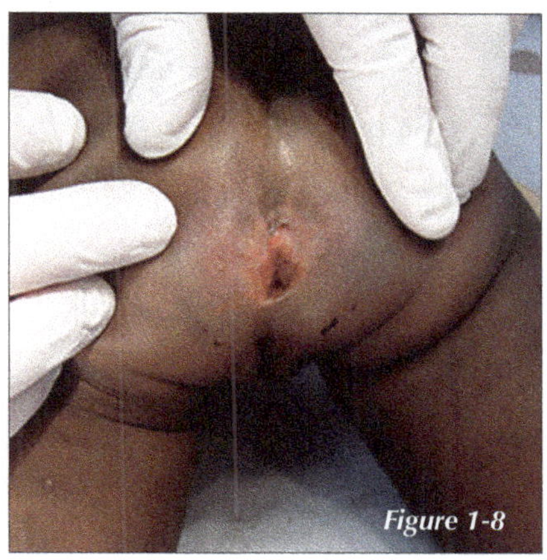

Figure 1-8. Rectum of 10-month-old girl showing acute lacerations.

tographically. Sections can be taken for microscopic examination. The presence of blood or other fluids within the pleural cavity, pericardial sac, or the abdominal cavity is noted, described, and documented photographically. If blood is present, an attempt to accurately measure the amount is made (**Figure 1-9**).

The parietal pleura are manually removed from the rib cage to view each rib. It should be noted that fresh rib fractures in young infants may not be visible on radiographs, so the actual bone must be inspected and more thoroughly examined. If there are numerous rib fractures, it is helpful to remove the entire rib cage and photographs can then demonstrate the fractures (**Figure 1-10-a** and **b**).

Before the head is opened for internal examination, the scalp should be closely inspected for any injury by shaving away the surrounding hair to expose the wound. When the scalp is reflected forward and backward in order to expose the underlying calvarium, the undersurface of the scalp is closely examined for hemorrhage. The injuries are measured, described, and documented, and sections are taken for microscopic examination. The calvarium is then closely examined for fracture and for blood present in the periosteum as it might be indicative of an underlying skull fracture. Then, the periosteum should be removed to directly view the underlying bone. Any identified fractures can then be described and documented (**Figure 1-11-a** and **b**).

As the calvarium is lifted off, the pathologist looks for the presence of subdural or epidural blood which can then be documented and photographed. Once the brain has been removed, the dura is stripped away from the inner surface of the calvarium and from the cranial fossae to inspect the bones for fracture. In the case of any suspected abusive head trauma, it is important to remove the brain with the spinal cord attached rather than separately, which can be done by either an anterior combined with posterior approach or a totally posterior approach for both (**Figure 1-12-a** and **b**).[2]

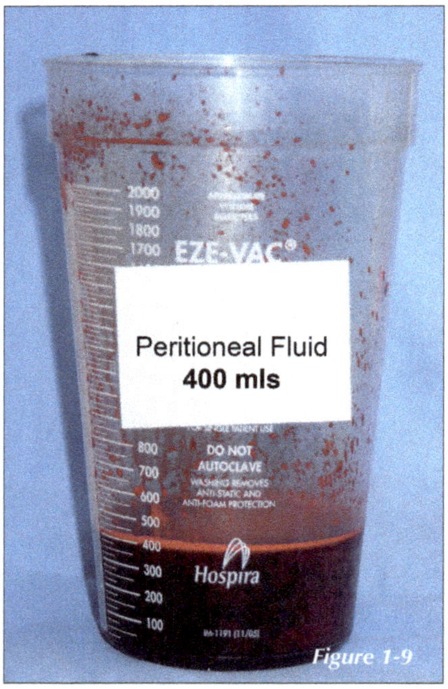

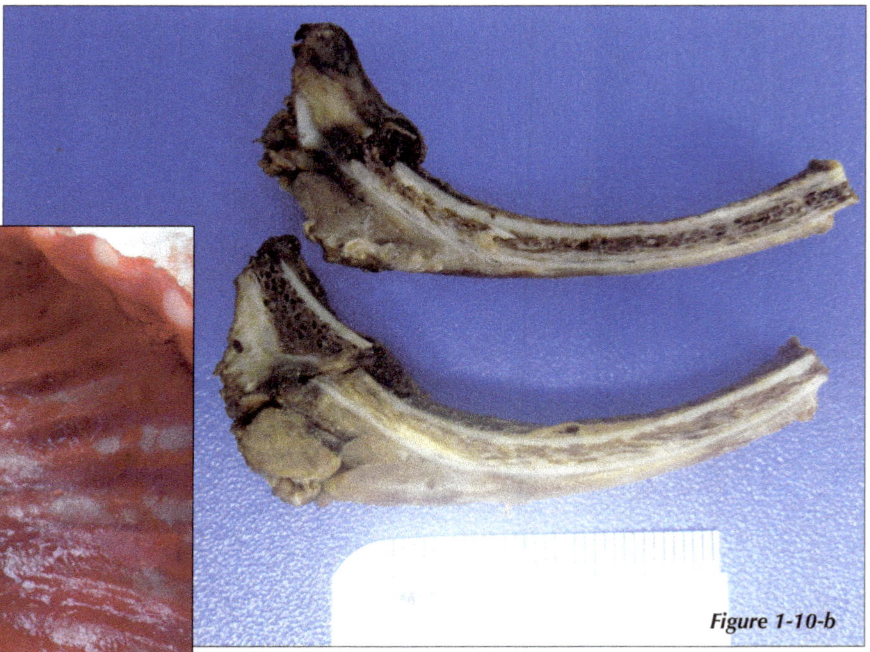

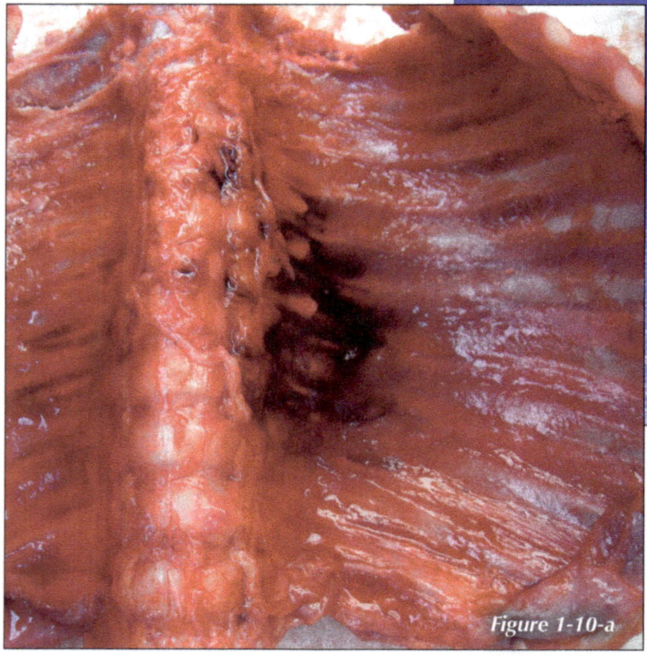

Figure 1-9. *Cup of blood from abdominal cavity to demonstrate measurement technique.*

Figure 1-10-a. *Rib cage removed to show multiple acute posterior fractures.*

Figure 1-10-b. *Individual fractured rib transected to submit for microscopic examination of aging.*

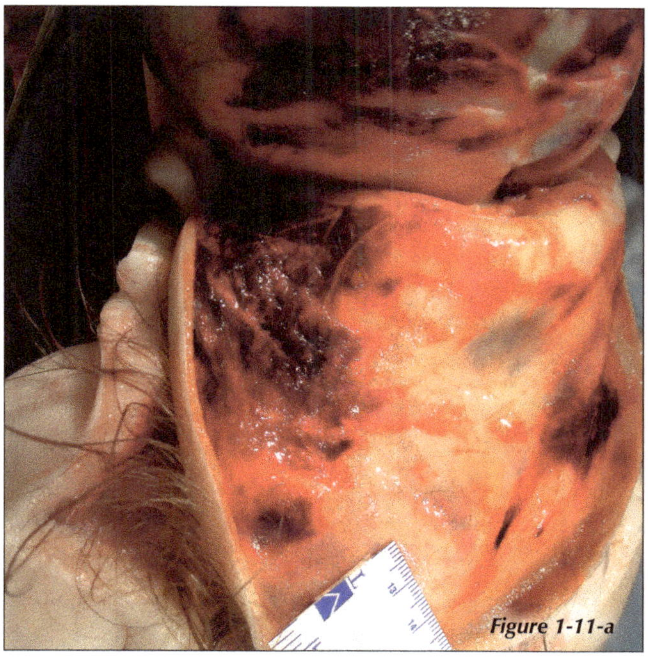

Figure 1-11-a

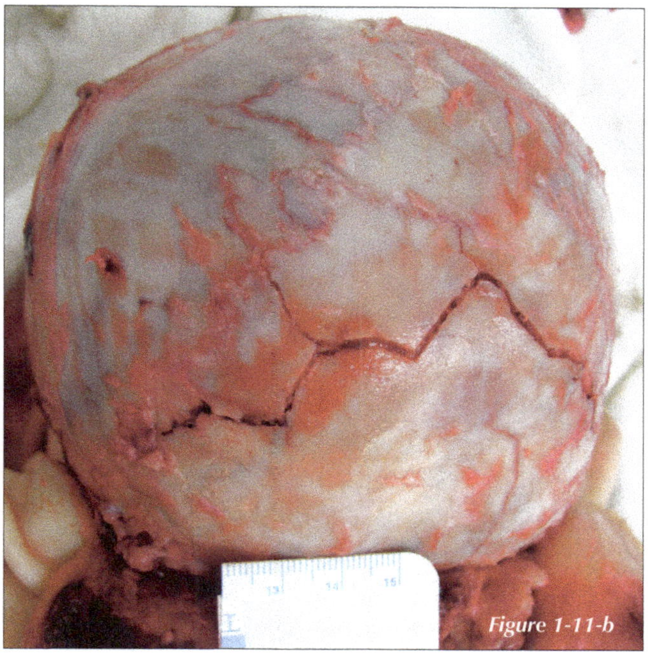

Figure 1-11-b

The spinal cord is then examined with the brain. The epidural compartment of the spine is distinctly different from the epidural space of the head in that the presence of spinal epidural blood does not necessarily imply trauma,[3,4] especially where in infants, it appears to be related to hemodynamic forces.

In child autopsies where there is any suspicion of abusive practice or injury, the body is turned into the prone position after the completion of the internal examination. The soft tissues of the back, buttocks, and extremities are examined by making incisions down the line of the back and then dissecting away the underlying soft tissues (**Figure 1-13-a** and **b**). It should be noted that even in children with pale complexions, deep hemorrhages in the buttocks and back may not be visible externally and that presence of dermal melanocytosis (previously known as Mongolian spots) may appear as a contusion externally but can be easily differentiated as a non-injury upon incision.

Figure 1-11-a. *Periosteal hemorrhage overlying fracture of occipital skull.*

Figure 1-11-b. *Periosteum has been removed to show underlying fracture of occipital skull.*

Figure 1-12-a. *Removal of brain and spinal cord together from a posterior approach.*

Figure 1-12-b. *Calvarium showing small amount of subdural blood in a case of abusive head trauma.*

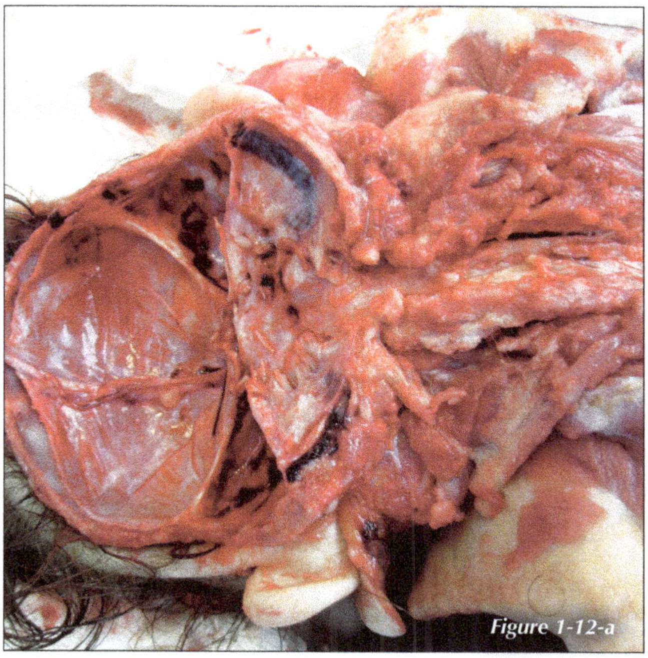

Figure 1-12-a

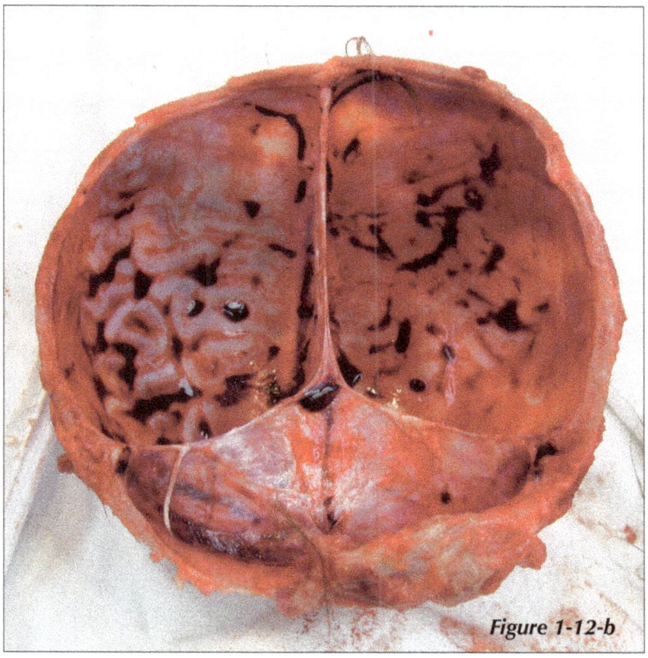

Figure 1-12-b

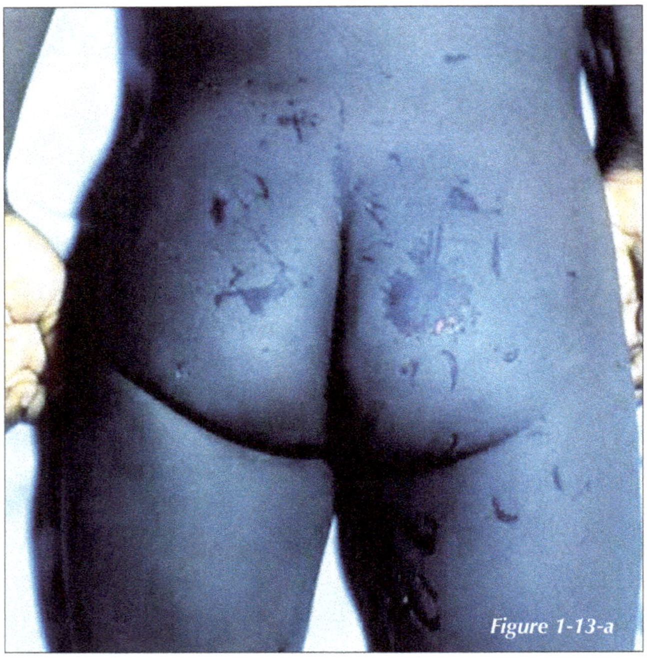

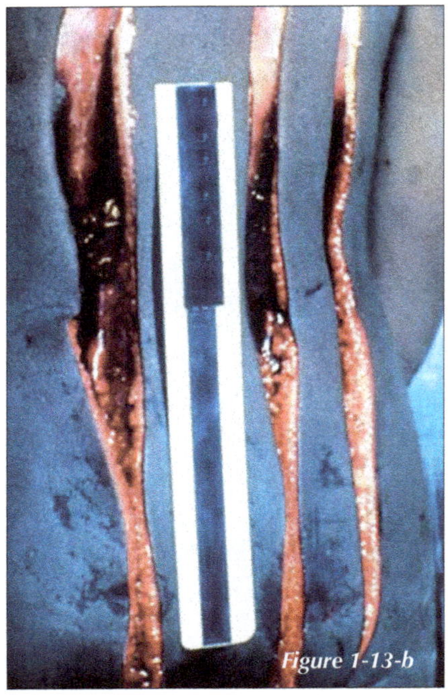

Figure 1-13-a. *Child with extensive contusions of the back and buttocks.*

Figure 1-13-b. *Incisions into soft tissue of the back and buttocks to demonstrate underlying hemorrhage in soft tissues.*

Toxicology

During the autopsy, specimens are taken of blood, urine, vitreous fluid, gastric contents, bile, liver, brain, and sometimes other organs for testing for the presence of alcohol, medications, poisons, or gases such as carbon monoxide. The forensic pathologist will consider the findings from toxicology in the overall evaluation of a child's death. In an effort to test for any of these substances or to check for a medication overdose, baby bottles or the medication itself can be seized and evaluated as well.

Histology and Aging of Injuries

As mentioned previously, during the autopsy, sections of tissues are taken from each major organ and from areas of possible injury or disease which are then processed into microscopic slides for examination. The findings on microscopic examination can diagnose tumors, infections, inflammation, and many other pathologic changes. In cases of child abuse, it is important to closely examine all organs for the possibility of disease because alternative causes of death may be claimed, and any source that might contribute to the ease with which an injury might occur should be considered. Additionally, one of the most important uses of histologic examination in child abuse cases is the evaluation and estimation of the age of injuries, mostly because the naked-eye examination is not precise. The initial phase of the inflammatory response, which is the body's response to any type of injury, occurs in the early hours after injury and extends over several days.[5]

The earliest change that is typically discernable after an injury is the influx of neutrophils into an area of injury. After about 24 hours, neutrophils can disintegrate or undergo lysis as they release their hydrolytic enzymes. In 2 to 3 days, mononuclear cells begin to move into the area and become more numerous in the following days. Once the inflammatory response has progressed for 5 to 7 days, a reparative phase ensues. During this phase, there will be a change in the ingrowth of endothelial cells to allow neovascularization of the healing tissue, and fibroblasts will become more numerous. The extent of the area of injury determines how long the healing process will last, but some tissues may take several months for the reparative process to be complete. Understanding the body's process of repair allows the pathologist to distinguish early injury from injury that is 2 to 3 days old, a week old, or older.

The aging of wounds, including the ability to look at microscopic changes in injuries, is important in the evaluation of the overall case and may be helpful when giving court testimony.

Other Laboratory Studies

The vitreous fluid can be analyzed for glucose, urea nitrogen, creatinine, and electrolytes and is informative in cases being evaluated for dehydration, diabetic states, and other metabolic conditions. In cases of suspected infection (eg, sepsis, pneumonia, meningitis), empyema fluid, swabs, blood, or cerebrospinal fluid may be obtained postmortem and sent for culture to a microbiology laboratory.

References

1. DiMaio V, DiMaio D. *Forensic Pathology*. 2nd ed. CRC Press; 2001.
2. Judkins AR, Hood IG, Mirchandani HG, Rorke LB. Techincal communication: rationale and technique for examination of nervous system in suspected infant victims of abuse. *Am J Forensic Med Pathol.* 2004;25(1):29-32.
3. Towbin A. Sudden infant death (cot death) related to spinal injury. *Lancet.* 1967;290(7522):940-942.
4. Harris LS, Adelson L. "Spinal injury" and sudden infant death: a second look. *Am J Clin Pathol.* 1969;52(3):289-295.
5. Perper JA, Wecht CH, eds. Histological estimation of age of injuries. In: *Microscopic Diagnosis in Forensic Pathology.* Charles Thomas; 1980:3-16.

Section III

PATHOLOGICAL EVALUATION

Chapter 2

Head Trauma

Objectives

After reviewing this chapter, the reader will be able to:

1. *Compare and categorize traumatic head injuries by mechanism of injury (ie, static and dynamic).*
2. *Explain the causes of subdural hemorrhages (SDH) and hygromas and their relation to one another.*
3. *Identify retinal hemorrhages and describe how they are related to or caused by head trauma.*

Introduction

In the United States, it is estimated that 2000 children die each year from abuse and neglect.[1] Medical examiners often see inflicted head trauma as the cause of death in infants and young children because abuse is the most common cause of severe traumatic brain injury. As many as 80% of lethal cases of child physical abuse are a result of injury to the head.[2] Not only does abusive injury account for 10% of all injuries in children younger than 5 years of age, but the younger an abused child is, the more likely it is that the most significant injuries are to the head, especially when under the age of 2.[3-8]

Fully comprehending traumatic head injury in young children requires an understanding that young children and infants have unique differences in the brain, skull, and neck related to the long period of developmental and anatomical maturation that occurs in the human species. In most animal species, these developmental periods are brief, some only a day or two. None are as long as the many years required for maturation in the human species, which have marked differences at the youngest ages and extend into middle childhood, making young children particularly susceptible to injuries from acceleration-deceleration forces (eg, the causation of shearing injuries to the brain and adnexal vascular structures). The skull of the young child is thin and pliable, features that assist the fetus in moving through the birth canal, but are of less help in reducing the force of a blow to the head, allowing force to cause skull fractures or to be transmitted through the skull to the brain.

The brain is a large, heavy organ at birth and grows rapidly after birth to reach 75% of its full weight by age 2 years (although the brain is far from mature at this age). An adult's head is about 2% to 3% of the body's weight, while an infant's head may be as much as 20% to 30%. In young childhood, the head may be as much as 10% to 15% of the body's weight.[9] The brain of the young child is very soft in consistency because of the high water content, immaturity in the number of and development of the glial cells, immaturity of the myelination of axons, and the small size of the axons. A thin or absent layer of myelin facilitates axonal damage resulting from strain, as most axonal damage occurs at the node of Ranvier where myelin is discontinuous.[10,11] Lastly, the neck muscle of a young child is weak, underdeveloped, and offers little support to the head or ability to prevent movement of the head on impact or impulse (ie, movement of the body that causes the head to move). The young child's head is free to move with any impact or impulse.

Mechanisms of Injury

Traumatic brain injury can be classified into static and dynamic injuries on the basis of the rate at which force is loaded to the head. ***Static injuries*** are relatively rare and occur over longer periods of time, usually longer than 200 milliseconds, and cause crushing head injury. Crushing head injuries are seen in children in the context of a head being run over by a motor vehicle wheel or a heavy object falling onto the child's head. ***Dynamic head injuries*** account for the vast majority of head injuries at all ages and occur when a force is rapidly loaded onto the head in less than 200 milliseconds. Dynamic head injuries are caused by impulse loading, such as shaking, or impact loading.

Impulse loading may impart inertial movement of the brain within the cranial cavity, wherein the brain moves and is displaced away from the skull. The unsupported head will rotate at the point where it joins the cervical spine, which creates differential motion of the brain and skull because of the differing rigidities between the brain and skull. Because the dura is attached to the skull, differential motion between the skull and brain may strain and tear bridging veins (eg, the source of subdural bleeding), which begins within the interhemispheric sulcus and spreads out over the cerebral convexities. The inertial movement of the brain as it rotates within the cranial cavity results in traumatic axonal injury and is greatest in the brain's periphery. With greater force, brain motion extends deeper into the center of the brain to the basal ganglia and thalamus and down into the brainstem.

Brain injuries may also be classified into focal and diffuse injuries. ***Focal injuries*** (also known as contact injuries) result from direct impact to the head and can be seen with the naked eye. These injuries include scalp lacerations and contusions, skull fractures, epidural hemorrhage, focal SDH, and brain contusions. ***Diffuse injuries*** result from inertial loading of the head and include interhemispheric subdural hemorrhage and traumatic diffuse axonal injury.[16-19.]

In 1971, a British neurosurgeon, Guthkelch,[20] postulated that SDHs in infants could be created by whiplash forces, which tore bridging veins. Referencing the research of Ommaya et al[21] in the 1960s on the effects of rotational movement of the head on the neck producing concussion and hemorrhages over the surface of primates' brains, Guthkelch suggested that the injuries to infants with SDHs might be caused by these acceleration-deceleration forces rather than direct impact. In 1972, Caffey[22] used the term "whiplash shaken baby syndrome" to describe infants with SDH or subarachnoid hemorrhages (SAH), retinal hemorrhages, and little or no external marks of trauma to the head. In the following years, the concept of shaking as a mechanism of injury to young children became generally known and has generated great interest in continued study and research.

In 1987, in a landmark paper, Duhaime et al[23] questioned whether shaking without impact could create the rotational acceleration and velocity to reach the thresholds of concussion, SDH, or axonal injury. Duhaime looked at a group of 48 children with SDH or SAH, retinal hemorrhages, and a history suggestive of abuse. All of the children who died had evidence of head impact at autopsy, and 63% of the living children had evidence of impact. Using a doll model that could be shaken or impacted, Duhaime found that shaking alone did not reach the thresholds of rotational acceleration for significant injury, while impact did generate forces above the thresholds for SDH and axonal injury. Intense scrutiny of these findings led to a corollary question: whether abusive head injury that lacks external marks of trauma can be recognized as trauma (eg, marks of impact are visible on the inner surface of the scalp).[24,25]

Thresholds established for concussion, SDH, and axonal injury were derived from animal studies rather than human studies. In the 1940s, Holbourn[26] hypothesized that smaller brains would require more force than larger brains to produce similar injury and that the critical factor for brain injury is angular acceleration. Ommaya's[21] research on nonhuman primates confirmed Holbourn's hypotheses and found that the increasing risk for brain injury in larger brains was related to an inverse two-thirds power of the brain mass known as the scaling relationship.[27] Because of the physiological factors in the young child that were noted above, it seems likely that the young child brain would be more vulnerable than the adult brain to acceleration-deceleration forces as predicted by the scaling relationship. The 1987 Duhaime et al[23] study relied on the scaling relationship to calculate the thresholds used in the study, but more recent biomechanical studies have provided evidence that the traditional approach of scaling by brain mass does not explain the vulnerability of the infant porcine brain model to inertial injury compared with the toddler-age porcine brain.[13] Raghupathi and Margulies[12] found that rotational head injuries in infant piglets resulted in more injured axons per unit area than in adults. There is also clinical evidence to support that age significantly affects the response of the brain to trauma. There are more severe cognitive and motor function deficits in younger brain-injured children than in older children.[28] Closed head trauma in infants often results in diffuse brain atrophy, which is seldom seen after head injury in older children.[29]

At the present time, there is no conclusion to the discussion of whether shaking is a plausible mechanism of injury to the young brain. Much of the controversy surrounding shaking is media generated and not science based. Gilliland and Folberg[31] examined autopsy findings in a group of 80 children from which they then defined that evidence of shaking had to include at least 2 of the following findings: (1) fingermarks and/or rib fractures, (2) SDH and/or SAH, and (3) a history of vigorous shaking. From their study, 3 categories emerged: (1) shaking, (2) combined shaking and impact injuries, and (3) impact injuries. Of the total number of abusive head injuries that they examined, 11% accounted for shaking; therefore, the authors concluded that shaking was a valid mechanism of lethal injury.

Some medical examiners state that they have never seen an abusive head injury without evidence of an impact. In looking at the series of cases studied by the author from 1975 to 1985 and 1986 to 1999, there were a total of 40 abusive head trauma cases, of which 11 were likely caused by shaking because there was no evidence of impact. The confidence with which the diagnosis is made by a medical examiner may contribute to a difference in findings, particularly in difficult cases wherein no marks are found on the head or body but a thin layer of subdural blood, with or without retinal hemorrhages, is present. Minns[32] notes that across the literature of cases of abusive head trauma, approximately 33% are thought to be due to shaking.

Two cases of shaken adult syndrome have been noted in the literature. Pounder[33] described a 30-year-old prisoner who was shaken by a much larger prison guard as a form of torture. The prisoner became unconscious and then died after one of the multiple shakings carried out over a 3-day period. The autopsy showed SDH, retinal hemorrhages, diffuse axonal injury, and bruising over the chest and shoulders. Carrigan et al[34] reported a similar case of a 34-year-old woman who was the victim of domestic violence and had SDH, retinal hemorrhages, and bruising, demonstrating that these types of injuries affect people of all ages.

Skull Fracture

The skull is about 1 mm thick at birth and increases to 3 to 4 mm in the young child then to 10 mm in the adult. The skull protects the brain from impact injury. In the adult skull, sutures act as shock absorbers and distribute force away from the point of impact. While not well studied, some research shows that infant cranial bones offer little resistance to external loading and will deform in structure to a much greater degree than fully calcified bone. The sutures of the infant lack the ability to absorb shock, leading to skull fracture when the strength of the bone fails to resist the loaded force.[35]

Hobbs' seminal paper on skull fracture and the diagnosis of abuse reported findings in 89 children younger than 2 years of age with skull fractures, of which 29 were definite abusive injuries and 60 were accidental injuries.[36] There were 20 deaths, 19 of which were from the abuse group. The characteristics found more commonly in the abused group were: multiple or complex fractures, depressed fractures, fractures with a maximum width greater than 3 mm, growing fractures, involvement of more than 1 cranial bone, non-parietal fractures, and associated intracranial injuries. In the author's collection of abusive head trauma cases, fractures were seen in 40% of the cases.

A large body of literature on short falls in young children has been gathered to assist in the understanding of the types of injuries that occur in common household falls during childhood.[37-43] Short falls from distances of less than 4 to 5 feet seem to be primarily associated with focal contact injuries, such as scalp laceration or contusion, although the great majority of children suffer no injury at all. This literature reveals that about 1% to 3% of children sustain a skull fracture, generally without intracranial injury, in a short fall. In slightly less than 1% of the fracture cases, there is an associated epidural or focal SDH, and if these injuries are associated with significant increased intracranial pressure, they may have a lethal outcome.[44,45] Chadwick's study of the annual risk of death from short falls found a mortality rate of less than 0.48 deaths per 1 million young children per year, confirming the benign nature of most short falls.[46]

Weber[47-49] carried out 3 studies on fractures in infant cadavers that are puzzling when compared to observations in the living infant and child. Among his findings was that of 15 infant cadavers dropped from a horizontal position from a height of 82 cm, fractures occurred in all 15. Weber concluded that low-level falls can result in a skull fracture that may be asymptomatic and unknown to the caretakers. Because the infants studied by Weber were cadavers, the resiliency of the bone may have changed from the vital state.

Subdural Hemorrhage

The most common finding at autopsy in a case of abusive head trauma is the presence of subdural blood. Knowledge about the subdural space and SDH has changed over the last 30 years, and the current understanding is that there is not a true subdural space.[50] The dura is made up of fibroblasts and large amounts of extracellular collagen. The innermost cell layer is a continuous with the arachnoid outer barrier, so subdural space only exists when the weak dural border cell layer is dissected during traumatic cleaving. Because the dura is attached to the inner skull and the arachnoid is attached to the pia mater on the brain's surface, the dural border separates from the arachnoid during autopsy to create a subdural space. Bridging veins pass through the meninges, the pia, and the arachnoid as they exit the cortical surface of the brain and pass to the venous sinuses in the dura. While the walls of bridging veins attach to both the dural border cell layer and to arachnoid cells, their attachment to the arachnoid is stronger, so differential motion between the brain and skull causes the dura to move with the skull while the arachnoid moves with the brain. If the motion is great enough to strain the bridging veins, blood enters the intradural layer of the dural border cells and is seen as "subdural" blood. This discussion will continue to use that terminology, although it is understood that the subdural space is only a potential space.

SDH is present in 90% to 95% of cases of fatal inflicted head injury at autopsy and can be imaged in 40% to 55% of living children with such head injuries.[23,52,53] There is a difference in the numbers of cases with SDH at autopsy and in the living on computed tomography (CT) scan because a thin layer of subdural blood that is visible at autopsy may not be visible on CT imaging, while small amounts of interhemispheric blood can be seen on CT but not at autopsy.[54,55] Magnetic resonance imaging (MRI) is better able to detect small amounts of SDH than the CT scan, although many young children with abusive head trauma are too critically ill to undergo MRI.[14] In many cases, the subdural blood is a thin layer over both cerebral convexities (**Figure 2-1**).

In some cases, the SDH will be unilateral rather than bilateral, but it will be over the cerebral convexity rather than focally in an isolated location (**Figure 2-2**). The subdural bleeding is caused by the inertial brain motion, which separates the cortical surface from the overlying skull and attached dura, resulting in the tearing of bridging veins.[56,57] Inertial motion of the brain begins earliest in the posterior hemispheric fissure, so the earliest subdural blood appears there and then spreads anteriorly and outward.[58] Wells et al[59] looked at intracranial hemorrhage in 293 children younger than age 3 years. They found that interhemispheric SDH was the most common type of subdural bleeding, as it was seen in 49% of the cases, and 73% of the children with interhemispheric SDH had abusive head trauma. Accidental head trauma caused only 15% of the interhemispheric subdural bleeding and these were from relatively high force incidents. SDH over the convexities was seen in 47% of cases, and abusive head trauma accounted for 72% of the convexity SDH. Accidental head trauma accounted for 10% of the convexity SDH and again was from relatively high force incidents.

In cases with an associated skull fracture, the subdural blood is not always immediately adjacent to the fracture. The amount of subdural blood may be minimal, even less than 5 to 10 mL of blood. Because the amount of blood is so minimal, it is important that the pathologist is always the person who opens the calvarium of a child, so any subdural blood can be observed and documented (**Figure 2-3**). During this process, the venous sinuses will be disrupted, which will cause blood to be added to any subdural blood already present. Once the brain is removed, there is often subdural blood in the cranial fossae and the spinal subdural space. While the general opinion among forensic pathologists is that the spinal subdural blood has descended by gravity from the intracranial compartment, Rorke-Adams[60] notes that subdural blood that originates in the supratentorial space cannot gain access to the spinal subdural space. However, in many cases of abusive head trauma, the posterior fossa, along with the convexities, contains subdural blood possibly because blood in the posterior fossa has easy access to the spinal subdural space.[60]

SDH may occur in association with numerous causes and conditions, including inflicted head trauma, accidental head trauma, medical or surgical manipulation,

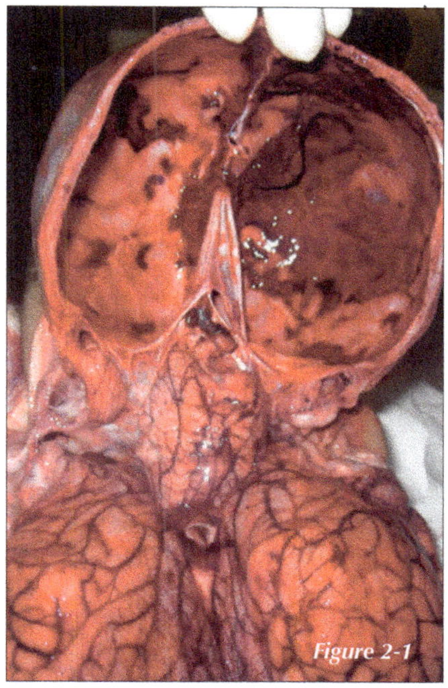

Figure 2-1. *Posterior dissection of brain and spinal cord. Child is face down. The skull cap is being retracted to show subdural blood over cerebral convexities; blood is greater on the left.*

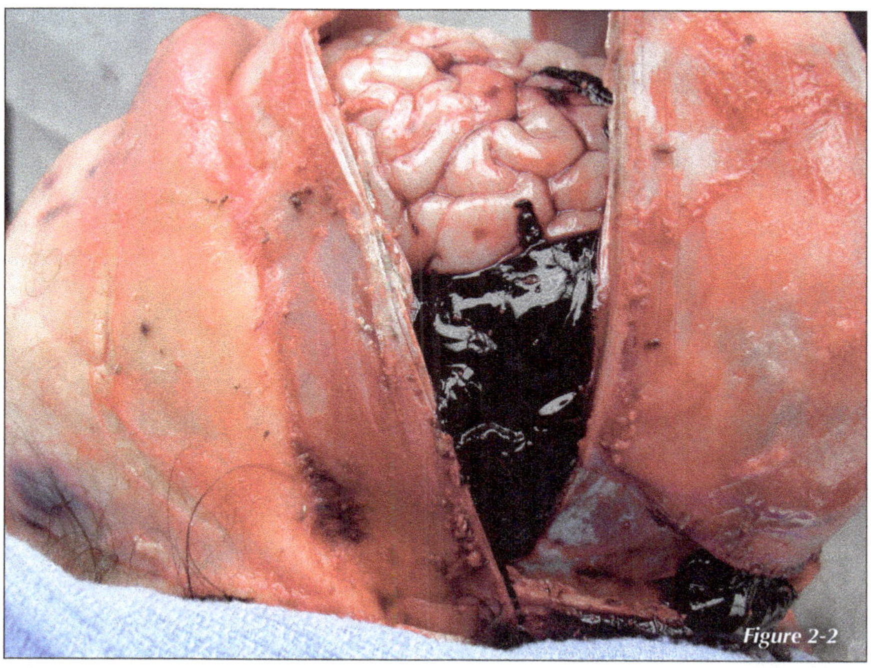

Figure 2-2. *The opened skull reveals subdural blood over left cerebral convexity.*

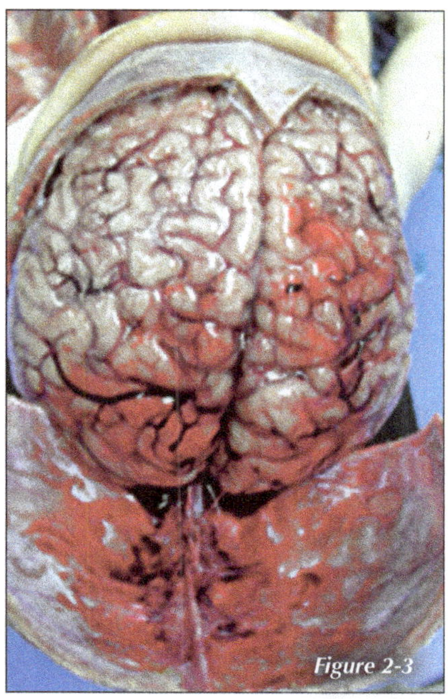

Figure 2-3. *Skull opened to demonstrate minimal subdural blood over cerebral convexities.*

metabolic diseases, birth trauma, tumors, genetic disorders, autoimmune diseases, clotting disorders, infectious diseases, long-term shunting for hydrocephalus, and other miscellaneous conditions. In cases of possible inflicted head trauma, other sources of subdural bleeding must be considered, and close attention must be given to the history, physical examination, radiological imaging, and laboratory studies before excluding other causes of the bleeding. Subdural blood isolated to the ventral surface of the brain or to a small focal area of the convexity requires close examination for another source of bleeding, as these locations are in variance with the mechanism of ruptured bridging vein bleeding.[61,62] Contact injury to the head can also produce subdural bleeding. Denton and Mileusnic[44] reported a 9-month-old boy who fell from 30 inches and sustained a right parietal fracture with a thin, adherent clotted 2 cm x 2 cm x 0.1 cm SDH underlying the fracture. This child survived without symptoms for 72 hours, but later, at autopsy, had severe brain edema and herniation.

Chronic Subdural Hematoma

Few cases of SDH evolve into chronic subdural hematomas, as most subdural blood will be resorbed over several weeks.[62-66] Experimental models are unable to reproduce a chronic subdural hematoma from acute subdural blood.[67] It has become clear that the majority of ***chronic subdural hematomas*** develop from subdural hygromas, which are caused by a traumatically induced tear of the arachnoid so that cerebrospinal fluid (CSF) can pass into the subdural space as an acute SDH is resolving.[68,70] A major factor promoting the resorption of acute subdural blood is the high levels of tissue thromboplastin in the brain and CSF.[71] Any pathologic process that causes cleavage of the dural border cell zone can induce proliferation of the dural border cells, which will produce a neomembrane. As an acute SDH resolves, the cleaved intradural zone may remain as a persistent space. A lowered intracranial pressure could promote persistence of an intradural space and allow CSF or remnants of the liquid portion of an acute SDH to pass into the cleaved space and create the hygroma. Intracranial pressure determines what happens to the hygroma. Normalizing of pressure leads to the resolution of the hygroma while continued lower pressure allows for hygromal expansion wherein the proliferating of dural border cells may develop a neomembrane. Neovascularization of the neomembrane is part of a process by which the membrane develops. Fragile vessels created in this neovascularization may tear with little or no trauma and result in microhemorrhages. The repeated microhemorrhage bleeding and repeated resolution of the hemorrhages leads to an enlarging hygroma that then transforms into a chronic enlarging subdural hematoma.[68,74,75]

The histopathology of subdural membranes in young children is similar to those described in adults. A chronic subdural hematoma is a liquefied hematoma with a membrane. The membrane consists of fibroblastic proliferation and neovascularization.[66] An acute SDH is a clot and does not have a membrane. The fluid in a subdural hygroma is a mixture of blood and CSF. In infants and younger children, it may be difficult to distinguish between a subdural hygroma and a chronic subdural hematoma. Because the infant's skull is deformable, posttraumatic brain atrophy may allow significant enlargement of a chronic subdural hematoma. Later, when the sutures fuse, an enlarging chronic subdural hematoma may cause a mass effect.

Figure 2-4. *Patches of fresh SAH in the right parasagittal region.*

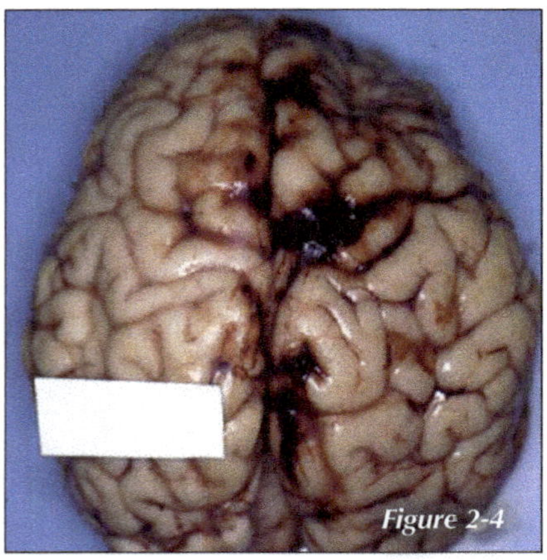

Subarachnoid Hemorrhage

SAH and SDH can both result from disruptions of the bridging veins, as these veins pass from the cortical surface through the arachnoid membrane. SAH occurs in roughly the same number of cases of abusive head injury as SDH but appears as patches over the cerebral convexities and within the interhemispheric surfaces, where it may be difficult to see. SAH is usually adjacent to or under areas of SDH (**Figure 2-4**). SAH is more difficult to visualize on CT images than SDH.

Retinal Hemorrhage

In cases of suspected or obvious abusive injury, forensic pathologists routinely remove the eyes and attached optic nerves by sawing away the bone of the orbital roofs and lifting out the globes with the attached optic nerves and surrounding fatty soft tissue. The eyes are fixed in formaldehyde and examined after at least 2 weeks of fixation. The external features of the eyes are noted, and any blood in the optic nerve sheath is described and documented. The eyes are then sliced open through a plane from the pupil to the optic nerve to expose the interior of the eye (**Figure 2-5**). The eyes are transilluminated and examined closely for the presence of retinal hemorrhages, retinoschisis, retinal folds, vitreous hemorrhage, or other abnormalities. Microscopic sections are taken from each eye. Usually retinal hemorrhages are easily seen, but retinal hemorrhages in small numbers can be present on microscopic examination instead.

In the gross examination, the pathologist should document features including the presence of retinal hemorrhages; the distribution of the hemorrhages within the retina, posterior, mid-retina, or peripheral retina extending to the ora serrata; the number of hemorrhages (numerous or few); the presence of retinoschisis cavities; and the presence or absence of blood in the optic nerve sheath. The microscopic examination should document the number of retinal hemorrhages, their distribution within the retina, and the layers of the retina involved in hemorrhage.

Retinal hemorrhages are common in abusive head trauma and occur in as many as 85% of cases.[76-78] The number of children who have retinal hemorrhages is higher in children who died than in unimpaired survivors.[79] The pattern of retinal hemorrhages associated commonly with abusive head trauma is numerous hemorrhages in multiple layers of the retina that are widely distributed from the posterior pole to the periphery as far as the ora serrata. The retinal hemorrhages tend to be bilateral and are often more numerous in one eye than in the other but may also only be in 1 eye. The side of unilateral hemorrhages does not necessarily correspond to the side of impact, fracture, or SDH, but it can. ***Retinoschisis***, the splitting of the layers of the retina with blood filling the cleaved cavity, results from vitreous traction on the retina during acceleration-deceleration motions of the head transmitted to the eye.[80,81] Retinoschisis is highly associated with acceleration-deceleration abusive head injury but has been reported in 2 cases of fatal crushing head injury,[82,83] a fatal motor vehicle accident,[84] and an 11-meter fall.[85] Although retinal folds originating at the optic nerve head and radiating outward in vertical folds across the retina may be postmortem artifacts, perimacular folds said to be characteristic of violent shaking appear as circumlinear traumatic retinal pleats that surround retinoschisis and can be identified and distinguished postmortem.[79,86]

Figure 2-5. *Eye sectioned to demonstrate numerous retinal hemorrhages throughout retina and blood in optic nerve sheath.*

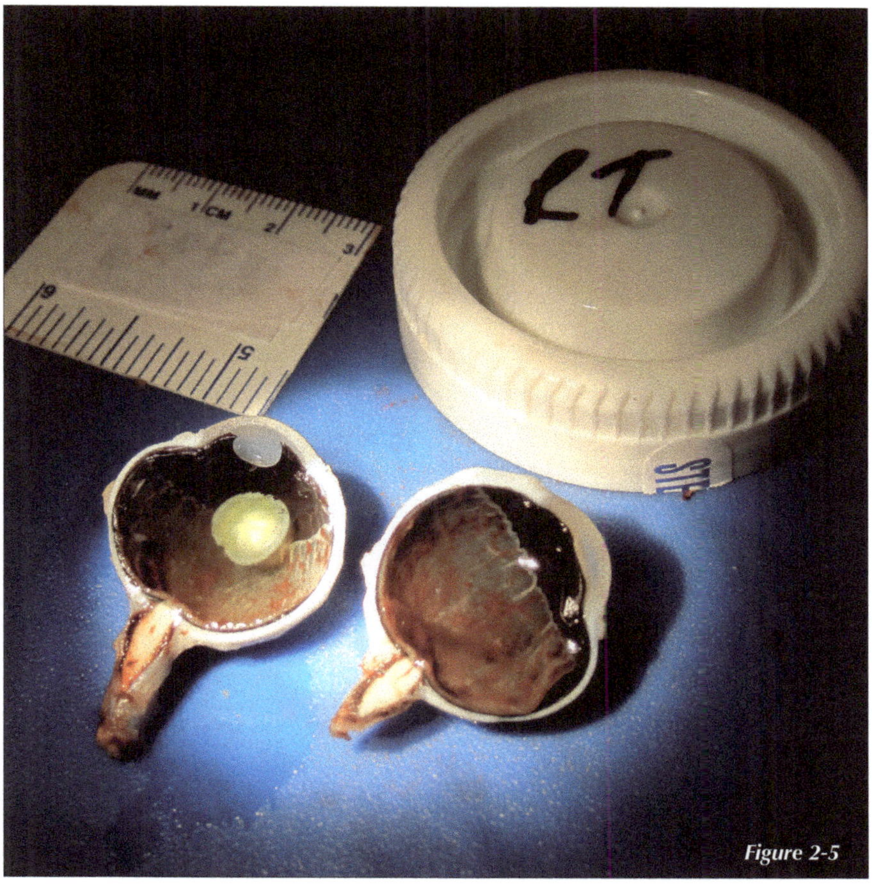

Figure 2-5

Along with abusive injury, retinal hemorrhages can be caused by bleeding disorders and coagulopathies, sepsis, meningitis, birth, certain genetic disorders, increased intracranial pressure, vasculopathies, vascular malformations, and more.[79,87-90] When retinal hemorrhages are seen in these conditions, they tend to be few in number and confined to the posterior pole and may have other unique characteristics. While resuscitation is sometimes mentioned as a cause of retinal hemorrhages, and many of the children who are found to have abusive head injuries underwent resuscitation, Gilliland and Luckenbach[91] found no support for the hypothesis that retinal hemorrhages are caused by resuscitation.

Retinal hemorrhages are seen in fewer cases of accidental trauma than inflicted head injury. Of 140 children injured by motor vehicle accidents, falls, assaults (eg, non-child abuse), and miscellaneous accidents, Johnson et al[92] found 2 children who had retinal hemorrhages in association with head trauma. Both were passengers in motor vehicle accidents. One of these children died and the other had cerebral contusions and SAH. Optic nerve sheath hemorrhage is also commonly associated with the retinal hemorrhages that accompany abusive head trauma in young children. Blood in the optic nerve sheath may also be seen in other causes of intracranial hemorrhage not associated with abusive injury.

Brain Contusions

The soft consistency of the young brain makes it less likely to contuse than the brain at later ages. Even in very young children, brain contusions may be seen adjacent to skull fractures and then are correctly categorized as fracture contusions. Neither coup nor contrecoup contusions are seen before the age of about 4 years. ***Contrecoup contusions*** are caused by a moving head falling from a standing position in such a manner as to cause a torque action and accelerate the head. Because young children begin close to the ground, they do not fall in this same manner as adults because they cannot torque when falling from standing. In young children, when brain contusions do appear, they tend to be rather faint and may appear almost as a blush on the surface of the cortex. In infants younger than 5 months, contusion tears may be seen. These lesions were described by Lindenberg and Freytag[93] as a manifestation of diffuse axonal injury. ***Contusion tears*** are slits or splits within the junction of the cortex and white matter or within the lamina of the cortical layers (**Figure 2-6**). These tears may vary in dimension from thin, small splits to larger, gaping defects. Similar defects may be produced by handling the brain, so caution is needed when diagnosing these lesions. The diagnosis of a contusion tear is a gross diagnosis that can be confirmed microscopically, but a tear first visualized microscopically is an artifact of handling.

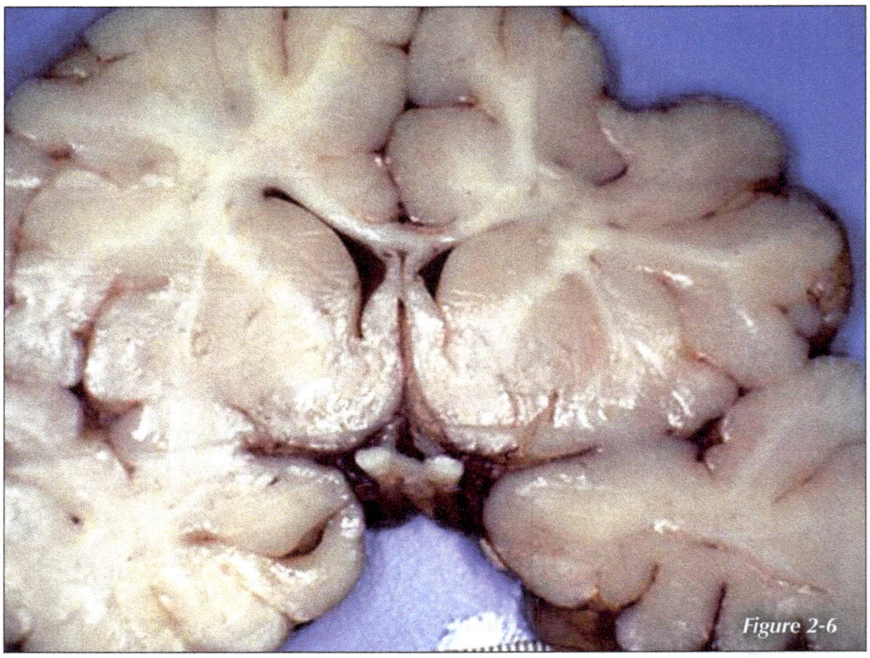

Figure 2-6. *A 4-month-old male with shaking head injury. A contusion tear is seen in the right side of the corpus callosum.*

Diffuse Axonal Injury

Severe angular acceleration-deceleration forces on the head can create diffuse shearing injury of the brain, resulting in widespread damage to axons, small blood vessels, and even tissue tears as described above. The inertial brain motion causes differential rotational movement of the brain beginning at the periphery of the brain and extending centrally with increasing force. As the tissues encountered are of differing consistencies and structure, shearing is facilitated at these points.[94,95]

Adams[95] proposed the following grading system for traumatic diffuse axonal injury (tDAI):

— ***Grade 1:*** Microscopic damage to axons without gross hemorrhage

— ***Grade 2:*** Microscopic damage to axons with hemorrhage in the corpus callosum

— ***Grade 3:*** Microscopic damage to axons with hemorrhage in the dorsal aspect of the brainstem

The hemorrhages described in association with tDAI are streak and punctuate hemorrhages that occur in the same locations as the axonal damage. These hemorrhages range from 1 mm to several centimeters when there has been survival for many days, and the hemorrhages enlarge over this time.[94] In young children, tDAI is seldom associated with these hemorrhages, possibly because the blood vessels are elastic and tend not to tear as readily as axons on tissue deformation. Damaged axons may be visible on light microscopy after 18 to 24 hours using hematoxylin-eosin (HE) staining. Damaged axons appear as retraction bulbs where the axoplasm has accumulated at points of axonal injury. On HE staining, the retraction bulbs are pink. In young children, the axons are very thin, and the resulting small retraction bulbs are difficult to see. To better study axonal injury, it is helpful to use special staining techniques. ***Beta-amyloid precursor protein*** (BAPP) is an immunohistochemical stain that is helpful in viewing damaged axons. BAPP staining can demonstrate damage to axons within 2 hours of injury.[96,97]

The axonal damage that is elucidated by BAPP immunohistochemistry is not specific as to the type of axonal damage. Patterns of axonal damage related to trauma (tDAI), hypoxic/ischemic (VAI), or metabolic, may be discerned using BAPP immunohistochemistry. To study the neuropathology of axonal injury requires protocols for sampling techniques and interpretation of the slides to distinguish and to diagnose these patterns of axonal injury.[98,99] In some cases, BAPP expression may be absent in damaged axons even when there has been a length of survival, and reactive changes would be expected if the cerebral circulation is halted rapidly at the time of injury.

Geddes and colleagues[100,101] studied the neuropathology of 53 cases of inflicted head injury using the BAPP technique. In one study,[100] 37 of the 53 were younger than 9 months of age and 16 were between 13 months and 8 years. The sampling protocol for BAPP staining used many sections, including several sections of hemispheric white matter, corpus callosum, internal capsule, cerebellum, midbrain, pons, medulla, and spinal cord. BAPP staining identified 2 patterns of axonal damage, VAI and tDAI.

The VAI pattern is characterized as broad geographic areas of BAPP expression that is often related to vessels. The tDAI pattern is identified as individual BAPP positive axons or small groups of scattered BAPP positive axons (**Figure 2-7-a** and **b**). Geddes et al[101] reported only 3 of 53 cases as having evidence of tDAI, an 8-year-old boy and 2 infants, both of whom had severe head injuries with bilateral skull fractures. Geddes found damaged axons in the corticospinal tracts of the medulla and pons in 8 cases and concluded that focal axonal damage to the craniocervical junction was probably more frequent and significant than tDAI. Geddes suggested that this type of damage was secondary to stretch injury from cervical hyperextension/flexion. Although

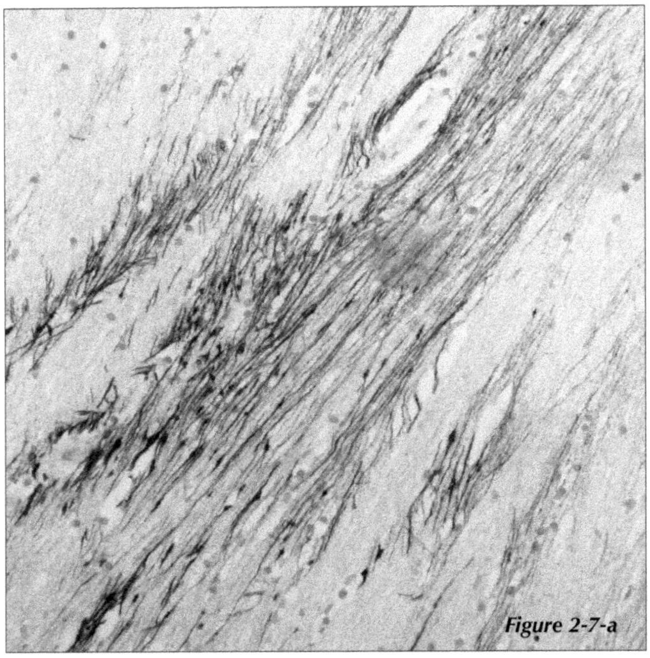

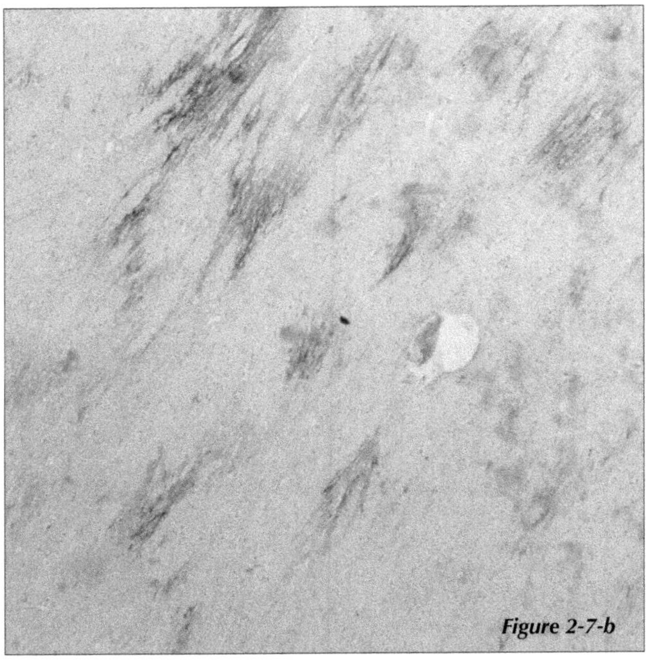

Figure 2-7-a. *Photomicrograph of vascular pattern of axonal injury with broad areas of BAPP expression.*

Figure 2-7-b. *Photomicrograph of traumatic pattern of axonal injury showing scattered individual axons with positive staining with BAPP.*

Geddes found that tDAI was rare in infants, it was noted that their control group of non–head-injured infants who had suffered respiratory abnormalities did not show the same evidence of VAI as did the group with inflicted head injury.

The author carried out a study similar to the Geddes 2001 studies.[102] The study included 34 cases of inflicted head trauma, with 18 cases involving children younger than 1 year and 16 children aged 13 months to 8 years. Nineteen control cases of non–head-injured children ranged from 5 weeks to 10 years.

In some cases of head injury studied by the author,[102] both VAI and tDAI were present together and could be distinguished. Many infants and children with inflicted head injury have such global hypoxic damage, which means that it may be difficult to recognize the pattern of tDAI when there is extensive VAI because the tDAI pattern is much less pervasive compared to the VAI pattern.

Table 2-1. Geddes and Colleagues Findings

Case Study Age Groups

— 37 of 53 were younger than 9 months

— 16 of 53 were between 13 months and 8 years

Finding	*Frequency*
Skull Fractures	36%
Acute SDH	72%
Retinal Hemorrhages	71%
Additional Injuries (eg, non-head fractures, abdominal injuries, bruises, burns)	51%
Impact at the Head with Scalp Bruising or Skull Fracture	85%
Cortical Contusions	9% (all cases younger than 4.5 months)
Global Neuronal Hypoxia-Ischemia	84% (infants), 63% (older children)

Table 2-2. Author Findings

Finding	*Frequency*
Multiple Bruises	50%
Burns	5%
Rib Fractures	20%
Laceration of Liver	5%
Torn Frenulum	5%
Laceration of Mesentery	2%
Healing or Healed Skull Fracture	5%
Healed Clavicle Fracture	8%
Long Bone Fractures	29%
Subgaleal Contusions	76%
Skull Fractures	20%
SDH	91%
Retinal Hemorrhages	80%
VAI pattern of BAPP Expression	27%
tDAI Pattern of BAPP Expression	73%
BAPP Expression in cord/Corticospinal Tracts of the Medulla	73% of cases including cervical spinal cord
Contusion Tears	6% of cases in head injury group

Figure 2-8. *Calvarium opened to show small atrophic brain following 13 years of survival after severe abusive head trauma.*

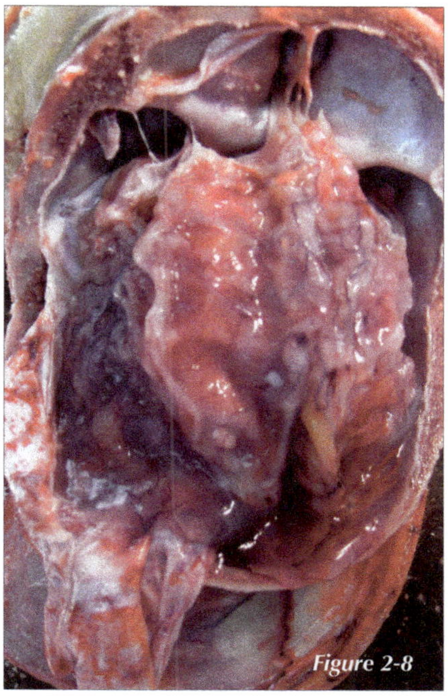

Brain Swelling

Brain swelling is a common finding in the autopsies of young children who died from inflicted head injury if there is survival for some period of time. If the child dies shortly after the injury, there may be little swelling of the brain. Brain swelling is recognizable by the flattening of the gyral surfaces and narrowing of the sulci, along with the appearance of the brain filling the cranial cavity when the brain is removed. Brain weight is also a good indicator of swelling if the weight is 10% to 15% greater than the expected value. Brain swelling is hypothesized by some investigators to be caused by hypoxia that follows the apnea that commonly accompanies these head injuries. Hypoxia does not fully explain the pathological findings, such as SDH, retinal hemorrhages, and the pattern of atrophy that develops in surviving children (**Figure 2-8**).

Head Trauma Case Studies

Case Study 2-1

This mother left her 14-month-old daughter with her boyfriend when she went to work. When she returned home in the morning, she did not see the child and woke up the boyfriend who said the child was on the floor. The mother then found the child unresponsive in a prone position on the floor next to her bed. A soiled fitted bed sheet was found wedged between the bed and the wall. The boyfriend said the space heater, which sat on a dresser above the bed, had fallen onto the child in the middle of the night and her screaming woke him up. When the mother left for work that night, the child was wearing a onesie, but when she came home, the child was only wearing a diaper. The child's clothes were found and had blood on the neck, crotch, and right arm area. In an interview, the mother became very upset and shouted, "He killed my baby."

Cause of Death: Closed head trauma

Other Significant Conditions: Blunt Thoracoabdominal Trauma

Manner of Death: Homicide

Table 2-3-a. Autopsy Results

Injuries

Head

Type	*Measurement*
Fresh abrasions on the nose:	
— Right	10 mm x 8 mm
— Left	9 mm x 7 mm
Abrasion on nose tip	4 mm x 3 mm
Philtrum abrasion	13 mm x 4 mm
Contusion on inner mucosal surface of upper lip	15 mm x 15 mm
Tear of right upper lip	1 mm
Large, fresh tear of frenulum	15 mm x 8 mm
Abrasion on chin	8 mm x 5 mm
Left cheek, upper crescent contusion	35 mm
—Lower crescent contusion consistent with bite mark	30 mm

Extremities

2 punctate abrasions on left shoulder	1 mm each
5 burns with a grid pattern from portable heater on right arm	11 mm x 20 mm, 50 mm x 47 mm, 60 mm x 35 mm, 55 mm x 20 mm, 40 mm x 20 mm
Abrasion on right wrist	2 mm
3 round scars on right thigh	2 mm
Patterned burn on right thigh	55 mm x 35 mm

Chest/Abdomen

3 areas of burn in grid pattern	80 mm x 25 mm, 85 mm x 90 mm, 55 mm x 25 mm
Bite mark contusion on abdomen	35 mm and 41 mm crescents
Multiple contusions:	
— 23 contusions on left upper abdomen	10 to 20 mm
— 6 contusions on midline chest	5 to 15 mm
— 8 contusions on right upper abdomen	10 to 15 mm

Anus

Fresh deep tears:	
— 12 o'clock	8 mm
— 8 o'clock	4 mm
— 5 o'clock	4 mm
— 6 o'clock	5 mm
Rectum was removed and found to have extensive soft tissue hemorrhage sounding serosal surface of the rectum and soft tissue of the rectum	3 cm x 4 cm area
Hemorrhages and tears were found within the mucosal surface of the rectum	

(continued)

Table 2-3-a. Autopsy Results *(continued)*

INJURIES *(CONTINUED)*

Back

TYPE	*MEASUREMENT*
4 patterned grid burns	90 mm x 50 mm, 10 mm x 70 mm, 45 mm x 10 mm, 65 mm x 50 mm
Multiple contusions:	
— Right mid-back had 4 contusions	5 mm each
— Midline back had 10 to 12 contusions	10 to 15 mm each
— Left mid- and lower back had 12 contusions	10 to 20 mm x 10 mm

Chest

- — Fresh hemorrhage was present in the subcutaneous tissue beneath contusions
- — Clear serous fluid tinged with blood in the left pleural cavity
- — Fractures of left ribs 5 through 9 posteriorly
- — Hemorrhages beneath the pleura of the left rib cage covering fresh fractures

Abdomen

Liquid blood in the peritoneal cavity	100 mL
Extensive fresh hematoma adjacent to the cecum	5 cm x 4 cm
Fresh hemorrhage in the mesentery of the small bowel	4 cm

INTERNAL EXAMINATION

Lungs

Small hemorrhages within the parenchyma, contusions	8 mm

Liver

Large area of subcapsular hemorrhage	80 cm x 20 cm
Laceration between the right and left lobes	15 mm x 5 mm

Pancreas

Fresh hemorrhage within middle portion	10 mm x 10 mm

Adrenals

Extensive hemorrhage in soft tissue surrounding the right kidney and adrenal

Kidneys

Fresh hemorrhage within the pelvis of both kidneys

Uterus and Adnexa

Extensive fresh hemorrhage in the soft tissues surrounding the vagina, similar to the hemorrhage around the rectum

Cranial Cavity

Subgaleal hemorrhages, right parietal	15 mm x 10 mm, 20 mm x 10 mm, 5 areas of 5 mm and 10 mm
Thin layer of subdural blood over cerebral convexities and fresh subdural blood over posterior fossa	
Eyes were negative for retinal hemorrhages	

(continued)

Table 2-3-a. Autopsy Results ***(continued)***

MICROSCOPIC EXAMINATION

- ***Lung:*** Focal edema, aspirated materials, postmortem growth of bacteria, large areas of contusion and hemorrhage
- ***Liver:*** Large areas of acute subcapsular hemorrhage and acute laceration and hemorrhage
- ***Mesentery:*** Acute hemorrhage
- ***Pancreas:*** Acute hemorrhage in multiple sites
- ***Rectum:*** Laceration of the mucosal surface with early neutrophilic reaction and extensive acute hemorrhage in the muscle wall and rupturing through serosa
- ***Vagina:*** Acute hemorrhage in soft tissue between rectum and vagina with early neutrophilic response
- ***Scalp:*** Right parietal showed acute subgaleal hemorrhage with very early neutrophilic response
- ***Back:*** Acute hemorrhage in subcutaneous tissue underlying burn
- ***Ribs:*** Acute fractures with acute subperiosteal hemorrhage
- Right adrenal showed acute hemorrhage in surrounding soft tissue
- ***Brain:*** Increased mononuclear cells in leptomeninges
- BAPP staining is negative
- Dura showed acute subdural blood

Figure 2-9-a. *Back with 4 areas of patterned grid burn and contusions.*

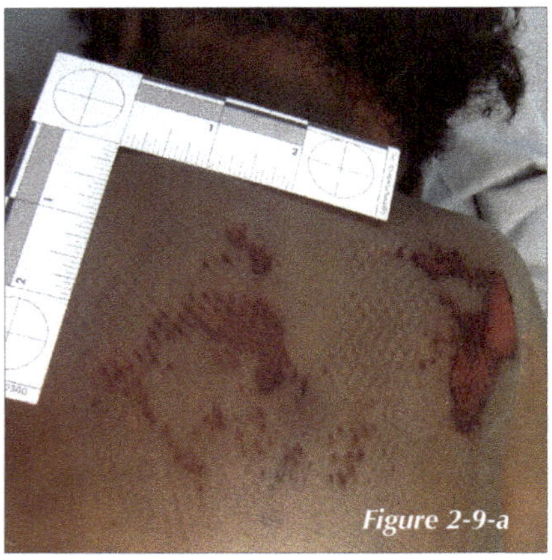

Figure 2-9-a

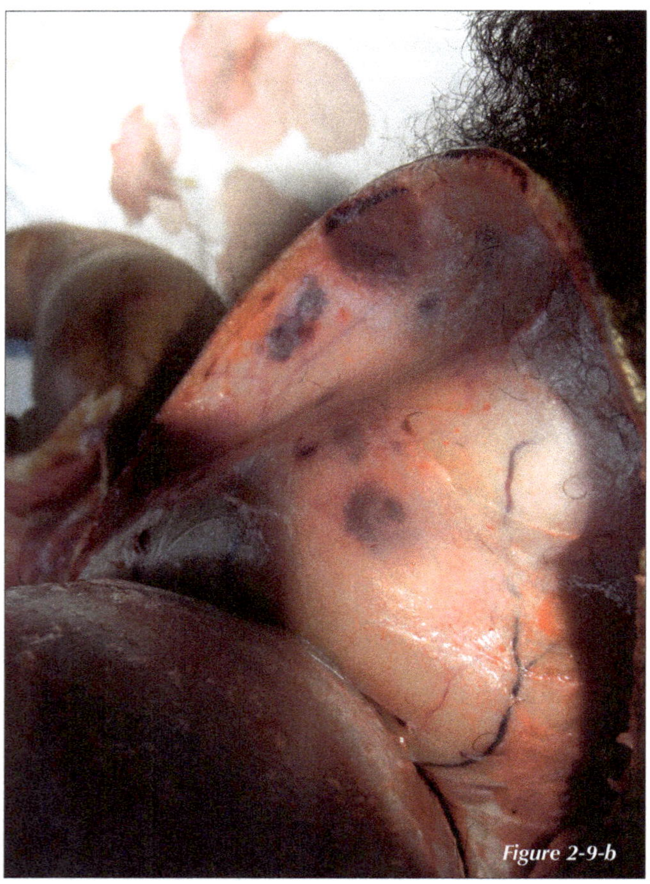

Figure 2-9-b

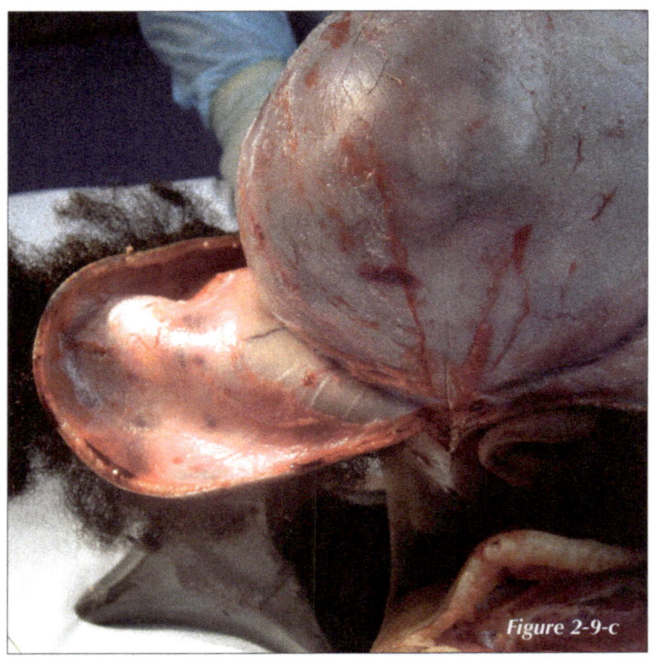

Figure 2-9-c

Figure 2-9-b and c. *Multiple subgaleal hemorrhages, right parietal scalp.*

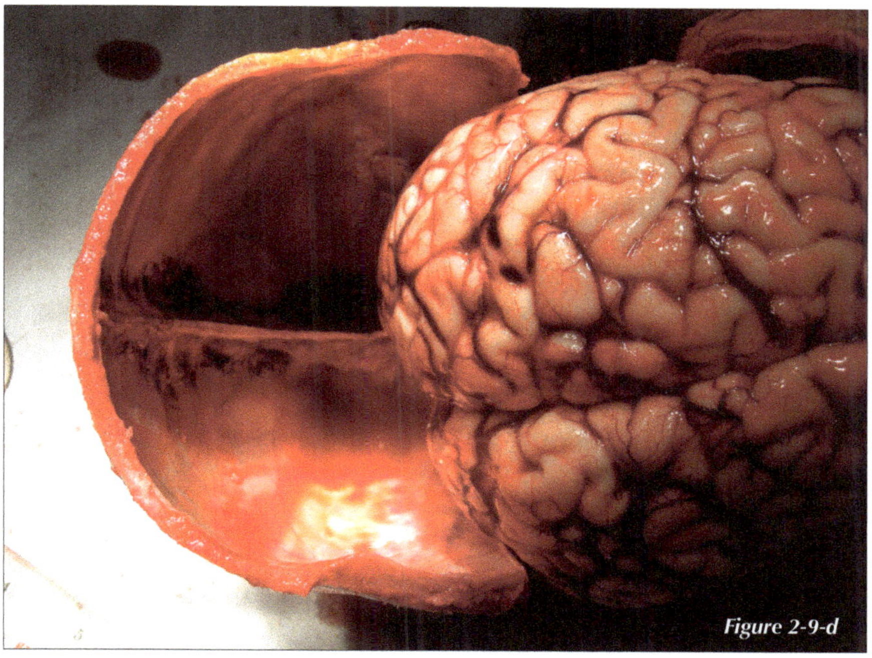

Figure 2-9-d. Subdural blood over cerebral convexities.

Figure 2-9-e. Fractures of left ribs 5 through 9.

Figure 2-9-f. Liver with large area of subscapular hemorrhage and laceration between right and left lobes.

Figure 2-9-g. Rectum removed and opened to show extensive soft tissue hemorrhage surrounding serosal surface of rectum.

Figure 2-9-h. Block of organs removed at autopsy, dorsal surface showing large area of hemorrhage around right kidney and adrenal.

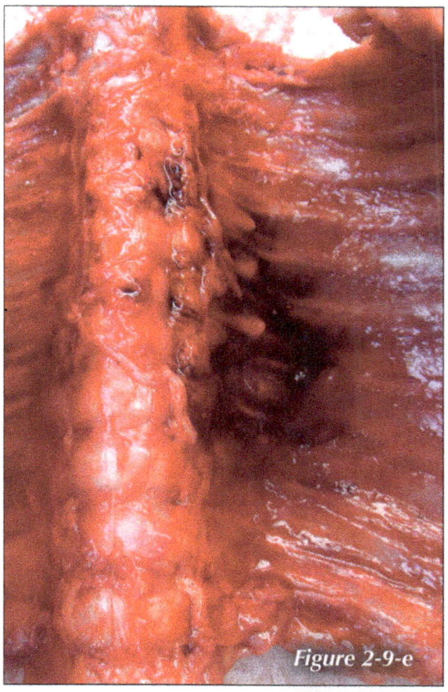

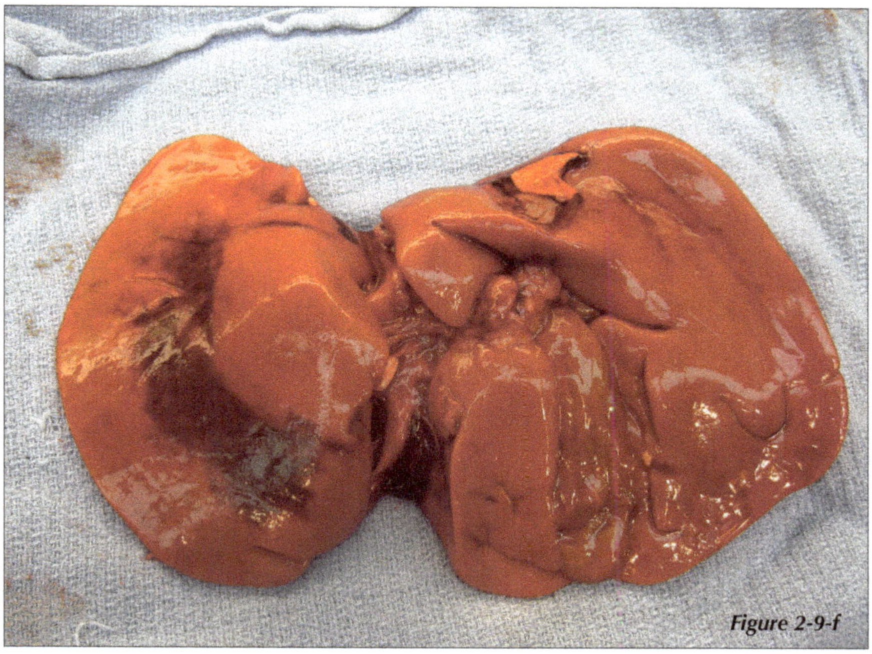

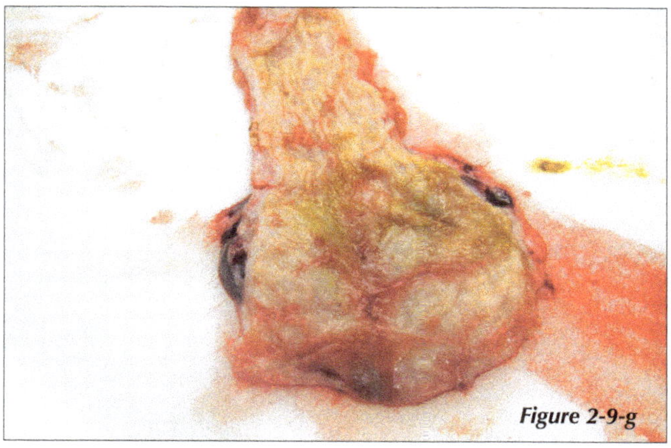

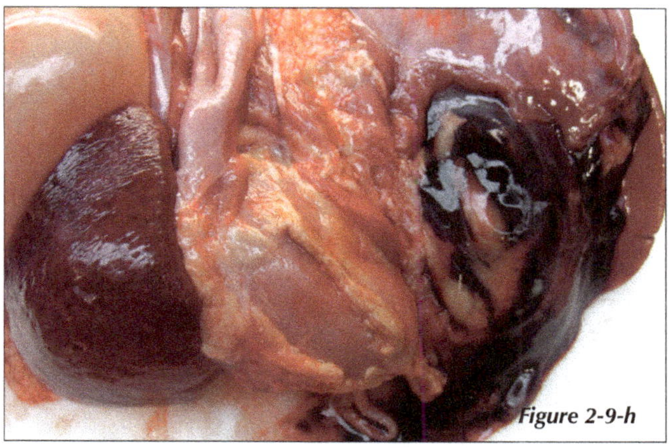

Case Study 2-2

The initial history given to the emergency department (ED) staff was that this 11-month-old girl was found sitting in a car seat unresponsive after the mother left her for a few minutes to use the restroom. When the mother returned, she saw her 4-year old son standing in front of the child and holding a flashlight. At this time, a friend showed up at the home. Seeing that the child was unresponsive, the friend placed her under the shower to try to get a response. There was no response to the water, so the mother ran to the house next door to call 911. The mother lived in a townhouse with no electricity, so it was also very warm. There were 5 other children living at the residence. The child abuse hotline had 3 prior reports for this child, all against the mother, for malnourishment, untreated illness and injury, and a newborn crisis assessment. There were also 2 other prior reports against the mother for her other children, 1 for unsanitary living conditions and the other for a skull fracture. The child was in full arrest in the ED and was pronounced dead.

Cause of Death: Blunt Thoracoabdominal and closed head trauma

Manner of Death: Homicide

Table 2-4-a. Autopsy Results

External Examination

— Child appeared younger than stated age

— Weighed 12 pounds and measured 26 inches

Injuries

Head

Type	*Measurement*
Scabbed abrasion on right orbit below brow	4 mm
Fresh abrasion on right chin	2 mm
Left anterior neck contusion	4 mm x 3 mm
Thin, fresh SDH over both cerebral convexities and over right and left middle and posterior cranial fossae	
SAH over the brain	
Hemorrhage in fat tissue surrounding the left eye	
Both eyes contained optic nerve sheath hemorrhage	
SDH over the entire spinal cord	

Chest/Abdomen

13 purple contusions on mid to right lower chest to right upper abdomen	10 to 20 mm each, in an area of 10 mm x 7 cm
Fresh blood in the peritoneal cavity	110 mL
Left pelvic gutter hemorrhage into the muscle	3 cm x 3 cm
Hemorrhage in the abdominal cavity from liver laceration between the left and right lobes on ventral surface and soft tissue hemorrhage extending to the soft tissue of the pancreas	36 mm x 17 mm
Massive maceration and laceration of the internal parenchyma of the liver	60 mm x 35 mm area
Multiple contusions on thymus	
Multiple fresh contusions on right lower lobe	

Extremities

Scars on left thigh	1 mm (2), 6 mm x 3 mm, 4 mm x 5 mm
Brown pigmentation surrounding the anus	3 cm x 5 cm
Scar on right thigh	10 mm x 15 mm
Internally fresh hemorrhage in the soft tissue surrounding the rectum	

(continued)

Table 2-4-a. Autopsy Results *(continued)*

MICROSCOPIC EXAMINATION

- ***Lungs:*** Fresh hemorrhage in right lower lobe with tearing of alveolar walls and hemorrhage into the parenchyma
- ***Liver:*** Acute laceration and maceration of the capsule and parenchyma with associated acute hemorrhage
- ***Thymus:*** Contusional hemorrhages
- ***Perirectal soft tissue:*** Acute hemorrhage without inflammatory response
- ***Right upper abdominal wall contusions:*** Fresh hemorrhage within the fat of the subcutis

NEUROPATHOLOGY EXAMINATION

- ***Dura:*** Fresh, thin acute subdural blood; 1 mm thick old subdural membrane
- Subarachnoid hemorrhage over cerebral convexities
- Mild ventricular dilatation
- Thin layer of subdural hemorrhage over entire spinal cord
- Bilateral optic nerve sheath hemorrhages
- Heavy retinal hemorrhages in posterior portion of left eye
- No retinal hemorrhages in right eye

NEUROPATHOLOGIC MICROSCOPIC EXAMINATION

- Medulla, midbrain, pons, and cervical cord BAPP positive for traumatic axonal injury

Table 2-4-b. Diagnoses - Multiple Traumatic Injuries

CLOSED HEAD TRAUMA

- Acute SDH, cerebral convexities and cranial fossa
- SAH over cerebral convexities
- Bilateral optic nerve sheath hemorrhages
- Retinal hemorrhages, left eye
- Mixed patterns of diffuse traumatic and hypoxic axonal injury
- SDH over spinal cord
- Old, thin subdural membrane
- Mild ventricular dilatation

BLUNT THORACOABDOMINAL TRAUMA

- Contusions, right chest and abdomen (13)
- Contusions, thymus, right lower lobe
- Massive liver laceration
- Hemoperitoneum, 110 mL
- Contusion, left pelvis

OTHER TRAUMA

- Healed abrasion, right orbit
- Abrasion, right chin
- Contusion, left anterior neck

Figure 2-10-a. Multiple contusions on chest and onto right upper abdomen.

Figure 2-10-b. Chest and abdomen opened to show contusion of right lower lobe of lung and laceration of liver.

Figure 2-10-c. Calvarium retracted to demonstrate bilateral SDH over cerebral convexities and patches of parasagittal SAH.

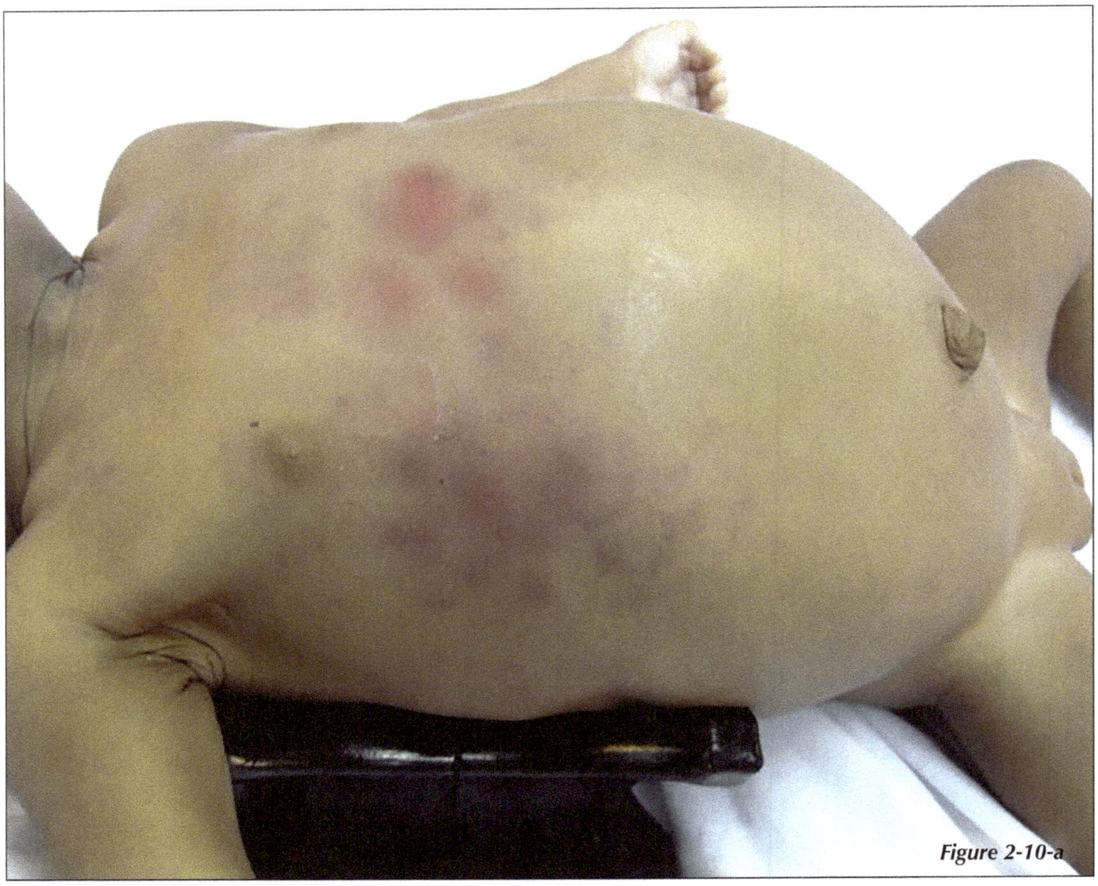

Figure 2-10-a

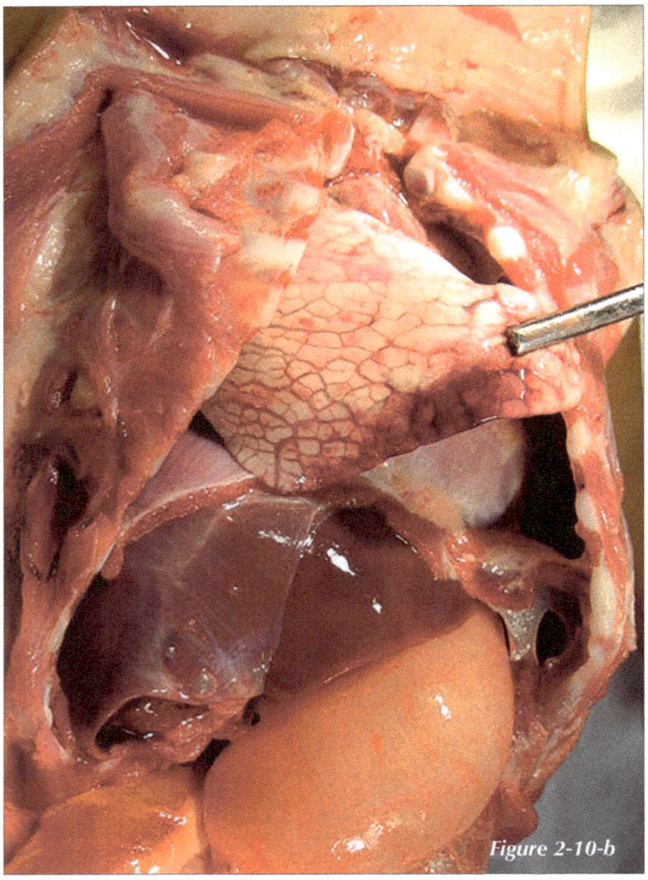

Figure 2-10-b

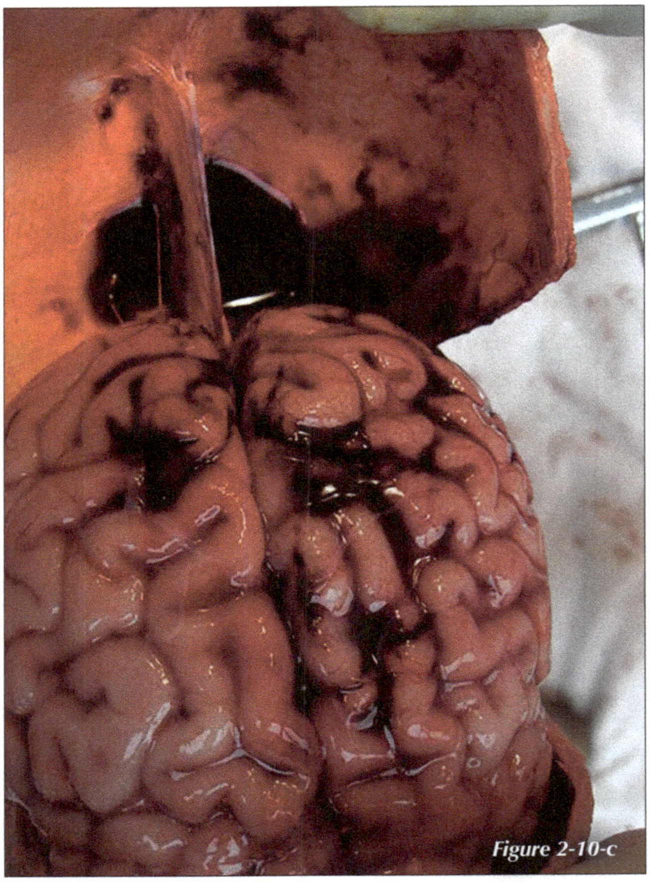

Figure 2-10-c

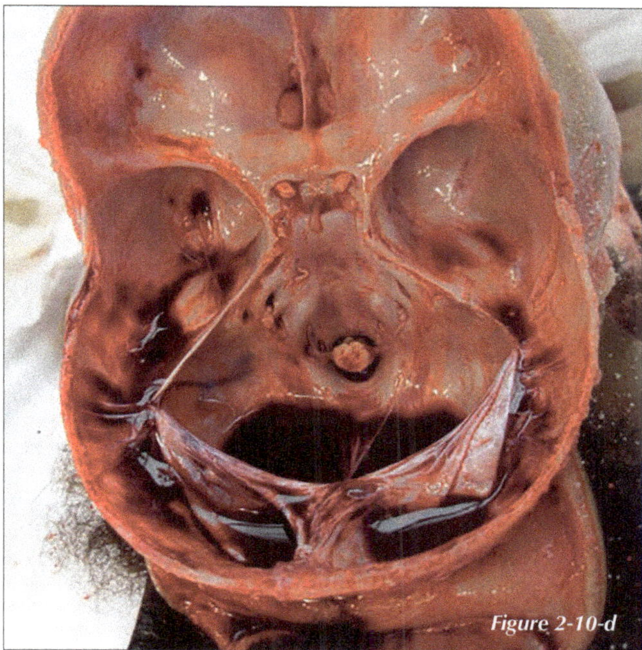

Figure 2-10-d

Figure 2-10-d. *Base of skull showing subdural blood in right and left middle and posterior fossae.*

Figure 2-10-e. *Brain after fixation demonstrating patches of parasagittal SAH.*

Figure 2-10-f. *Dura after fixation showing thin, old subdural membrane.*

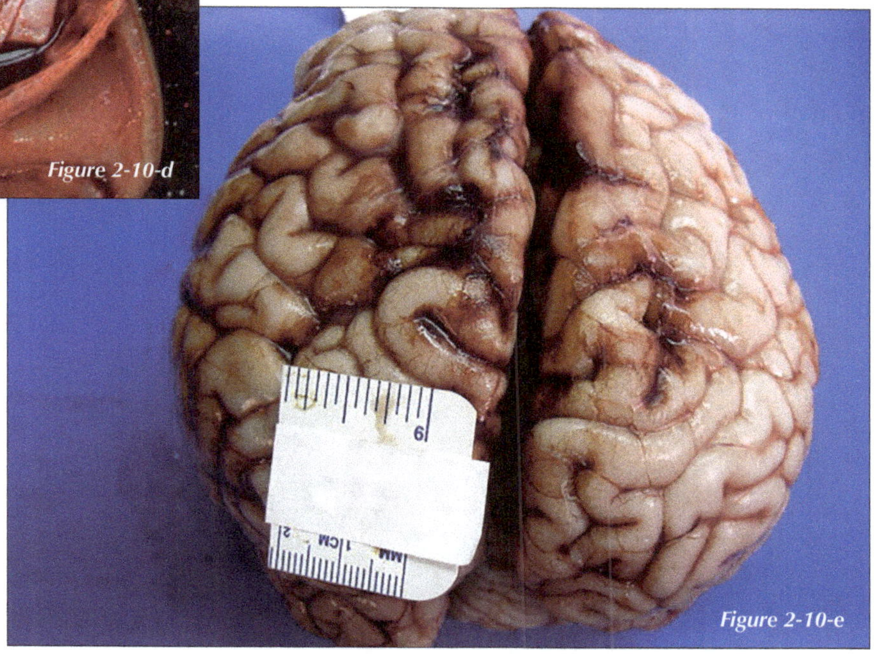

Figure 2-10-e

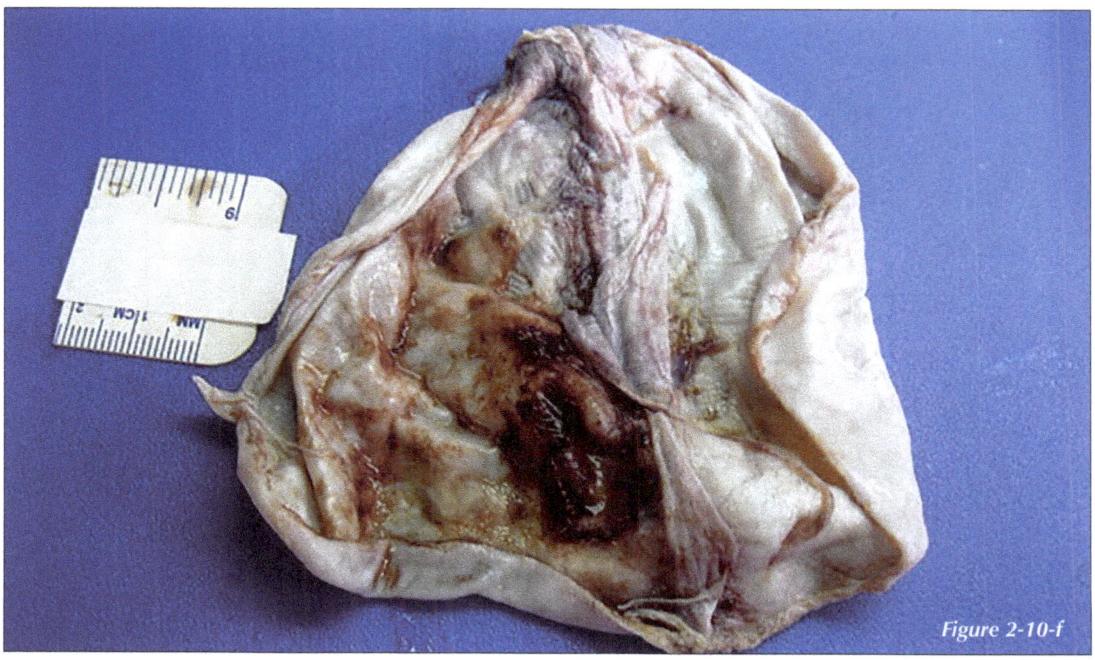

Figure 2-10-f

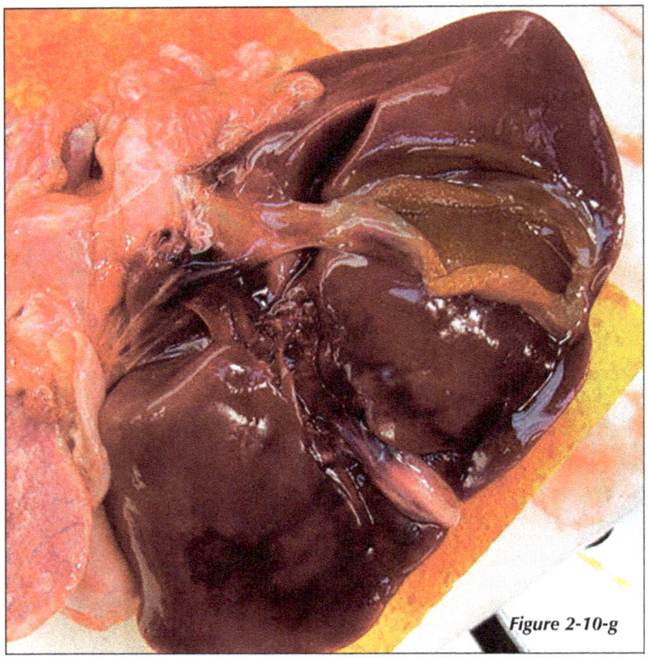

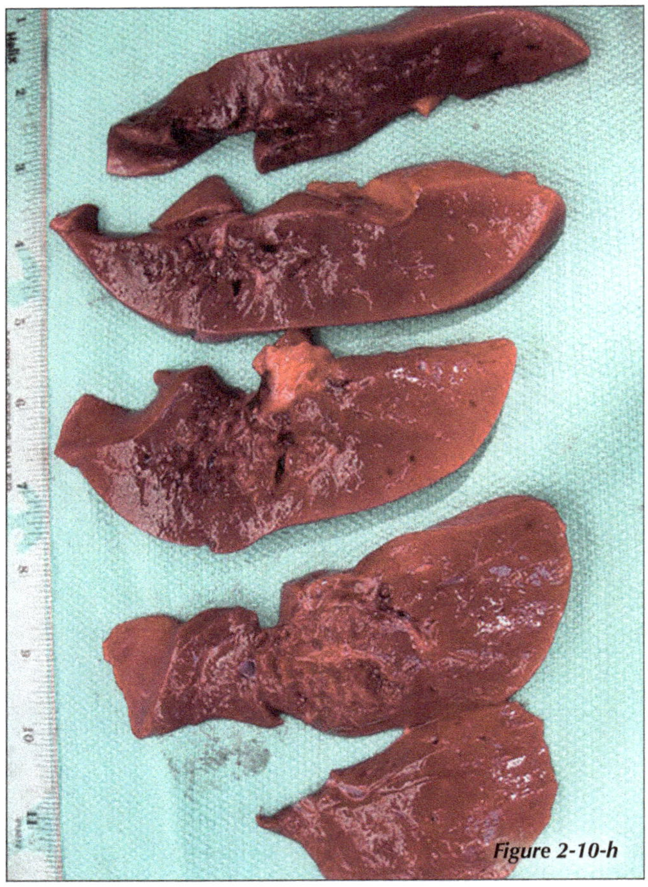

Figure 2-10-g. *Inferior surface of liver showing laceration between right and left lobes.*

Figure 2-10-h. *Sections of liver showing maceration of parenchyma by laceration.*

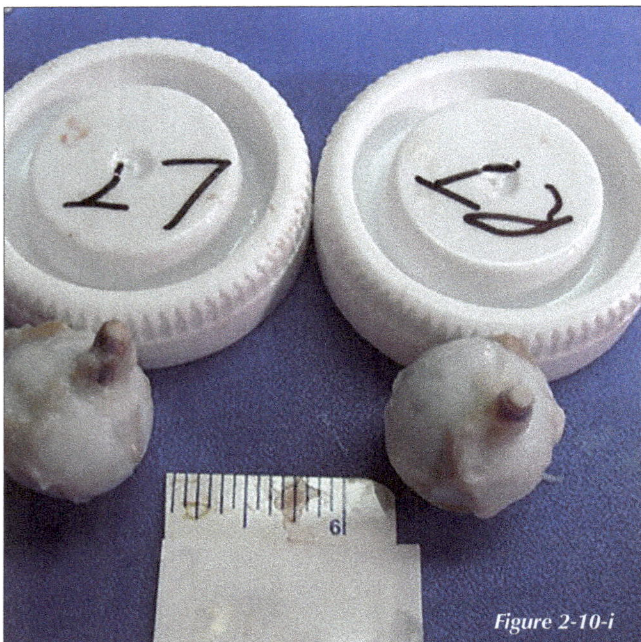

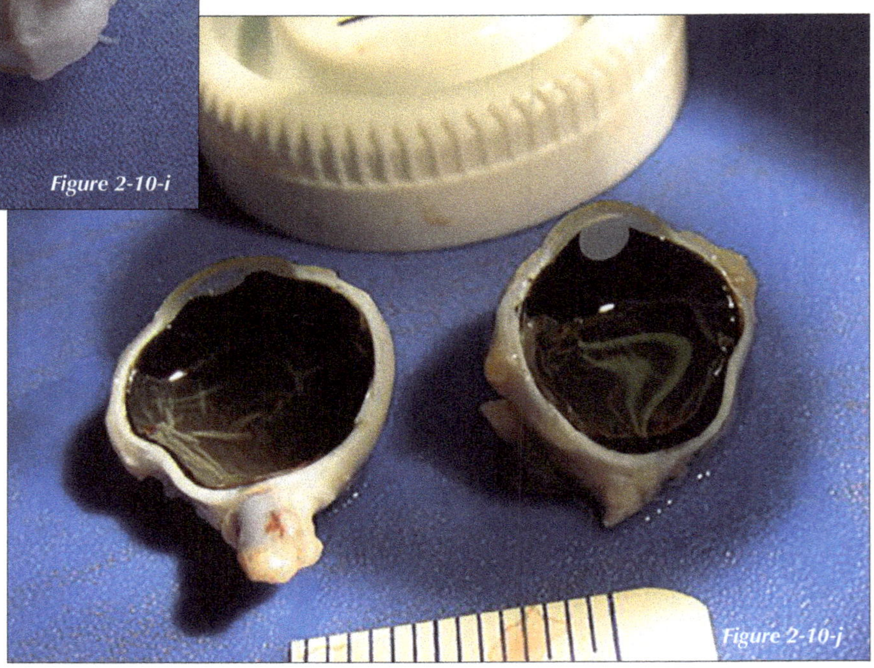

Figure 2-10-i. *Right and left eyes showing optic nerve sheath hemorrhages.*

Figure 2-10-j. *Sections of eyes showing a few retinal hemorrhages in the posterior pole of the right eye and none in the left eye.*

Case Study 2-3

This 18-month-old boy was left at his babysitter's home in the morning. The first provided history was that the babysitter placed the child on a blanket on the floor to go to sleep. She then went to put her own children to sleep when she heard the child scream. When she returned, she found him lying next to the coffee table with a red bump on his head. She laid him down again. The child started breathing irregularly and eventually stopped breathing, so she called 911. The second history given by the babysitter was that she was carrying the child while he was sleeping, and he slipped out of her arms and hit his head on vinyl-covered hardwood floor. The child was unconscious at the scene, and 911 was called. The child was unresponsive in the ED and died in the hospital.

Cause of Death: Blunt craniocerebral trauma

Manner of Death: Homicide

Table 2-5-a. Autopsy Results

Injuries

Type	***Measurement***
Multiple contusions along each side of face/upper neck:	
— Right	25 to 30 cm
— Left	20 mm
Contusion, right retroauricular scalp	20 mm
Small contusions in the right occipitoparietal area	20 mm x 20 mm area
4 contusions on right occipitoparietal scalp	70 mm x 10 mm linear area, 5 to 10 mm each
Ecchymotic areas scattered across the anterior chest	5 mm
Contusion, right nipple	15 mm x 10 mm
Contusion, lower sternal area	15 mm x 10 mm

Mild hemorrhage in these areas of the reflected scalp

Lungs

— Increased firmness and decreased crepitance, congestion and edema

Cranial Cavity

— Bilateral thin layer of SDH over the cerebral convexities, more prominent on the left

— Thin film of SDH overlying the floor of the left anterior and middle cranial fossae

Microscopic Examination

— ***Lung:*** Focal acute bronchopneumonia

— ***Brain:*** SAH, cerebral edema, axonal retraction bulbs

— ***Dura:*** Acute SDH

— ***Eyes:*** Retinal hemorrhages

Table 2-5-b. Diagnoses

Shaken Infant Syndrome

— Brain, axonal retraction bulbs

— Subarachnoid space

— SDH

— Cerebral edema, transtentorial herniation

— Eyes, retina, hemorrhage

Contusions

— Skin and scalp

Bronchopneumonia

— Lungs

Case Study 2-4

This 4-month-old girl had a history of vomiting and congestion for the past 2 weeks. On the day of the child's death, the father was trying to feed her, but she would not stop crying and started "breathing funny." The father stated that he shook the child to try to get her to breathe. 911 was called. She was unresponsive in the ED and died inpatient. The father was eventually charged with murder after admitting to potentially causing harm from CPR and shaking the child.

Cause of Death: Closed head injury; shaken infant syndrome

Manner of Death: Homicide

Table 2-6-a. Autopsy Results

CRANIAL CAVITY

— SDH overlying each cerebral hemisphere and within the base of the skull; hemorrhage is less than 2 to 3 mm thick

— Patchy SAH on convexities

NEUROPATHOLOGY EXAMINATION

— Mild, patchy SAH on the inferior surface of the temporal lobes

Table 2-6-b. Diagnoses

SHAKEN INFANT SYNDROME

— Bilateral SDH

— SAH

— Brain, diffuse axonal injury

— Cerebral edema

— Brain death

Case Study 2-5

This 10-year-old boy was found on the ground with an overturned bicycle. He had been riding the bicycle and was not wearing a helmet. At the scene, he was combative and became somnolent in the ED. A CT of the head showed fracture of the right temporal calvarium. The child became unresponsive in the ED. Neurosurgery was consulted, and observation of the boy was recommended. He died 2 days later.

Cause of Death: Craniocerebral Trauma

Manner of Death: Accident

Table 2-7-a. Autopsy Results

— Right temporal scalp contusion

— Fracture, right temporal skull

— Epidural hemorrhage over right parietal lobe

— Contrecoup contusions, left temporal lobe

Table 2-7-b. Diagnoses

CRANIOCEREBRAL TRAUMA

— Contusion, right temporal scalp

— Fracture, right temporal skull

— Epidural hemorrhage, right parietal lobe

— Contrecoup contusions, left temporal lobe

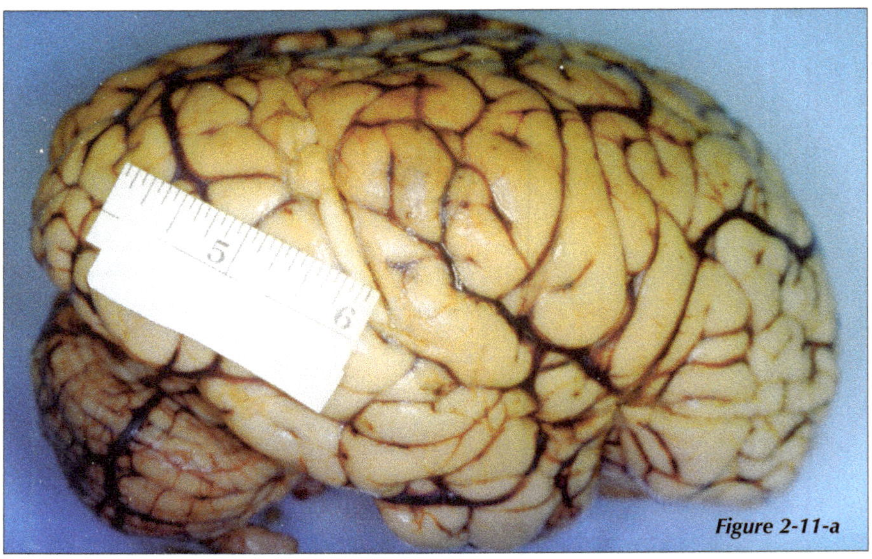

Figure 2-11-a

Figure 2-11-a. *Brain after fixation showing the lateral surface of the right hemisphere with marked flattening of the temporal lobe because of the epidural hemorrhage.*

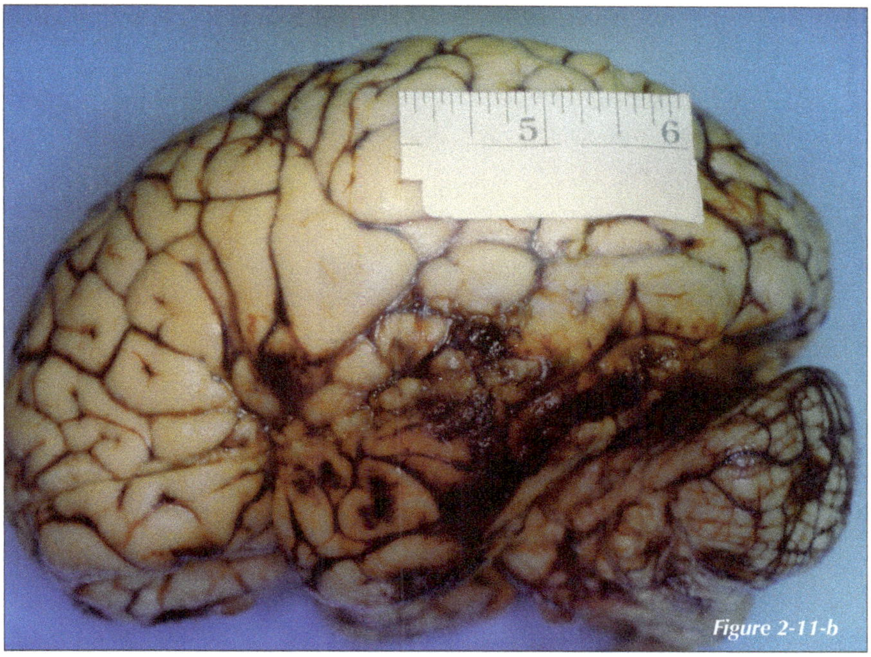

Figure 2-11-b

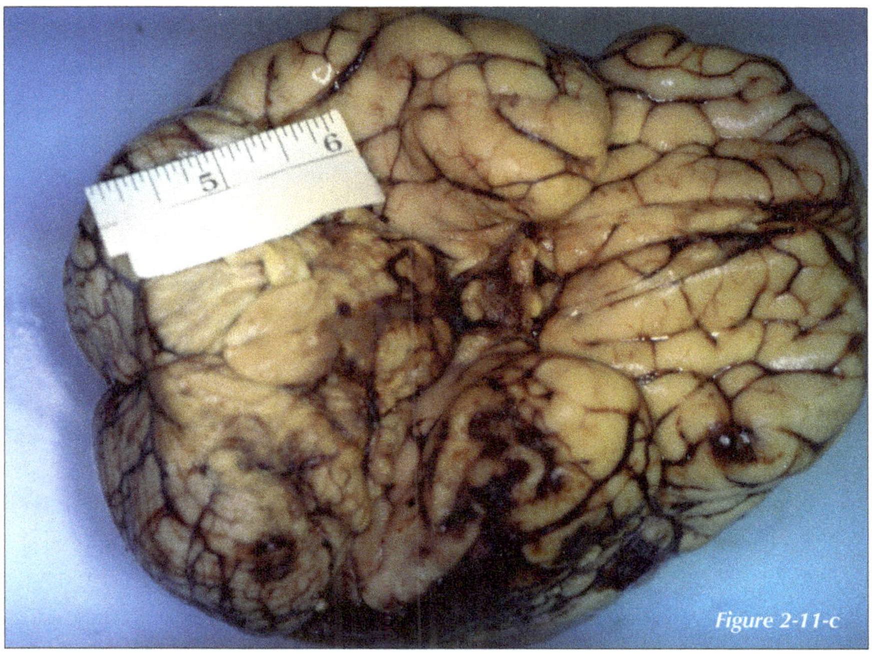

Figure 2-11-c

Figure 2-11-b. *Brain after fixation showing contrecoup contusions of the left superior, middle, and inferior temporal gyri.*

Figure 2-11-c. *Brain after fixation showing the ventral surface with bilateral tentorial herniation.*

References

1. McClain PW, Sacks JJ, Froehlke RG, Ewigman BG. Estimates of fatal child abuse and neglect, United States, 1979 through 1988. *Pediatrics*. 1993;91(2):338-343.
2. DiMaio V, DiMaio D. *Forensic Pathology.* 2nd ed. CRC Press; 2001.
3. McClelland CQ, Rekate H, Kaufman B, Persse L. Cerebral injury in child abuse: a changing profile. *Childs Brain*. 1980;7(5):225-235.
4. Christian CW, Taylor AA, Hertle RW, Duhaime AC. Retinal hemorrhages caused by accidental household trauma. *J Pediatr*. 1999;135(1):125-127.
5. Case ME, Graham MA, Handy TC, Jentzen JM, Monteleone JA; National Association of Medical Examiners Ad Hoc Committee on Shaken Baby

Syndrome. Position paper on fatal abusive head injuries in infants and young children. *Am J Forensic Med Pathol.* 2001;22(2):112-122.

6. Salehi-Had H, Brandt JD, Rosas AJ, Rogers KK. Findings in older children with abusive head injury: does shaken-child syndrome exist? *Pediatrics.* 2006;117(5):e1039-e1044.

7. Duhaime AC, Christian CW, Rorke LB, Zimmerman RA. Nonaccidental head injuries in infants—the "shaken baby syndrome." *N Engl J Med.* 1998;338:1822-1829.

8. Keenan HT, Runyan DK, Marshall SW, Nocera MA, Merten DF, Sinal SH. A population-based study of inflicted traumatic brain injury in young children. *JAMA.* 2003;290(5):621-626.

9. Soames RW. Cranial characteristics at different ages. In: Williams PL, ed. *Gray's Anatomy.* 38th ed. Churchill Livingston; 1995:607-609.

10. Gennarelli TA, Tipperman R, Maxwell WL, Graham DI, Adam JH, Irvine A. Traumatic damage to the nodal axolemma: an early secondary injury. *Acta Neurochir Suppl.* 1993;57:49-52.

11. Maxwell WL, Watt C, Graham DI, Gennarelli TA. Ultrastructural evidence of axonal shearing as a result of lateral acceleration of the head in non-human primates. *Acta Neuropathol.* 1993;86(2):136-144.

12. Raghupathi R, Margulies SS. Traumatic axonal injury after closed head injury in the neonatal pig. *J Neurotrauma.* 2002;19(7):843-853.

13. Ibrahim NG, Ralston J, Smith C, Margulies SS. Physiological and pathological responses to head rotations in toddler piglets. *J Neurotrauma.* 2010;27(6):1021-1035.

14. Gean AD. Pediatric trauma. in: Gean AD, ed. *Imaging of Head Trauma.* Raven Press; 1994:367-426.

15. Cantu RC. Biomechanics of head trauma. In: Cantu RC, ed. *Neurologic Athletic Head and Spine Injuries.* WB Saunders; 2000:2-5.

16. Graham DI, McIntosh TK, Maxwell WL, Nicoll JA. Recent advances in neurotrauma. *J Neuropathol Exp Neurol.* 2000;59(8):641-651.

17. Margulies SS, Thibault LE. An analytical model of traumatic diffuse brain injury. *J Biomech Eng.* 1989;111(3):241-249.

18. Ommaya AK. Biomechanics of head injury: experimental aspects. In: Ommaya AK, ed. *The Biomechanics of Trauma.* Appleton-Century-Crofts; 1985:245-269.

19. Stålhammar D. Experimental models of head injury. *Acta Neurochir Suppl.* 1986;36:33-46.

20. Guthkelch AN. Infantile subdural haematoma and its relationship to whiplash injuries. *Br Med J.* 1971;2(5759):430-431.

21. Ommaya AK, Faas F, Yarnell P. Whiplash injury and brain damage: an experimental study. *JAMA.* 1968;204(4):285-289.

22. Caffey J. On the theory and practice of shaking infants. Its potential residual effects of permanent brain damage and mental retardation. *Am J Dis Child.* 1972;124(2):161-169.

23. Duhaime AC, Gennarelli TA, Thibault LE, Bruce DA, Margulies SS, Wiser R. The shaken baby syndrome. A clinical, pathological, and biomechanical study. *J Neurosurg.* 1987;66(3):409-415.

24. Geddes JF, Plunkett J. The evidence base for shaken baby syndrome: we need to question the diagnostic criteria. *BMJ.* 2004;328(7442):719-720.

25. Donohoe M. Evidence-based medicine and shaken baby syndrome: part I: literature review, 1966-1998. *Am J Forensic Med Pathol.* 2003;24(3):239-242.

26. Holbourn AHS. Mechanics of head injury. *Lancet.* 1943;242(6267):438-441.

27. Ommaya AK, Hirsch AE. Tolerances for cerebral concussion from head impact and whiplash in primates. *J Biomech.* 1971;4(1):13-21.

28. Agran PF, Anderson C, Winn D, Trent R, Walton-Haynes L, Thayer S. Rates of pediatric injuries by 3-month intervals for children 0 to 3 years of age. *Pediatrics.* 2003;111(6 pt 1):e683-e692.

29. Duhaime AC, Raghupathi R. Age-specific therapy for traumatic injury of the immature brain: experimental approaches. *Exp Toxicol Pathol.* 1999;51(2):172-177.

30. Gill JR, Goldfeder LD, Armbrustmacher V, Coleman A, Mena H, Hirsch CS. Fatal head injury in children younger than 2 years in New York City and an overview of the shaken baby syndrome. *Arch Pathol Lab Med.* 2009;133(4):619-627.

31. Gilliland MG, Folberg R. Shaken babies—some have no impact injuries. *J Forensic Sci.* 1996;41(1):114-116.

32. Minns RA. Shaken baby syndrome: theoretical and evidential controversies. *J R Coll Physicians Edinb.* 2005;35(1):5-15.

33. Pounder DJ. Shaken adult syndrome. *Am J Forensic Med Pathol.* 1997;18(4):321-324.

34. Carrigan TD, Walker E, Barnes S. Domestic violence: the shaken adult syndrome. *J Accid Emerg Med.* 2000;17(2):138-139.

35. Margulies SS, Thibault KL. Infant skull and suture properties: measurements and implications for mechanisms of pediatric brain injury. *J Biomech Eng.* 2000;122(4):364-371.

36. Hobbs CJ. Skull fracture and the diagnosis of abuse. *Arch Dis Child.* 1984;59(3):246-252.

37. Chadwick DL, Salerno C. Likelihood of the death of an infant or young child in a short fall of less than 6 vertical feet. *J Trauma.* 1993;35(6):968.

38. Chadwick DL, Chin S, Salerno C, Landsverk J, Kitchen L. Deaths from falls in children: how far is fatal? *J Trauma.* 1991;13(10):1353-1355.

39. Helfer RE, Slovis TL, Black M. Injuries resulting when small children fall out of bed. *Pediatrics.* 1977;60(4):533-535.

40. Kravitz H, Driessen G, Gomberg R, Korach A. Accidental falls from elevated surfaces in infants from birth to one year of age. *Pediatrics.* 1969;44(suppl 5):869-876.

41. Lyons TJ, Oates RK. Falling out of bed: a relatively benign occurrence. *Pediatrics.* 1993;92(1):125-127.

42. Nimityongskul P, Anderson LD. The likelihood of injuries when children fall out of bed. *J Pediatr Orthop.* 1987;7(2):184-186.

43. Williams RA. Injuries in infants and small children resulting from witnessed and corroborated free falls. *J Trauma.* 1991;31(10):1350-1352.

44. Denton S, Mileusnic D. Delayed sudden death in an infant following an accidental fall: a case report with review of the literature. *Am J Forensic Med Pathol.* 2003;24(4):371-376.

45. Case ME. Accidental traumatic head injury in infants and young children. *Brain Pathol.* 2008;18(4):583-589.

46. Chadwick DL, Bertocci G, Castillo E, et al. Annual risk of death resulting from short falls among young children: less than 1 in 1 million. *Pediatrics.* 2008;121(6):1213-1224.

47. Weber W. Experimental studies of skull fractures in infants [Article in German]. *Z Rechtsmed.* 1984;92(2):87-94.

48. Weber W. Biomechanical fragility of the infant skull [Article in German]. *Z Rechtsmed.* 1985;94(2):93-101.

49. Weber W. Predilection sites of infantile skull fractures following blunt force [Article in German]. *Z Rechtsmed.* 1987;98(2):81-93.

50. Haines DE. On the question of a subdural space. *Anat Rec.* 1991;230(1):3-21.

51. Haines DE, Harkey HL, al-Mefty O. The "subdural" space: a new look at an outdated concept. *Neurosurgery.* 1993;32(1):111-120.

52. Gilles EE, Nelson MD Jr. Cerebral complications of nonaccidental head injury in childhood. *Pediatr Neurol.* 1988;19(2):119-128.

52. Hymel KP, Rumack CM, Hay TC, Strain JD, Jenny C. Comparison of intracranial computed tomographic (CT) findings in pediatric abusive and accidental head trauma. *Pediatr Radiol.* 1997;27(9):743-747.

54. Kleinman PK. Diagnostic imaging in infant abuse. *AJR Am J Roentgenol.* 1990;155(4):703-712.

55. Dias MS, Backstrom J, Falk M, Li V. Serial radiography in the infant shaken impact syndrome. *Pediatr Neurosurg.* 1998;29(2):77-85.

56. Gennarelli TA. Animate models of human head injury. *J Neurotrauma.* 1994;11(4):357-368.

57. Yamashima T, Friede RL. Why do bridging veins rupture into the virtual subdural space? *J Neurol Neurosurg Psychiatry.* 1984;47(2):121-127.

58. Gennarelli TA, Spielman GM, Langfitt TW, et al. Influence of the type of intracranial lesion on outcome from severe head injury: a multicenter study using a new classification system. *J Neurosurg.* 1982;56(1):26-31.

59. Wells RG, Vetter C, Laud P. Intracranial hemorrhage in children younger than 3 years: prediction of intent. *Arch Pediatr Adolesc Med.* 2002;156(3):252-257.

60. Rorke-Adams, LB. Neuropathology of Abusive head trauma. In: Jenny C, ed. *Child Abuse and Neglect: Diagnosis, Treatment and Evidence.* Elsevier; 2010:413-428.

61. Prahlow JA, Rushing EJ, Barnard JJ. Death due to a ruptured berry aneurysm in a 3.5-year-old child. *Am J Forensic Med Pathol.* 1998;19(4):391-394.

62. Weissgold DJ, Budenz DL, Hood I, Rorke LB. Ruptured vascular malformation masquerading as battered/shaken baby syndrome: a near tragic mistake. *Surv Ophthalmol.* 1995;39(6):509-512.

63. Cuatico W, Yamamoto R, Howeiler B, Smith R. Spontaneous resolution of subdural hematomas. *J Neurosurg Sci.* 1991;35(3):139-145.

64. Dolinskas CA, Zimmerman RA, Bilaniuk LT, Gennarelli TA. Computed tomography of post-traumatic extracerebral hematomas: comparison to pathophysiology and responses to therapy. *J Trauma.* 1979;19(3):163-169.

65. Lee KS, Doh JW, Bae HG, Yun IG. Relations among traumatic subdural lesions. *J Korean Med Sci.* 1996;11(1):55-63.

66. Parent AD. Pediatric chronic subdural hematoma: a retrospective comparative analysis. *Pediatr Neurosurg.* 1992;18(5-6):266-271.

67. Goodell CL, Mealey J Jr. Pathogenesis of chronic subdural hematoma. Experimental studies. *Arch Neurol.* 1963;8:429-437.

68. Lee KS, Bae WK, Doh JW, Bae HG, Yun IG. Origin of chronic subdural haematoma and relation to traumatic subdural lesions. *Brain Inj.* 1998;12(11):901-910.

69. Borzone M, Capuzzo T, Perria C, Rivano C, Tercero E. Traumatic subdural hygromas: a report of 70 surgically treated cases. *J Neurosurg Sci.* 1983;27(3):161-165.

70. Murata K. Chronic subdural hematoma may be preceded by persistent traumatic subdural effusion. *Neuro Med Chir.* 1993;33(10):691-696.

71. Astrup T. Assay and content of tissue thromboplastin in different organs. *Thromb Diath Haemorrh.* 1965;14(3-4):401-416.

72. Dierckx RA, Bruyland M, Nuyens Z, Stadnik T, Solheid C, Ebinger G. Non-traumatic subdural hygroma. *Acta Neurol Belg.* 1989;89(5):352-357.

73. Mayfrank L, Laborde G, Lippitz B, Reul J. Bilateral chronic subdural haematomas following traumatic cerebrospinal fluid leakage into the thoracic epidural space. *Acta Neurochir.* 1993;120(1-2):92-94.

74. Kleinman PK, Barnes PD. Head trauma. In: Kleinman PK, ed. *Diagnostic Imaging of Child Abuse.* 2nd ed. Mosby; 1998:285-342.

75. Wetterling T, Demierre B, Rama B, Nekic M. Protein analysis of subdural hygroma fluid. *Acta Neurochir.* 1988;91(1-2):79-82.

76. Kivlin JD. A 12-year ophthalmologic experience with the shaken baby syndrome at a regional children's hospital. *Trans Am Ophthalmol Soc.* 1999;97:545-581.

77. Levin A. The ocular findings in child abuse. *Am Acad Ophthalmol.* 1998;16:1-14.

78. Levin AV. Ocular manifestations of child abuse. *Ophthalmol Clin North Am.* 1990;3:249-264.

79. Levin AV. Retinal hemorrhage in abusive head trauma. *Pediatrics.* 2010;126(5):961-970.

80. Levin AV. Ophthalmology of shaken baby syndrome. *Neurosurg Clin N Am.* 2002;13(2):201-211.

81. Greenwald MJ, Weiss A, Oesterle CS, Friendly DS. Traumatic retinoschisis in battered babies. *Ophthalmology.* 1986;93(5):618-625.

82. Lueder GT, Turner JW, Paschall R. Perimacular retinal folds simulating nonaccidental injury in an infant. *Arch Ophthalmol.* 2006;124(12):1782-1783.

83. Lantz PE, Sinal SH, Stanton CA, Weaver RG Jr. Perimacular retinal folds from childhood head trauma. *BMJ.* 2004;328(7442):754-756.

84. Kivlin JD, Currie ML, Greenbaum VJ, Simmons KB, Jentzen J. Retinal hemorrhages in children following fatal motor vehicle crashes: a case series. *Arch Ophthalmol.* 2008;126(6):800-804.

85. Moran K, Reddie I, Jacobs M. Severe haemorrhagic retinopathy and traumatic retinoschisis in a 2 year old infant after an 11 metre fall onto concrete. *Acta Paediatr.* 2008;97(suppl 459):149.

86. Massicotte SJ, Folberg R, Torczynski E, Gilliland MG, Luckenbach MW. Vitreoretinal traction and perimacular retinal folds in the eyes of deliberately traumatized children. *Ophthalmology.* 1991;98(7):1124-1127.

87. Doherty WB, Trubek M. Significant hemorrhagic retinal lesions in bacterial endocarditis (Roth's spots). *JAMA.* 1931;97(5):308-313.

88. Emerson MV, Pieramici DJ, Stoessel KM, Berreen JP, Gariano RF. Incidence and rate of disappearance of retinal hemorrhage in newborns. *Ophthalmology.* 2001;108(1):36-39.

89. Fraser SG, Horgan SE, Bardavio J. Retinal haemorrhage in meningitis. *Eye.* 1995;9(pt 5):659-660.

90. Clark RS, Orr RA, Atkinson CS, Towbin RB, Pang D. Retinal hemorrhages associated with spinal cord arteriovenous malformation. *Clin Pediatr.* 1995;34(5):281-283.

91. Gilliland MG, Luckenbach MW. Are retinal hemorrhages found after resuscitation attempts? A study of the eyes of 169 children. *Am J Forensic Med Pathol.* 1993;14(3):187-192.

92. Johnson DL, Braun D, Friendly D. Accidental head trauma and retinal hemorrhage. *Neurosurgery.* 1993;33(2):231-234.

93. Lindenberg R, Freytag E. Morphology of brain lesions from blunt trauma in early infancy. *Arch Pathol.* 1969;87(3):298-305.

94. Adams JH, Graham DI, Scott G, Parker LS, Doyle D. Brain damage in fatal nonmissile head injury. *J Clin Pathol.* 1980;33(12):1132-1145.

95. Adams JH, Doyle D, Ford I, Gennarelli TA, Graham DI, McLellan DR. Diffuse axonal injury in head injury: definition, diagnosis and grading. *Histopathology.* 1989;15(1):49-59.

96. Sherriff FE, Bridges LR, Sivaloganathan S. Early detection of axonal injury after human head trauma using immunocytochemistry for beta-amyloid precursor protein. *Acta Neuropathol.* 1994;87(1):55-62.

97. Hortobágyi T, Wise S, Hunt N, et al. Traumatic axonal damage in the brain can be detected using beta-APP immunohistochemistry within 35 min after head injury to human adults. *Neuropathol Appl Neurobiol.* 2007;33(2):226-237.

98. Dolinak D, Reichard R. An overview of inflicted head injury in infants and young children with a review of beta-amyloid precursor protein immunohistochemistry. *Arch Pathol Lab Med.* 2006;130(5):712-717.

99. Reichard RR, White CL 3rd, Hladik CL, Dolinak D. Beta-amyloid precursor protein staining in nonhomicidal pediatric medicolegal autopsies. *J Neuropathol Exp Neurol.* 2003;62(3):237-247.

100. Geddes JF, Hackshaw AK, Vowles GH, Nickols CD, Whitwell HL. Neuropathology of inflicted head injury in children. I. Patterns of brain damage. *Brain.* 2001;124(pt 7):1290-1298.

101. Geddes JF, Vowles GH, Hackshaw AK, Nickols CD, Scott IS, Whitwell HL. Neuropathology of inflicted head injury in children. II. Microscopic brain injury in infants. *Brain.* 2001;124(pt 7):1299-1306.

102. Case ME. Inflicted traumatic brain injury in infants and young children. *Brain Pathol.* 2008;18(4):571-582.

Editor's note: All references were used in the creation of the original work, *Forensic Pathology of Child Death,* but may not be cited directly in this chapter.

Chapter 3

Injuries of the Spine and Spinal Cord

Objectives

After reviewing this chapter, the reader will be able to:

1. *Describe the relationship between epidural hemorrhages of the cervical spine and abusive head trauma.*
2. *Define distraction injury of the cervical spine and identify the mechanism by which it is caused.*
3. *Recognize an artifact that may resemble a cervical cord contusion or distraction injury of the spinal cord.*

Epidural Hemorrhage of the Cervical Spine

In 1967, Towbin[1] detected the presence of epidural hemorrhages in the cervical spine of 5 children who seemingly died suddenly and unexpectedly. He suggested that these hemorrhages might be both traumatic and related to the cause of death of these children (ie, producing mechanical injury to the spinal cord). Two years later, in 1969, Harris and Adelson[2] observed 19 infants, aged younger than 1 year, who also died suddenly and unexpectedly. They found that:

— 5 of the infants died of natural causes from diseases noted at autopsy.

— 14 of the deaths were unexplained by findings at autopsy and were considered to have died from sudden infant death syndrome (SIDS).

— 18 of the 19 infants had hemorrhage within the spinal epidural region, which was greatest in the cervical portion, that varied from venous congestion to hemorrhage within the adjacent soft tissues.

Together, these doctors made 3 conclusions: (1) these epidural hemorrhages were not traumatic; (2) the presence of blood was not damaging to the spinal cord; and (3) hemodynamic forces were probably responsible for this congestive phenomenon. However, it should be noted that these conclusions were made preceding the time when the diagnosis of inflicted head trauma was generally being made. At that time, no one was specifically looking at infants with abusive head injury to determine whether they also had hemorrhage in the spinal epidural space.

In 1989, Hadley and colleagues[3] observed 13 infants, aged 1.5 to 14 months, who were diagnosed as "shaken" infants. Eight of the infants died, and autopsies were done on 6 who had inflicted head injuries. The autopsies found that:

— 5 of the 6 infants had epidural hemorrhages in the cervical spine.

— 4 of the 6 infants had subdural hemorrhage (SDH) in the cervical spine.

— 4 of the 6 infants had contusions of the high cervical cord.

— 1 of 6 had none of these findings.

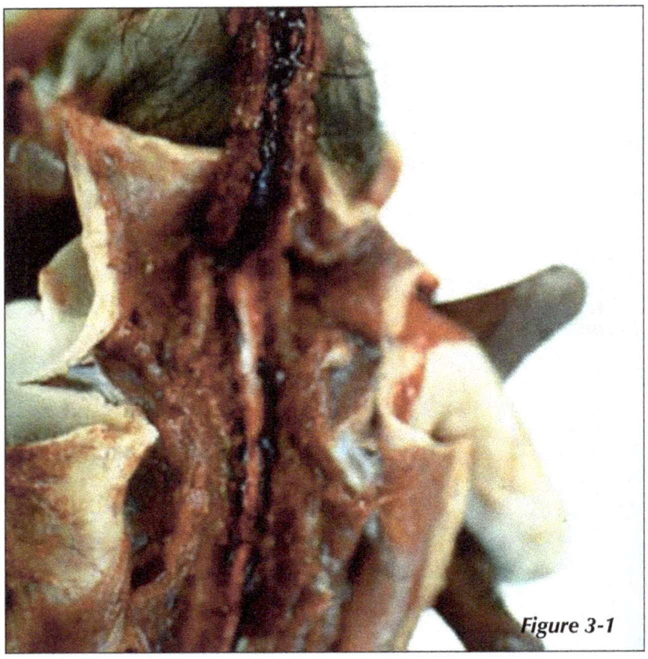

Figure 3-1. *Infant who died from SIDS demonstrating extensive epidural blood from the cervical to the thoracic regions of the spine.*

The subdural blood in the region of the cervical spine is not an unexpected finding because, in infants with abusive head trauma, the SDH in the posterior cranial fossa can descend by gravity into the spinal subdural space. Additionally, of the infants that had contusions of the high cervical cord, Hadley did not elaborate on the pathology of these contusions, so it is difficult to know if they were similar to those described by Geddes[4,5] in some of their cases—who were found to have focal axonal injury in the cervical region—or if they were truly contusional hemorrhages.

To elucidate the findings of hemorrhages in the spinal area of young children with and without abusive head injury, the author conducted a study from 1989 to 1992. She observed children younger than 3 years of age who died and were autopsied, specifically examining the spines of children in 50 cases of inflicted head trauma alongside control cases (eg, no head injury) for the presence of epidural blood. From this study, it was apparent that both groups frequently had spinal epidural hemorrhage and that no relationship could be established between head injury and spinal epidural hemorrhages (**Figure 3-1**).

When there is any possibility of head trauma, it is recommended that all autopsies in children younger than 3 years of age include a posterior neck dissection and examination of the vertebral bones and spinal cord.[6] Epidural hemorrhage of the cervical spine is not necessarily indicative of trauma.

Distraction Injury of the Cervical Spine

A ***distraction injury*** is defined as an extremely rare, abusive injury of the cervical cord.[7] Several cases have been examined throughout the years, and all involved shaking a child while grasping the child's head. As the child is grasped by the head, the weight of the unsupported suspended body will distract the upper cervical spinal cord and lower medulla.

In 1995, Piatt[8] described a 15-month-old child who presented to the emergency department (ED) with quadriplegia after reportedly falling from a couch. This child had linear bruises in front of the right ear and jaw, along with showers of petechial hemorrhages over the left side of the neck, over both ears, the right side of the jaw, and the upper chest. A magnetic resonance image (MRI) demonstrated fusiform swelling of the midcervical cord, representing hematomyelia. Two months later, a follow-up MRI demonstrated spinal cord atrophy, and the child's quadriplegia persisted.

Later, Parrish[9] reported a case of isolated spinal cord injury as a result of child abuse. This case involved a 2-month-old infant who was found, at autopsy, to have a contusion of the upper cervical spinal cord and lower medulla. The eyes were examined and found to have anterior chamber bleeding bilaterally, a dislocated left lens, and vitreous hemorrhage. These injuries were hypothesized to be the result of direct compressional force whereby the perpetrator picked up the child by the head with their thumbs positioned over the child's eyes and violently shook the child.

In the years following these reports, the author has seen 3 cases with findings that suggest a distraction mechanism of injury to the cervical cord and lower medulla.[10] Two of the cases were siblings. In the first of these 2 children, the father described that he had grasped the 3-month-old infant by the head and shook her body. That child survived with a central cord syndrome. A second sibling was found dead at the age of 3 months. Her autopsy demonstrated petechial hemorrhages of the right bulbar conjunctiva and hematomyelia of the upper cervical cord and medulla. It was suspected that the father had performed a similar abusive act, as with the first child, by grasping the head and shaking the body, causing a distraction injury of the cervical cord and medulla.

The third case of distraction injury seen by the author was a 25-day-old infant reported to have been found unresponsive in the morning after crying all night. He was dead on arrival at the ED. The autopsy demonstrated contusions of the right mandible, below the left lower lip, and on the right shoulder, left abdomen, posterior left arm, right thigh, and both legs. Several of the contusions on the extremities looked like gripping marks. There were petechial hemorrhages of the right preauricular area, left lateral forehead, and bulbar and palpebral conjunctivae. There was 1 small retinal hemorrhage and fracture of the right clavicle with early callus. The autopsy also revealed a separation of the C3-4 intervertebral disc and hematomyelia of the upper cervical cord and lower medulla (**Figure 3-2-a** and **b**). The mechanism of grasping a child by the head and violently shaking the body is suggested by these findings.

It should be noted that there is an artifact that may resemble a cervical cord contusion or distraction injury of the cord. This resemblance is seen in patients who become brain dead from brain swelling that cuts off the cerebral circulation and who are kept alive for several days in that state. These patients will begin to show fragmentation of the cerebellar tonsils. As the tonsils disintegrate and drop into the subarachnoid space, the material may descend downward into cervical spinal cord subarachnoid space, where it may compress and crowd the small vessels and result in ischemia of the cervical cord. Ischemic lesions of the cervical cord appear as hemorrhagic softening of the central cord, which resembles a contusion. Cerebellar detritus can be found within the subarachnoid space of the cervical cord in these cases. Identical lesions have been demonstrated in experimental animal models of brain death.[11]

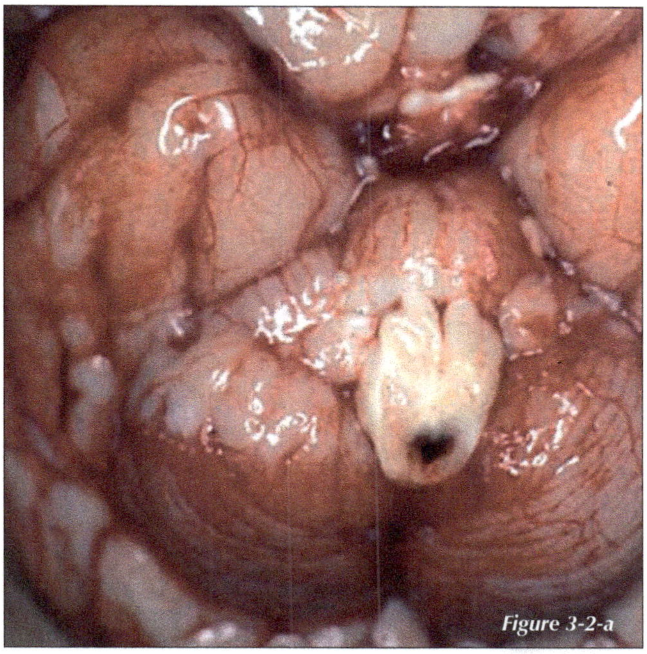

Figure 3-2-a

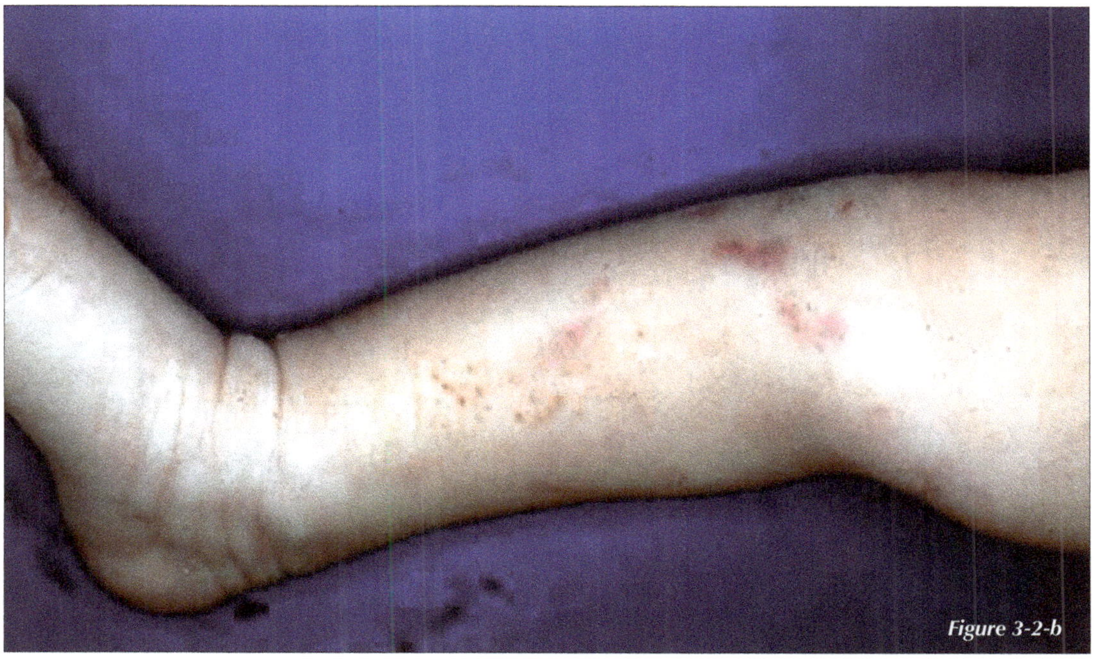

Figure 3-2-b

Figure 3-2-a. *Brain at autopsy with transverse section of caudal medulla showing a 4 mm area of hematomyelia.*

Figure 3-2-b. *A 3-month-old infant with distraction injury of the cervicomedullary region. Right leg shows gripping marks from grasping the leg with the fingers.*

Injuries of the Spine and Spinal Cord Case Studies

Case Study 3-1

This 3-month-old boy arrived in the ED at 7:11 AM in full arrest. His body temperature was 92.3°F. The father reported that the child had been restless all night and was crying much of the previous day. At 11:00 PM on the night before the child died, the father called the pediatrician and said the child was crying from gas. The doctor told the father to go to the ED if he felt there was a serious problem. The father was up with the child all night and would sleep only briefly before the child would start crying again. At 6:00 AM the child settled down and went to sleep. The father laid the child down on his left side on a full-size bed. The father then lay down across from the child and fell asleep. He woke up at 6:30 AM and noticed the child was not breathing. 911 was called. At 3:45 PM on the day preceding the child's death, the Department of Family Services received 1 hotline call from a professional who stated that the child was at high risk for abuse because the mother had a history of drug abuse. The mother had 1 prior child who died of SIDS, and she was not bonding with the current child. A scene investigation was carried out. The father stated that the child had been crying, and the mother went to another part of the house to get away. The father and child remained in the basement apartment.

Cause of Death: Cervicospinal blunt trauma

Manner of Death: Homicide

Note: This is a distraction injury from grasping the child's head and shaking the body.

Table 3-1. Autopsy Results

External Examination

- — Well-nourished infant
- — Child was 21 inches and 7 pounds
- — Eyes show 2 petechiae on left bulbar conjunctiva, multiple petechiae on the right bulbar and inferior palpebral conjunctivae, and a 5 mm confluent hemorrhage on the right lateral bulbar conjunctiva

Injuries

Type	*Measurement*
Contusion, inferior edge of middle third of right mandible	10 mm
Abrasion along vermilion border, left upper lip laterally	8 mm x 1 mm
Contusion, linear, below left lower lip	10 mm x 1 mm
Somewhat square area of petechiae on right preauricular area	20 mm x 20 mm
Some petechiae on left lateral forehead	
Contusion, anterior right shoulder medial to axillary line	20 mm x 5 mm
Punctuate contusions, lateral left abdomen, consisting of:	30 mm x 10 mm area
— An anterior contusion	3 mm
— A box of contusions	4 to 2 mm
— Posteriorly, 2 somewhat parallel linear contusions	4 mm x 1 mm
Contusion, posterior left arm	20 mm x 3 mm
Contusion, posterolateral right proximal thigh	20 mm x 4 mm
Curved contusion, right calf, continuing onto posteromedial right knee with S-shaped configuration	40 mm x 1 mm
Contusion, proximal anterior right thigh	30 mm x 12 mm
3 contusions, proximal anterior right thigh	2 mm (2), 3 mm
Contusion, proximal anteromedial left leg	20 mm x 4 mm
Contusion, left calf	20 mm

(continued)

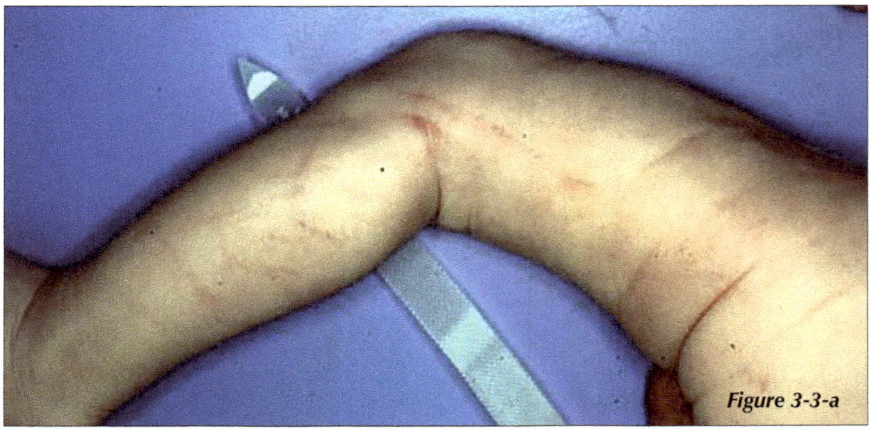

Figure 3-3-a. *Left leg of infant showing gripping marks from grasping the leg with the fingers.*

Table 3-1. Autopsy Results ***(continued)***

INJURIES ***(CONTINUED)***

TYPE	*MEASUREMENT*
Contusion	40 mm x 8 mm
— Consisting of 2 parallel linear marks separated by wide, pale area on posterolateral distal left thigh	5 mm
Approximately 3 to 9 other patchy contusions on left leg and knee	5 mm x 1 mm

All contusions were red-purple; incision into the contusions showed superficial hemorrhage

Fractures

— Diastasis of C3-C4 intervertebral disc

— Fracture of right clavicle with surrounding red/brown hemorrhage (microscopically, this is a healing fracture with superimposed refracture)

Internal Injuries

— Moderate hemorrhage in cervical perivertebral musculature

— Extensive hemorrhage within membrane of C1-C2 posteriorly

— Extensive hemorrhage in anterior prevertebral soft tissues including the distal pharyngeal soft tissues

— Mild hemorrhage in left paravertebral muscles

— Mild hemorrhage, 20 mm x 25 mm area, midoccipital periosteum

NEUROPATHOLOGY

— After fixation, the brain weighed 540 grams

— Cervical cord contusion with hematomyelia from upper cervical cord to lower medulla, 4 mm wide at greatest extent in the cord

EYES

— Single petechial retinal hemorrhage

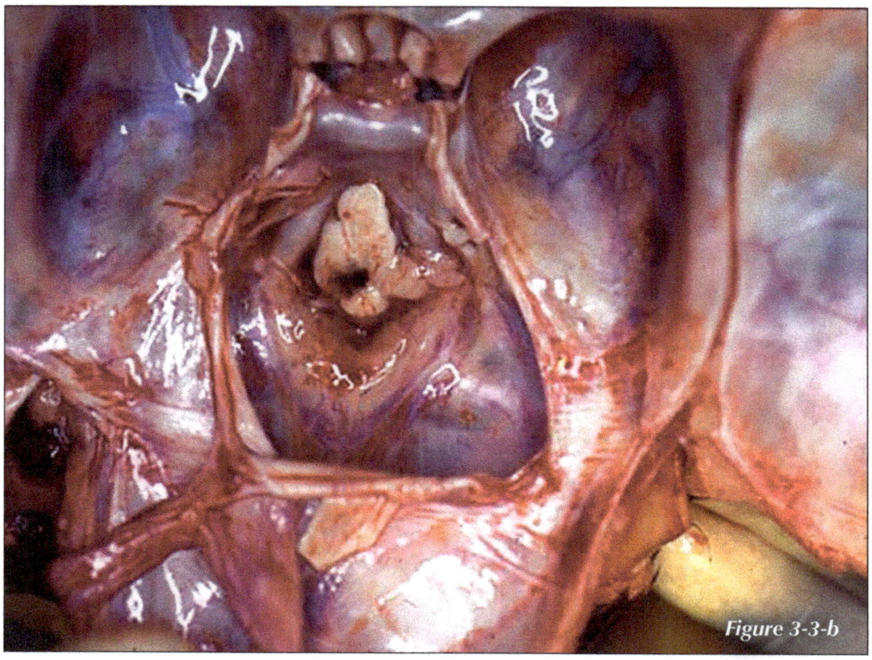

Figure 3-3-b

Figure 3-3-b. *At autopsy, when the brain is removed by sectioning between the cervical spinal cord and the medulla, an area of hematomyelia can be seen in the caudal medulla-cervical cord junction.*

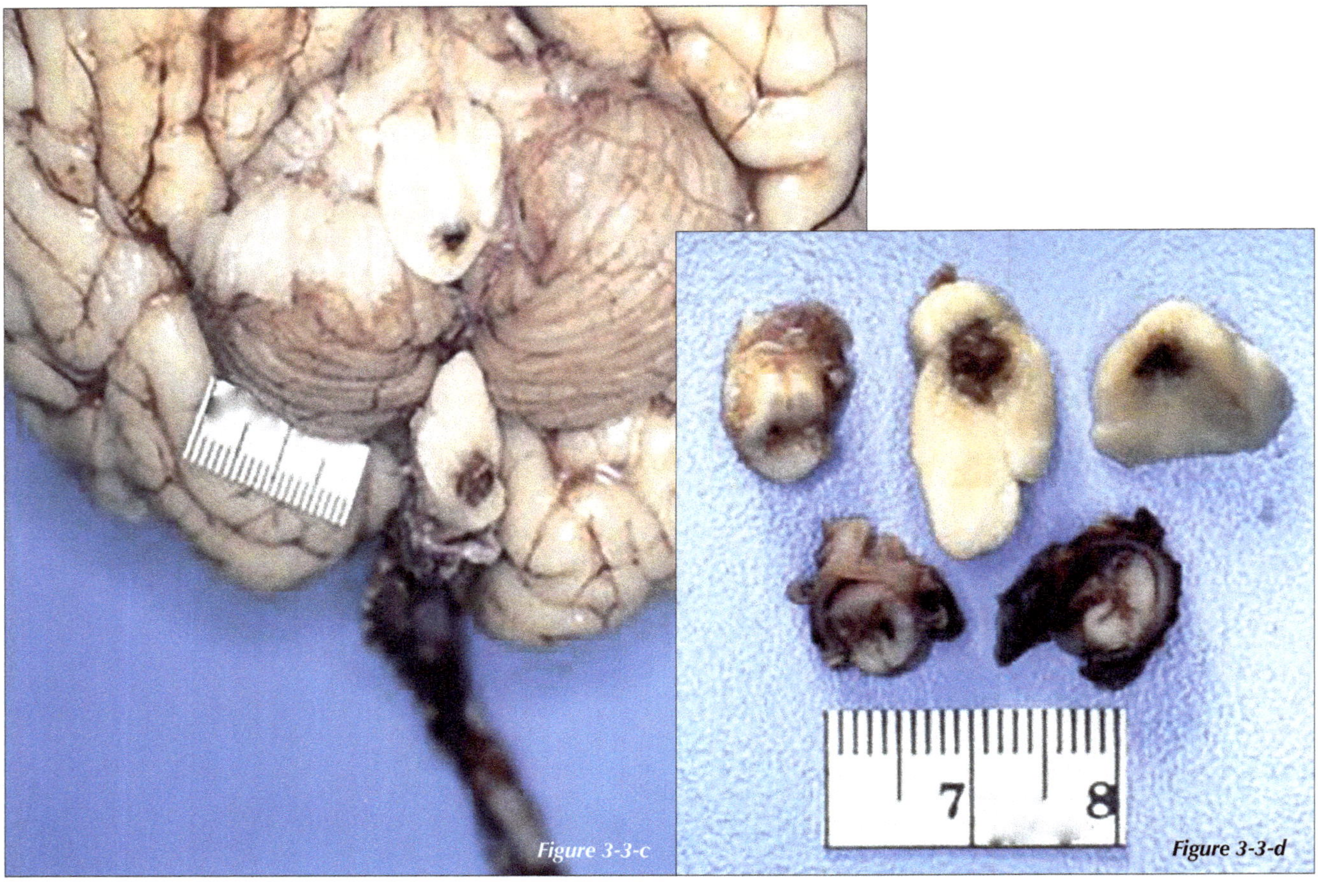

Figure 3-3-c. After fixation, an area of hematomyelia can be seen in both the medulla and upper cervical cord at their junction.

Figure 3-3-d. After fixation, the junction between the medulla and cervical cord is cut into transverse sections showing the area of hematomyelia extending from the medulla into the cord.

References

1. Towbin A. Sudden infant death (cot death) related to spinal injury. *Lancet.* 1967;290(7522):940-942.
2. Harris LS, Adelson L. "Spinal injury" and sudden infant death: a second look. *Am J Clin Pathol.* 1969;52(3):289-295.
3. Hadley MN, Sonntag VK, Rekate HL, Murphy A. The infant whiplash-shake syndrome: a clinical and pathological study. *Neurosurgery.* 1989;24(4):536-540.
4. Geddes JF, Hackshaw AK, Vowles GH, Nickols CD, Whitwell HL. Neuropathology of inflicted head injury in children. I: patterns of brain damage. *Brain.* 2001;124(pt 7):1290-1298.
5. Geddes JF, Vowles GH, Hackshaw AK, Nickols CD, Scott IS, Whitwell HL. Neuropathology of inflicted head injury in children. II: microscopic brain injury in infants. *Brain.* 2001;124(pt 7):1299-1306.
6. Judkins AR, Hood IG, Mirchandani HG, Rorke LB. Technical communication: rationale and technique for examination of nervous system in suspected infant victims of abuse. *Am J Forensic Med Pathol.* 2004;25(1):29-32.
7. Brink FW, Gold DL, Adler B, Letson MM. Distraction injury of the thoracic spine with spinal cord transection and vascular injury in a 5-week-old infant boy: a case of child physical abuse. *Pediatr Emerg Care.* 2017;33(3):192-197.
8. Piatt JH Jr, Steinberg M. Isolated spinal cord injury as a presentation of child abuse. *Pediatrics.* 1995;96(4 pt 1):780-782.
9. Parrish R. Isolated spinal cord injury in child abuse. *Pediatric Trauma Forensic Newsletter.* January 1996: Letter to the Editor.

10. Case ME, Graham MA, Wood J. Spinal cord injury in child abuse [abstract]. Presented at: National Association of Medical Examiners 1996 Annual Meeting; September 14, 1996.

11. Matakas F, Cervos-Navarro J, Schneider H. Experimental brain death. I: morphology and fine structure of the brain. *J Neurol Neurosurg Psychiatry.* 1973;36(4):497-508.

Chapter 4

Chest Trauma

Objectives

After reviewing this chapter, the reader will be able to:

1. *Recall the statistics surrounding traumatic chest injuries as well as the mechanisms of death.*
2. *Recognize rib fractures and other traumatic chest injuries as likely indicators of abuse.*
3. *Identify the procedures for and expected findings of a forensic autopsy examining chest trauma injuries.*

Chest Trauma

Thoracic injuries account for 25% of all traumatic deaths in the adult population.[1] Abusive trauma of the chest is common in young children, but it is rarely lethal. Cardiac lacerations in infants and young children are the result of severe blunt trauma (eg, from a motor vehicle accident, violent assaults, or large falls). These injuries do not occur from cardiopulmonary resuscitation or minor incidents in the home; therefore, if they are found, it is highly suspicious for abuse.

Rib fractures are common abusive injuries and account for 5% to 51% of all fractures in abused children.[2] Rib fractures are uncommon in accidental incidents to children[3] but are common abusive injuries in infants and may constitute 35% to 60% of fractures in infants compared to fractures in older children.[3,4] Rib fractures are highly correlated with abusive practices toward infants because of the mechanisms that result in these fractures. For example, holding an infant tightly around the chest with the strength of the adult hand can generate the forces necessary to fracture the anterior, lateral, and posterior aspects of the ribs. In addition, shaking an infant while holding a child tightly around the chest adds additional force that may injure the ribs as well.[2]

It should also be noted that rib fractures in infants and young children *may* be associated with cardiopulmonary resuscitation, but such fractures are much less frequent than rib fractures from resuscitation in adults.[5] In most cases, these fractures have been described in the anterior portions of the ribs. Since the institution of the newer method of infant cardiopulmonary resuscitation using 2 hands, forensic pathologists tend to find more resuscitation-associated rib fractures in infants, which are located in the anterior, lateral, and posterior aspects of the ribs and tend to be minimal. The fractures go through the cortex of the inner surface of the bone and are often associated with little hemorrhage (**Figure 4-1**).[6]

The entity of chest squeezing, in which an adult holds an infant with both hands or in their arms with the infant against their chest and then squeezes, is rare but has been seen. In one such case, the father noted that "she [the infant] liked to be held like that," because, when she was crying and then squeezed in this manner, she would stop crying. The father also noted that, on occasion, he could hear popping sounds as ribs broke.

Figure 4-1. *Rib cage removed to demonstrate 5 acute rib fractures from resuscitation. The fracture is through only the cortical surface of the inner surface of the bones.*

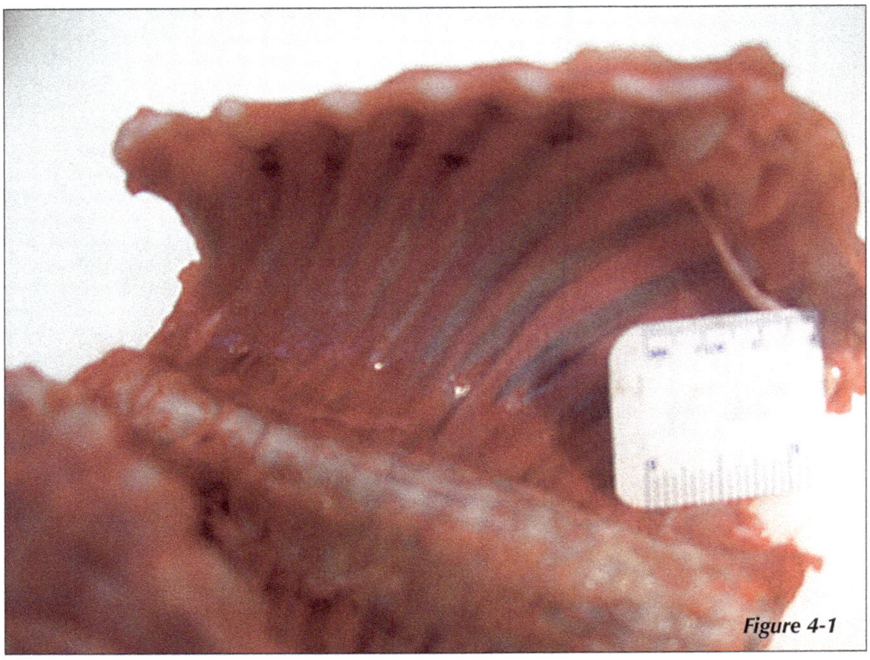

At autopsy, other infants killed in this manner were reported to have 27 to 36 rib fractures that ranged from acute to older and old. The mechanism of death for chest squeezing may either be compression asphyxia from the actual squeezing that is preventing the infant from excursing the chest, or from the effects of the many fractured ribs, causing instability of the rib cage and altered breathing. In all cases that have been personally seen by the author, the perpetrators were males who wished to stop the infant from crying.

Figure 4-2-a. *Rib cage removed to demonstrate multiple healing rib fractures with callus.*

Figure 4-2-b. *Single rib with callus transected and in cassette to be submitted for microscopic examination for aging of fracture.*

Forensic Autopsy of Chest Trauma Injuries

The forensic autopsy includes stripping the pleural membrane from the ribs to enable direct visualization of each bone. Radiographs do not always demonstrate acute rib fractures, especially in young infants. Acute rib fractures appear as a disruption of the cortex and adjacent bony trabeculae, often with hemorrhage around the fracture site or in the adjacent intercostal muscle. The pleural membrane may be intact or punctured by the displaced fractured bone, and any hemorrhage may persist for several weeks after the injury. In a living child, the body's fracture repair process begins very early. Microscopically, the earliest stage of healing is the inflammatory response, wherein there is an influx of neutrophils into the hematoma associated with the fractures, followed by

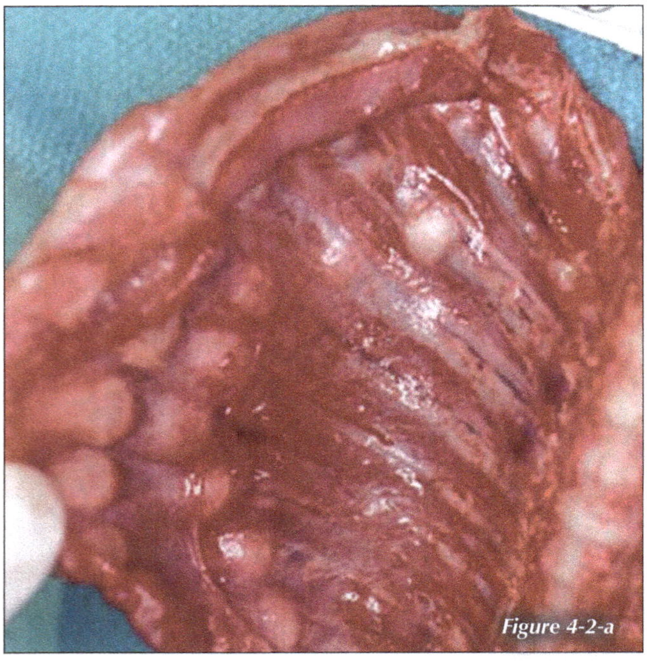

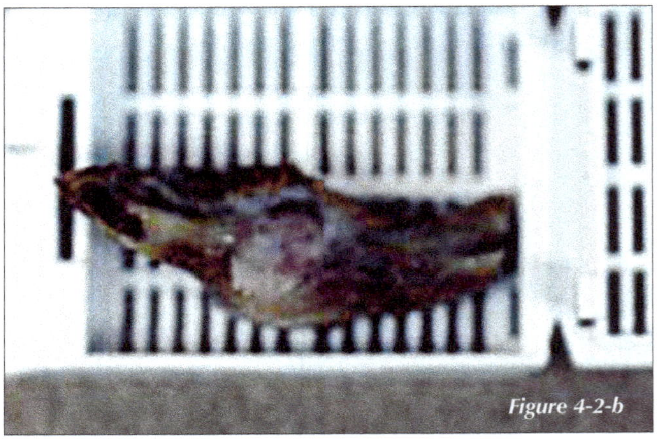

mononuclear cells. This change can be seen in the first or second day and proceeds for several days. Fibroblastic infiltration and granulation formation begins in 5 to 7 days and results in the formation of woven bone or soft callus, which binds the fracture site. Grossly, the appearance of callus is a white bulging knob on the bone (**Figure 4-2-a** and **b**). The soft callus is gradually remodeled into firmer hard callus, and then the hard callus is slowly further remodeled into normal trabecular bone. This process may take several weeks to several months to complete.[7]

References

1. Trunkey DD, Lewis FR. Chest trauma. *Surg Clin North Am.* 1980;60(6):1541-1549.

2. Kleinman PK. Bony thoracic trauma. In: Kleinman PK, ed. *Diagnostic Imaging of Child Abuse.* 2nd ed. Mosby; 1998:110-148.

3. Worlock P, Stower M, Barbor P. Patterns of fractures in accidental and non-accidental injury in children: a comparative study. *Br Med J (Clin Res Ed).* 1986;293(6539):100-102.

4. Kleinman PK, Marks SC Jr, Richmond JM, Blackbourne BD. Inflicted skeletal injury: a postmortem radiologic-histopathologic study in 31 infants. *AJR Am J Roentgenol.* 1995;165:647-650.

5. Bush CM, Jones JS, Cohle SD, Johnson H. Pediatric injuries from cardiopulmonary resuscitation. *Ann Emerg Med.* 1996;28(1):40-44.

6. Dolinak D. Rib fractures in infants due to cardiopulmonary resuscitation efforts. *Am J Forensic Med Pathol.* 2007;27(2):107-110.

7. Zumwalt RE, Fanizza-Orphanos AM. Dating of healing rib fractures in fatal child abuse. In: Fenoglio-Presiser C, ed. *Advances in Pathology.* Mosby; 1990:193-205.

Chapter 5

Abdominal Trauma

Objectives

After reviewing this chapter, the reader will be able to:

1. *Classify and define the different types of abdominal injury, including the differences seen between accidental and inflicted/abusive injury.*
2. *Interpret the correlation between abdominal organs and structures and the types of injuries inflicted.*
3. *Identify causes of increased susceptibility to abdominal injury in children.*

Introduction

Significant blunt abdominal trauma is a rare but deadly form of child abuse and ranks second only to head injury in causing abuse-related fatalities.[1] Only 1% of children hospitalized for child abuse have abdominal trauma, but 45% to 50% of these abdominal injuries are lethal.[2] Furthermore, of total child abuse deaths, about 12% are attributed to abdominal injuries.[3,4] Inflicted abdominal trauma has a high mortality rate compared to accidental injuries of the same magnitude.[5] In inflicted injuries, the perpetrator knows that the child has been injured, but they frequently delay seeking medical care until the child is morbid or dead to avoid arousing suspicion. By contrast, in accidental injuries, medical care is sought immediately.[2]

Inflicted abdominal injuries tend to terminate with severe peritonitis or hemorrhagic shock as a result of the untreated injuries. The anatomy of the young child's abdomen is distinct in that the abdominal wall has little or no muscle for protection against impact, and force can easily penetrate it. In addition, the rib cage is widely flared, and the ribs are flexible, so fewer organs are covered by this protective layer. Abdominal injuries are caused by direct blunt force from a punch or blow, or indirect forces of deceleration such as a child being thrown against a wall or object. In accidental circumstances, solid organs such as the liver, kidney, and spleen tend to be more commonly damaged than hollow organs. However, in inflicted abdominal trauma, the spleen and kidney are seldom injured, but the liver is frequently injured by both accidental and inflicted traumas.[6,7] Hollow viscus injury is more common in inflicted abdominal trauma than in accidental trauma, and it most commonly occurs in the proximal small bowel. Pancreatic and mesenteric injuries also occur. It is important to note that the abdominal wall may not demonstrate any area of contusion even when there has been significant impact and underlying lethal trauma (**Figure 5-1-a** and **b**). In some cases, however, prominent marks are present (**Figure 5-2-a** and **b**).[8]

The anatomy of the abdomen, in addition to being distinctly different in the young child, also has certain characteristics of importance in blunt abdominal trauma. The blood supply of the area most at risk of injury when an impact is made to the central abdominal area consists of the large arteries coming off the anterior side of the aorta, the celiac trunk, and the superior mesenteric artery. These 2 large arteries arise in close proximity to the area most commonly injured by inflicted trauma, and these arteries or their major branches may be transected.[9] Branches from the celiac artery supply the region around the stomach, pancreas, and proximal small bowel, while the superior mesenteric artery is the main supply for both the small and large bowels. These vessels travel within the mesentery, and in many cases of inflicted blunt trauma, the pathologist observes massive hemorrhage and actual tears or contusions within the mesentery at autopsy. These contusions then cause tears in branches of the superior mesenteric vessels. Typically, the pathologist does not dissect out the vessels to identify the precise damage, as might be done by the surgeon who is operating and making repairs to individual vessels. Isolated mesenteric lacerations may occur as a lethal injury with massive loss of blood from severed large vessels (**Figure 5-3-a** and **b**).

The most commonly injured organ in inflicted abdominal trauma is the small bowel.[8,10] In the author's series of lethal cases, however, liver lacerations outnumbered the duodenal injuries. Small bowel injuries occur in the proximal portion near the ligament of Treitz, where the bowel is relatively fixed. The bowel also has a rich blood supply at this point, so injuries tend to be lacerations or transection of the bowel, hematomas within the bowel wall or within the mesentery, or lacerations within the mesentery. The retroperitoneal location of the duodenum provides some degree of protection against blunt trauma, so that when injury does occur, it is the result of significant force applied to the abdomen. With significant force, the duodenum can be crushed between the spinal column and

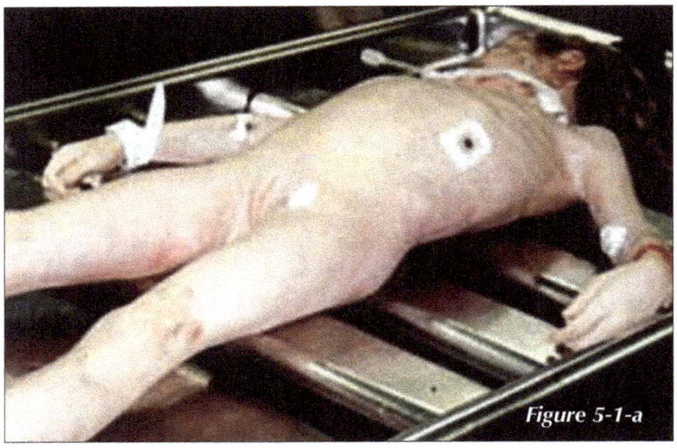

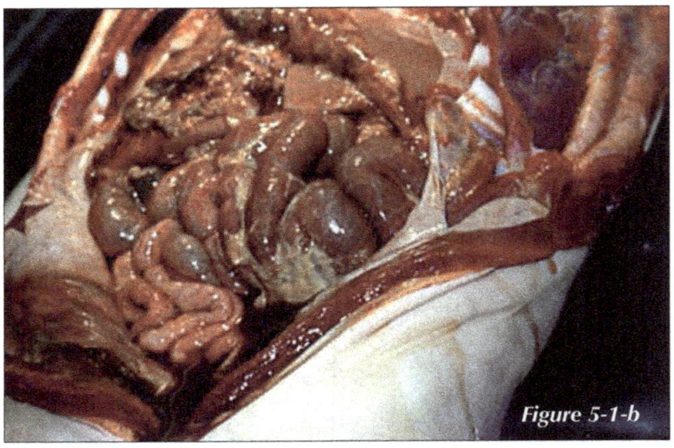

Figure 5-1-a. *A 6-year-old girl on autopsy table before autopsy showing that no marks are present on the abdomen. This child was kicked in the abdomen at noon by her aunt and died the following evening.*

Figure 5-1-b. *Abdomen opened to demonstrate extensive peritonitis with purulent exudate over the peritoneal surfaces and turbid brown fluid within the peritoneal cavity.*

Figure 5-2-a. *A 17-month-old girl showing prominent knuckle mark contusions on the chest and abdomen.*

Figure 5-2-b. *Abdomen opened at autopsy to show blood running out of peritoneal cavity from laceration of liver. Peritoneal cavity contained 400 mL of blood.*

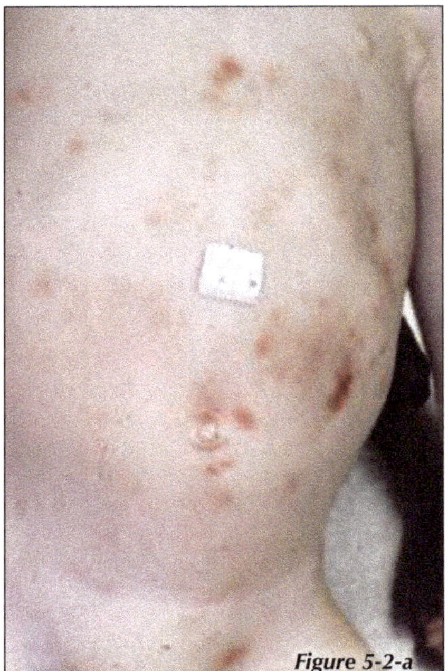

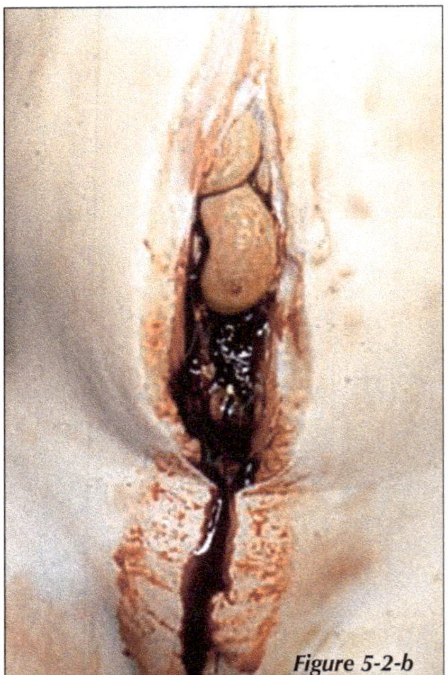

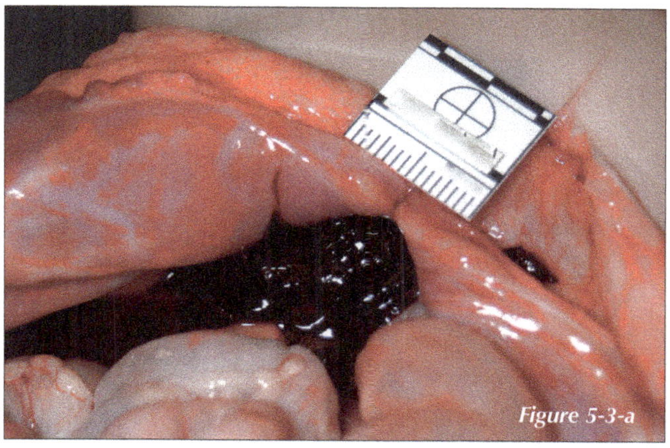

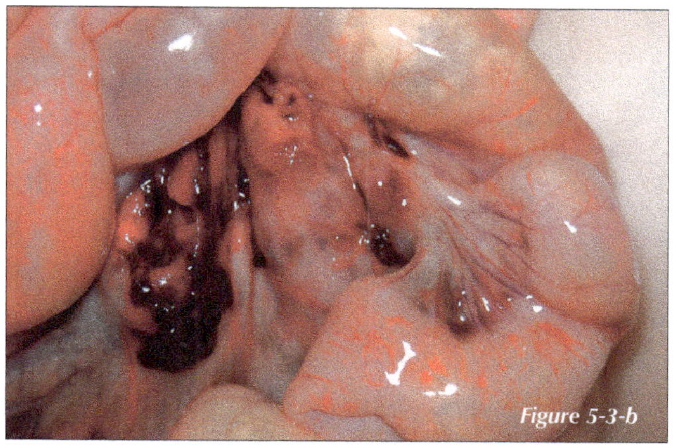

the striking force.[11] Although duodenal injuries are generally unusual in pediatric patients with trauma, physical abuse is the second most common cause of duodenal injury after motor vehicle accidents (MVAs). At autopsy, in cases of laceration of the duodenum, the peritoneal cavity contains purulent fluid, and the lacerated bowel tends to be necrotic and dark (**Figure 5-4**). Accidental injuries of the bowel tend to occur in MVAs but not in the home through minor falls or even in falls down stairs.[12,13]

Figure 5-3-a. *A 16-month-old boy with abdomen opened at autopsy showing large amount of blood in peritoneal cavity from laceration of mesentery.*

Figure 5-3-b. *Additional view of lacerations to the mesentery.*

Figure 5-4. *The 6-year-old girl from Figure 5-1 showing transection of duodenum with surrounding contusion of mesentery.*

Figure 5-5. *A 13-month-old boy with large laceration of greater curvature of stomach. This child was struck in the abdomen shortly after lunch at noon and died in the later afternoon.*

It is not unusual for the pathologist to find evidence of old injury to the bowel wall or mesentery in a child later dying of another form of abuse. These areas of old injury consist of firm, scarred, dark areas of the bowel wall or mesentery, often associated with adhesions and which, on microscopic examination, demonstrate granulation tissue and resolving hemorrhage. Children with inflicted abdominal trauma average 2.5 years of age, but some of the victims of lethal injury are as old as 4 to 6 years of age.[2] A notable finding is that younger children die more rapidly from inflicted abdominal trauma, from means such as peritonitis or homorrhagic shock, than older children. Additionally, the pancreas is situated near the small bowel and may be injured at the same time. Although it is not unusual to find hemorrhage surrounding the pancreas in association with adjacent duodenal or mesenteric trauma, the pancreas is not a site of lethal injury as an isolated injury.[14] Trauma is the leading cause of pancreatitis and pseudocysts of the pancreas, and about one-third of pancreatic trauma is related to abuse.[15,16]

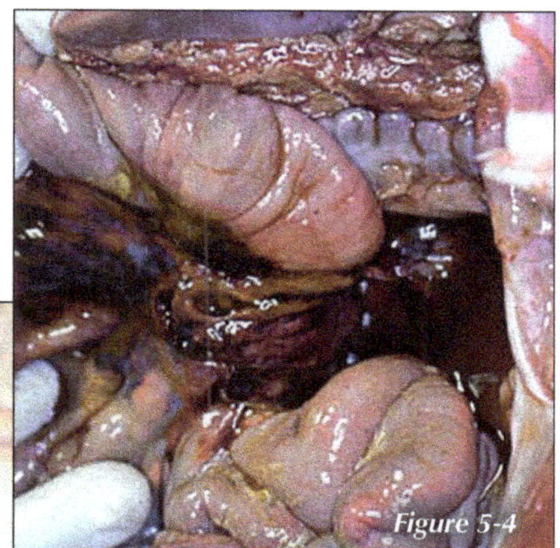

In rare cases, laceration of the stomach can occur from inflicted injury (**Figure 5-5**).[17] At autopsy, undigested food remains within the peritoneal cavity, and acute peritonitis may be present. Lacerations of the stomach typically occur in older children as a result of motor vehicle or biking accidents involving significant forceful impact to the abdomen. They are rarely seen in pediatric trauma patients.

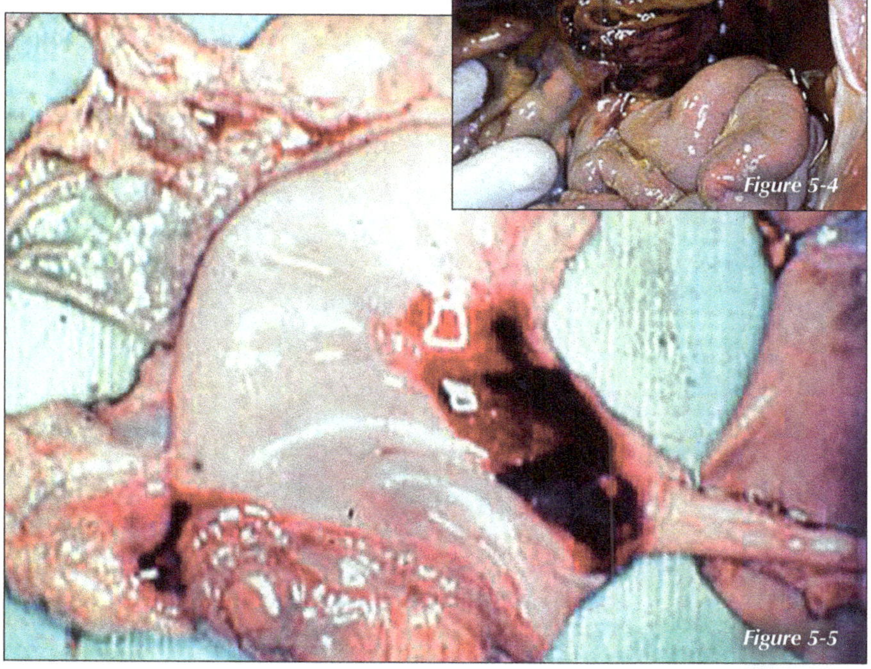

Inflicted liver injuries vary from small, subcapsular hematomas of little significance to lacerations that may transect portions of the liver or macerate the parenchyma. Depending on the age of the child and the amount of injury to the liver, hemorrhage from the injury may occur slowly or very rapidly, and the clinical appearance will be determined by the amount of blood loss. Large liver lacerations may cause rapid death in as little as 15 to 30 minutes. Old, resolving liver injury is also sometimes seen in children dying from another inflicted injury; these areas appear grossly as reddish-yellow areas in the liver and microscopically will demonstrate resolving hematoma that may be aged by the progression of the inflammatory response. Liver injury of significant amounts may rarely result from resuscitation in adults. An incidence of less than 1% of cases of adult resuscitation demonstrate such liver lacerations.[18] In contrast, cardiopulmonary resuscitation (CPR) efforts in infants and young children do not appear to result in significant liver laceration.[19,20]

Abdominal Trauma Case Studies

Case Study 5-1

This 15-month-old girl's mother's boyfriend reported that he was playing with her on the swing set when she fell off, hit a play truck, and groaned but did not cry. The boyfriend then put her back into the swing. Soon after, the mother came outside and picked up the girl who went limp in her arms. The child was unresponsive and died in the emergency department (ED). The girl lived with her mother, her mother's boyfriend, and a 6-year-old sibling. At trial, the boyfriend admitted that the injuries were a result of him swinging the child around in the yard and letting go, causing her to hit the pole of the swing set. He then tripped and fell on top of her. The mother told the doctors that her daughter had no bruises on her the night before, except for 1 on her finger. However, daycare workers indicated the child began coming in with bruises when the mother started dating her boyfriend. Two weeks before the child's death, the boyfriend was with the child when "she slipped down between the foot of the bed and the mattress" and fractured her left tibia and fibula.

Cause of Death: Blunt abdominal trauma

Manner of Death: Homicide

Table 5-1. Autopsy Results

External Examination

— Appears younger than stated age

Injuries

Type	*Measurement*
Chest has multiple punctate contusions on right and left sides, 10 on right and 15 to 18 on left	3 to 5 mm each
Multiple punctate contusions on abdomen, left side 21 to 25 in upper quadrant	3 to 5 mm each
2 patterned area contusions around umbilicus and left upper quadrant (double oval pattern)	4 cm across
Dried abrasion around umbilicus	3 cm x 1.5 cm
Right second finger swollen with contusion	2.5 cm x 1 cm
Left hand, 4 contusions	5 to 6 mm each
3 contusions in left pelvic area	1.5 cm x 1 cm, 1 cm, 5 cm
Left suprapubic area, 5 ecchymoses	1 to 1.5 cm
Left lateral back, 3 yellow abrasions	1 cm x 1.5 cm, 3 cm x 0.7 cm, 1 cm x 0.5 cm
2 dried abrasions on right back	1.5 cm x 0.7 cm, 1 cm
9 contusions on midline back	5 to 6 mm
Right leg, 2 contusions	4 cm x 5 cm each
Swelling and angulation of left wrist	
Fresh hemorrhage in subcutaneous tissue over fracture of left distal radius	

Internal Examination

Fractures

— Left distal radius, acute

— Left leg covered in cast with tibia and fibula fractured, recent

— Left tenth and eleventh ribs

Body Cavities

— Intercostal muscle hemorrhage

— 5 mL of blood diluted with serous fluid in pericardial sac

— Hemorrhage in soft tissue surrounding inferior vena cava extending into the pericardial sac and leaking blood

(continued)

Table 5-1. Autopsy Results *(continued)*

INTERNAL EXAMINATION

Abdomen

Fresh blood in peritoneal cavity	greater than 100 mL
Tear in transverse mesocolon on the greater curvature of the stomach	9 cm
3 tears of the mesentery of the small bowel	2 cm (2), 3 cm
Tear in the mesentery and lymph nodes near the head of the pancreas	3 cm
Subcapsular hemorrhage in right lobe of liver	3 cm x 1 cm
— Extending into the left lobe	3 cm x 2 cm x 4 cm in greatest dimensions
Fresh hemorrhage in abdominal wall fat under areas of contusion	
Large amount of retroperitoneal soft tissue hemorrhage	

Neck Organs

TYPE	*MEASUREMENT*
Laceration of tongue, right side, with large hemorrhage into the muscle	1 cm
Laceration at tip of tongue	5 mm

Lungs

— Multiple focal areas of contusion in the inferior portion of both lungs

— Hemorrhage in the parenchyma

Pancreas

— Fresh hemorrhage

GI Tract

— Soft tissue hemorrhage and contusion on the serosal surface of the greater curvature of the stomach

— Extensive contusional injury on the serosal surface of the duodenum

Uterus and Adnexa

— Soft tissue hemorrhage surrounding organs of the pelvis

Cranial Cavity

— 2 areas of subgaleal hemorrhage in left parietal region, 1 cm and 3 cm

Brain

— Gyri flattened and sulci narrowed

Buttocks

— Soft tissue hemorrhage within the fat of the left buttock, 3 cm

MICROSCOPIC EXAMINATION

— ***Left fibula:*** Healing fracture with thick bony callus formation

— ***Left radius:*** Fresh fracture with disruption of cortex and acute hemorrhage

— ***Left tenth and eleventh ribs:*** Fresh fractures with hemorrhage and cortex disruption

— ***Tongue:*** Bites on tongue with hemorrhage to deep muscle

— ***Scalp:*** Fresh subgaleal hemorrhage

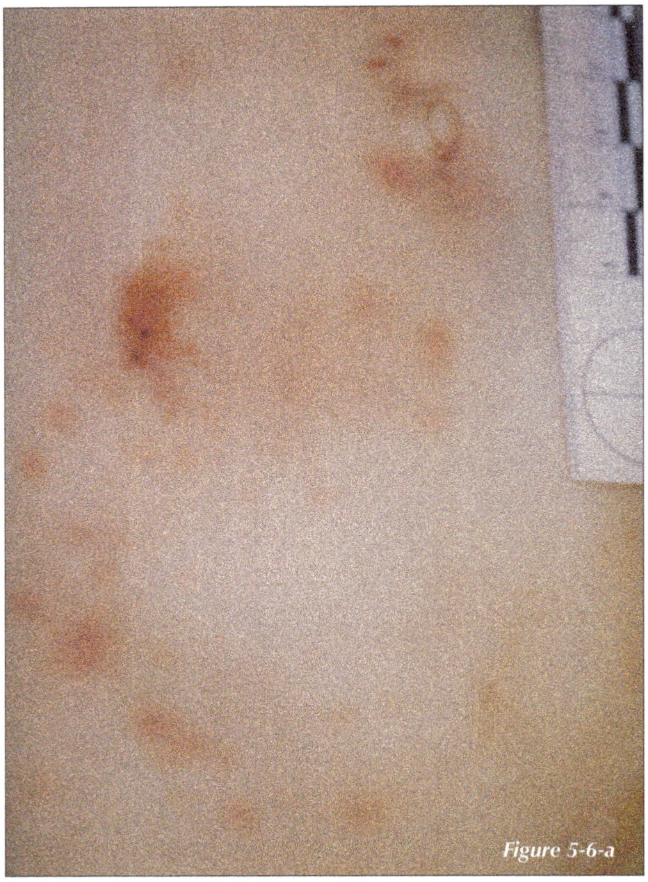
Figure 5-6-a

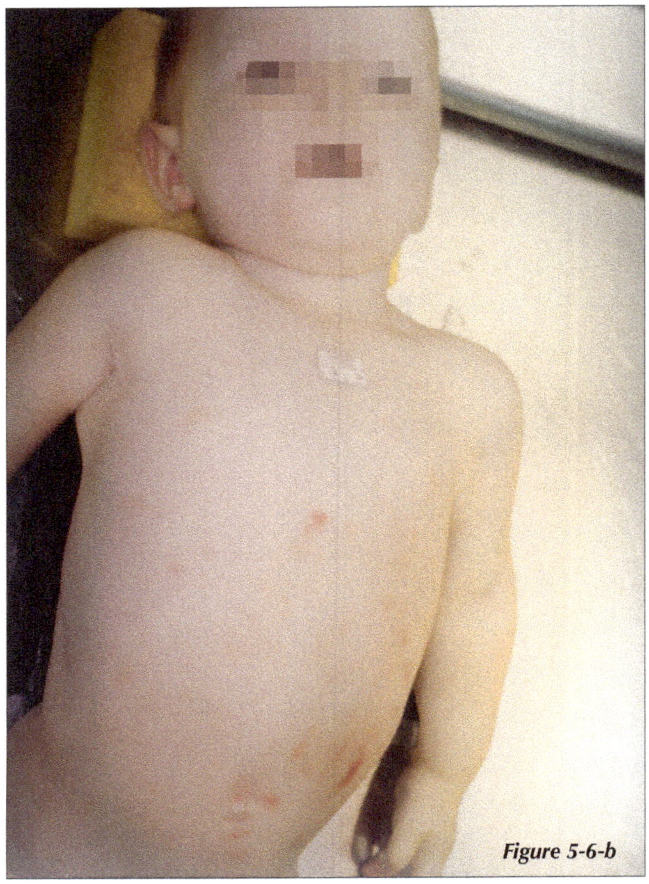
Figure 5-6-b

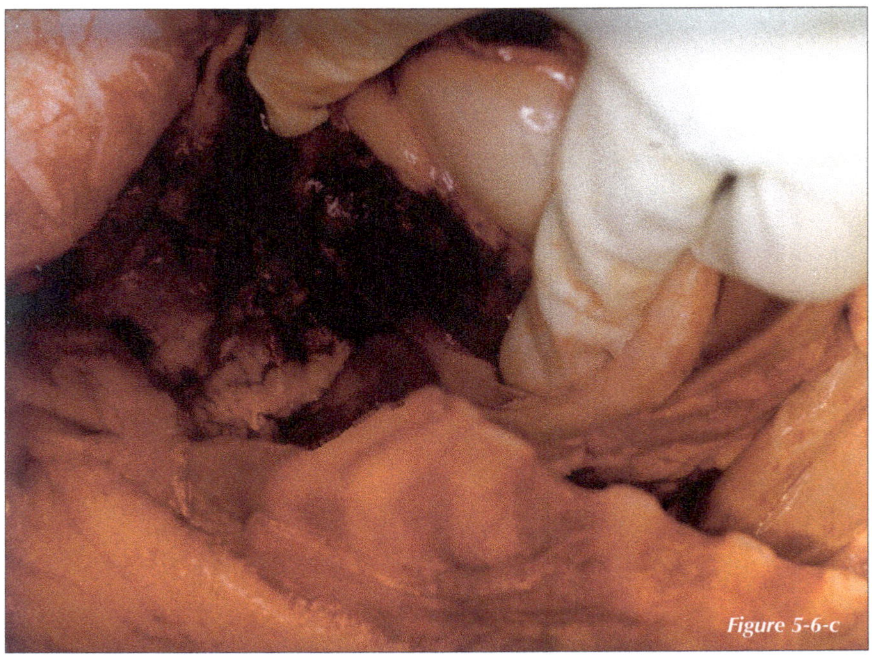
Figure 5-6-c

Figure 5-6-a. *Child at autopsy with contusions on abdomen.*

Figure 5-6-b. *Multiple punctate contusions apparent on the chest and abdomen.*

Figure 5-6-c. *Hemorrhage in laceration of transverse mesocolon over the greater curvature of the stomach.*

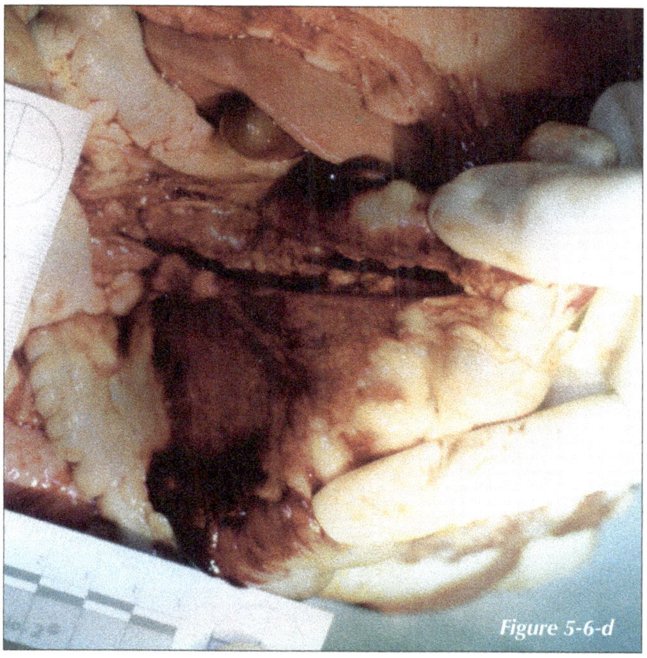

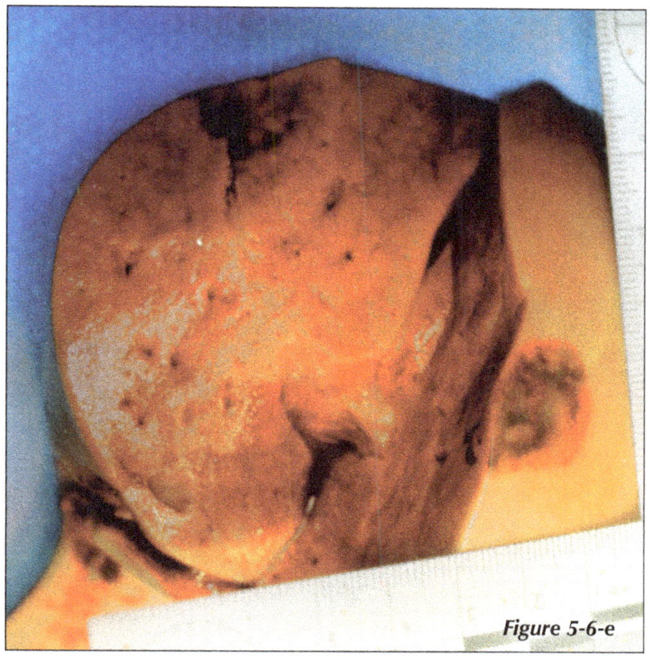

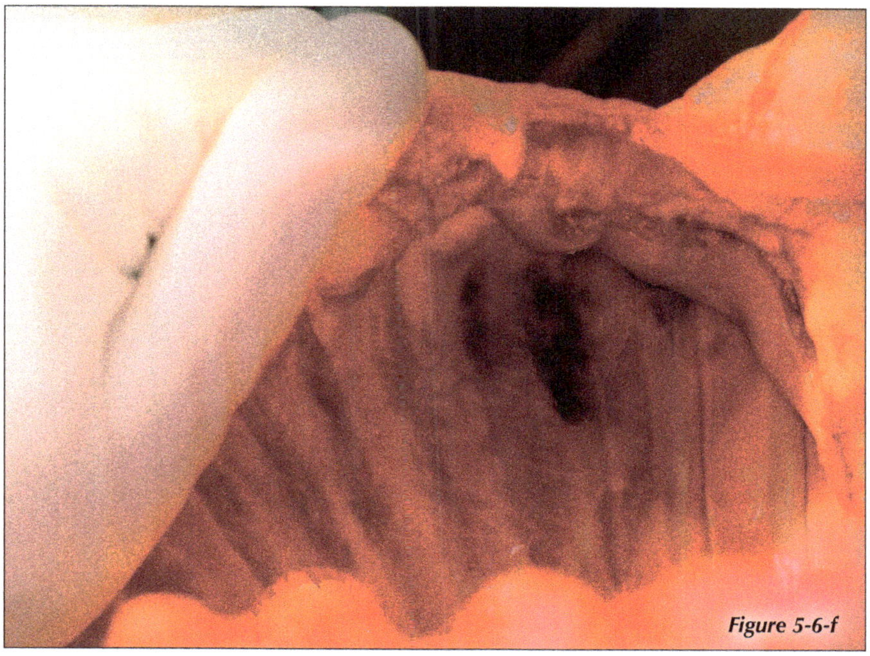

Figure 5-6-d. *Hemorrhage in mesocolon.*

Figure 5-6-e. *Liver showing subcapsular hemorrhage of right lobe.*

Figure 5-6-f. *Fractures of left tenth and eleventh rib.*

Figure 5-6-g. *Left distal radius removed with hemorrhage in periosteum over fracture.*

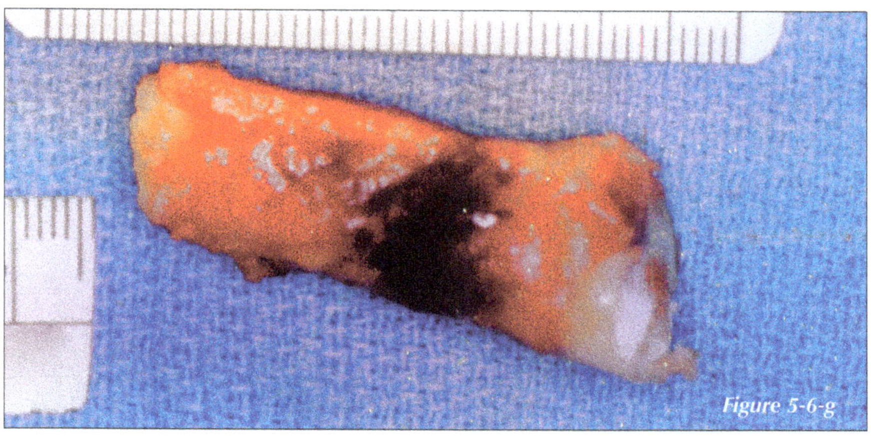

Abdominal Trauma Case Studies

Case Study 5-2

This 2-year-old child was kept home from daycare because he was not feeling well and had vomited the previous day at daycare and at home. When the child's 9-year-old brother arrived home from school, he went to check on the child and found him unresponsive. The child was in full arrest in the ED and was pronounced dead. On the day of death, he was in the care of the mother's boyfriend. The child abuse hotline indicated 2 previous reports for the child's brother concerning educational needs and unsanitary living conditions. The boyfriend admitted to striking the child several times over the past week. He admitted to hitting the child on the head, abdomen, and buttocks.

Cause of Death: Blunt abdominal trauma

Manner of Death: Homicide

Table 5-2-a. Autopsy Results

External Examination

Type	*Measurement*
Right cheek scar	30 mm x 5 mm
Left cheek scars	40 mm x 10 mm, 3 mm
Right back scar	40 mm x 5 mm
Left back scar	40 mm x 10 mm
Right buttock scars	20 mm, 50 mm (2), 40 mm (2)
Left shin, patterned scars	40 mm x 30 mm, 50 mm x 35 mm
Left thigh and knee scars	60 mm x 15 mm each

Injuries

Head

Right eyebrow contusions	15 mm, 5 mm
Left eyebrow contusions	5 mm, 10 mm
Left eyebrow abrasion/contusion	3 mm x 1 mm
Left mandible contusion	10 mm
Upper and lower lip lacerations and abrasions	5 to 8 mm
Reflected scalp showed scattered subgaleal hemorrhages on left scalp	5 to 150 mm in diameter

Dried blood on upper and lower lips

Chest/Abdomen

Contusions over midline and left side	4 to 40 mm in diameter
Blood in abdominal cavity	160 mL
Small bowel mesentery laceration	90 mm x 50 mm
Left lobe of liver, contusion	60 mm x 50 mm

Hemorrhage in peritoneal soft tissues

Back/Extremities

Lower back, subcutaneous hemorrhage	70 mm x 40 mm
Left buttock, soft tissue hemorrhage	50 mm x 40 mm
Soft tissue hemorrhage, right knee	120 mm x 60 mm

Internal Injuries

Lungs

— Patchy hemorrhage on visceral pleura of all lobes

— Small intestinal serosal patchy hemorrhages

— Small intestinal wall showed hemorrhages in the areas of contusion

Microscopic Examination

— ***Liver:*** Parenchymal hemorrhage

— ***Skin:*** Scalp, abdomen, back, and thigh show fresh hemorrhage within the contusions

— ***GI tract:*** Fresh mesenteric hemorrhage

Table 5-2-b. Diagnoses

Blunt Abdominal Trauma

— Hemoperitoneum

— Small bowel mesentery, lacerations

— Liver, left lobe contusion

— Peritoneal soft tissue hemorrhage

Integument and Soft Tissue

— Contusions and abrasions on scalp, abdomen, back, buttock, upper and lower extremity

— Lacerations and abrasions on upper and lower lips

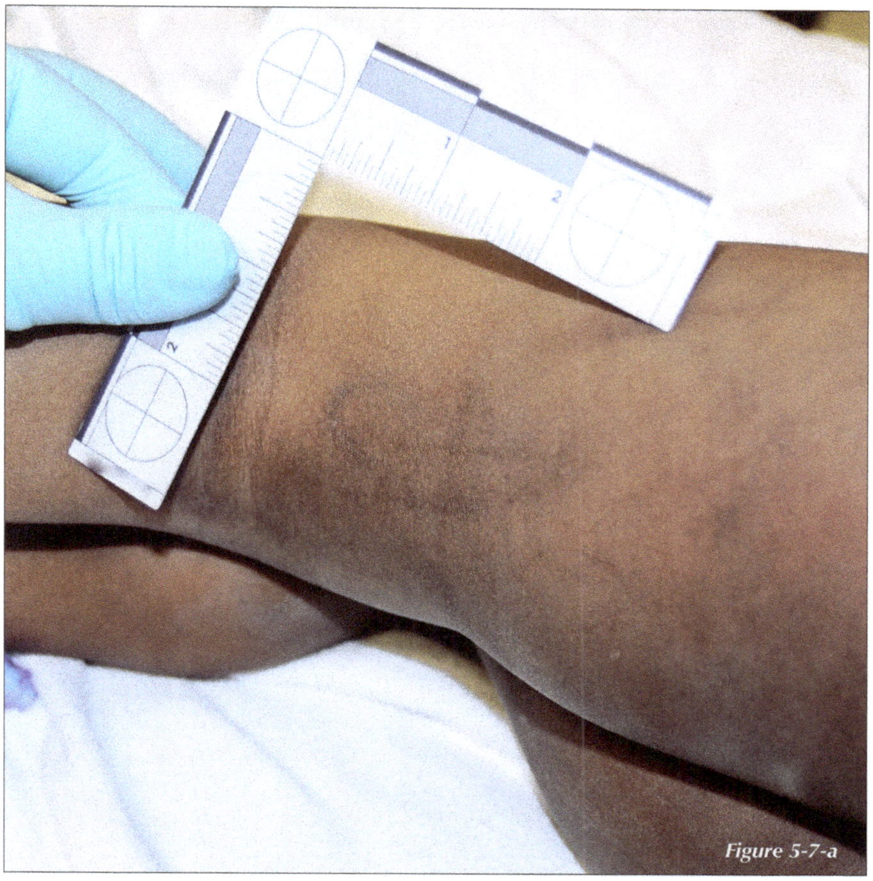

Figure 5-7-a. *Scars on left thigh.*

Figure 5-7-b. *Scars on left thigh.*

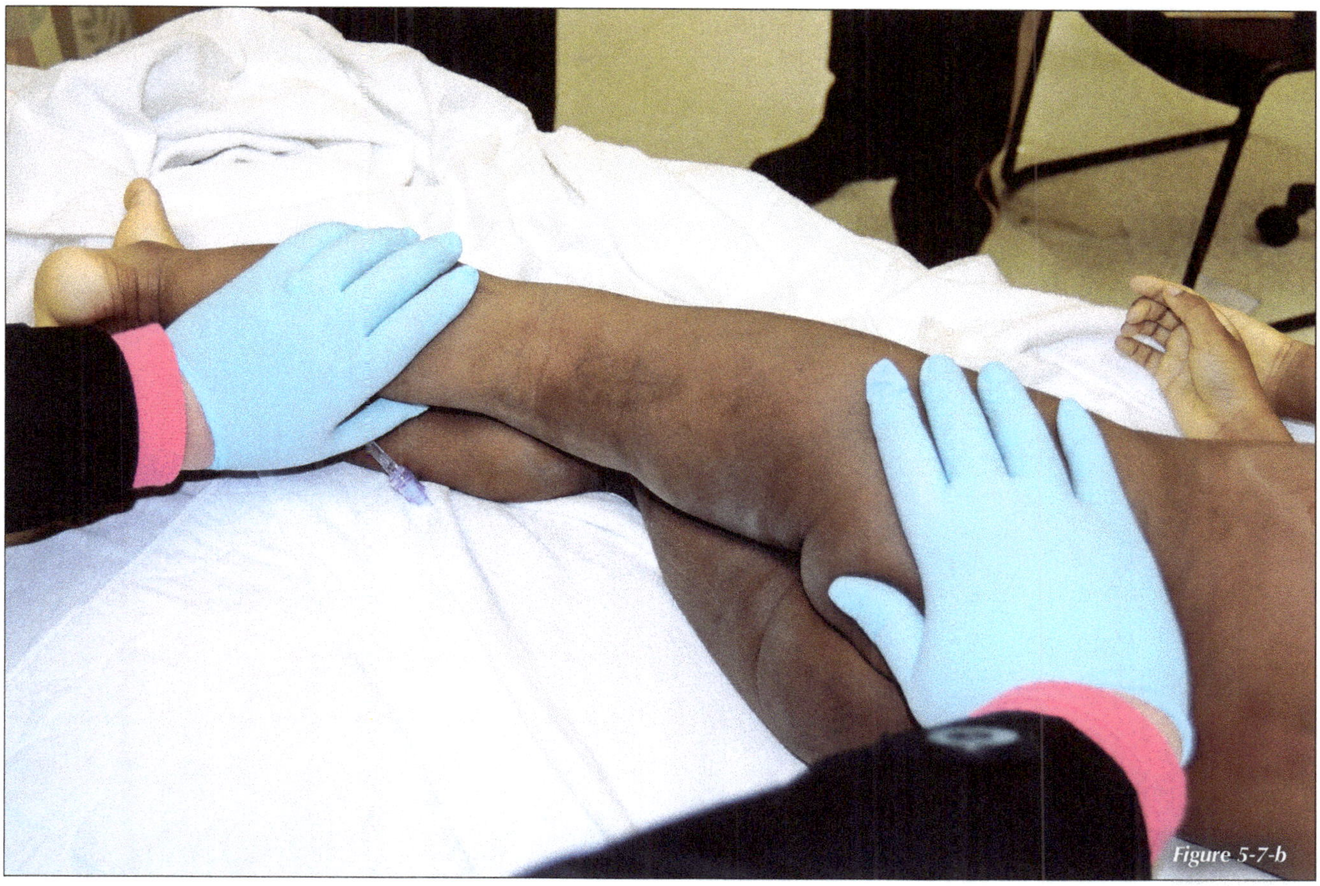

Figure 5-7-c. Abdomen showing contusions on midline and left side.

Figure 5-7-d. Back of body showing contusions on lower back and left buttock.

Figure 5-7-e and f. Scars on right back.

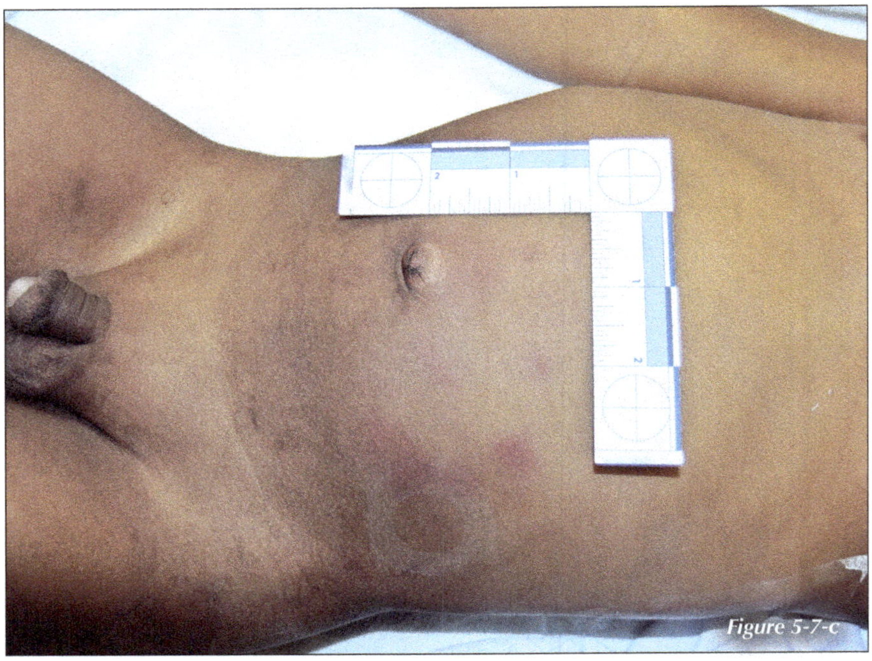

Figure 5-7-c

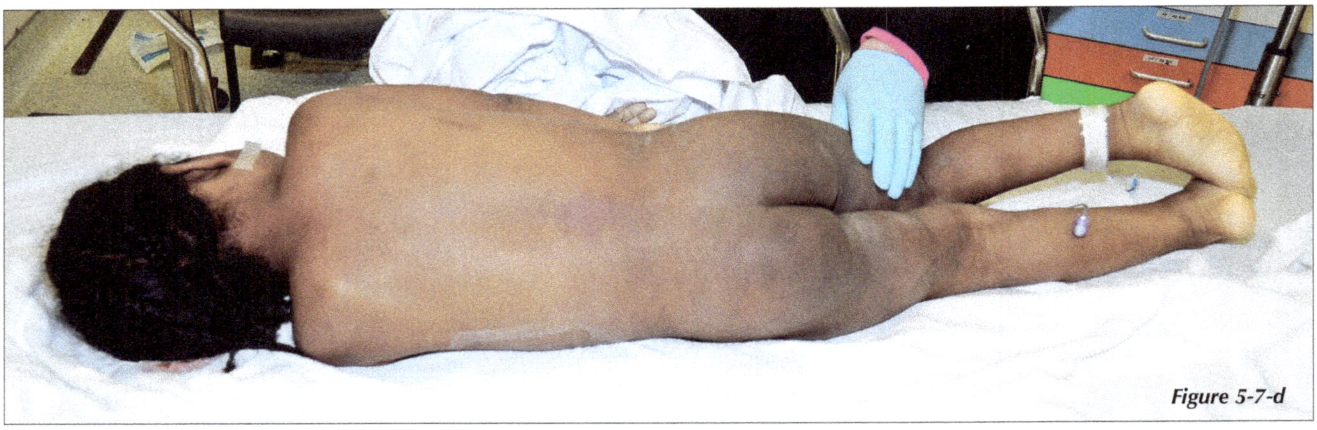

Figure 5-7-d

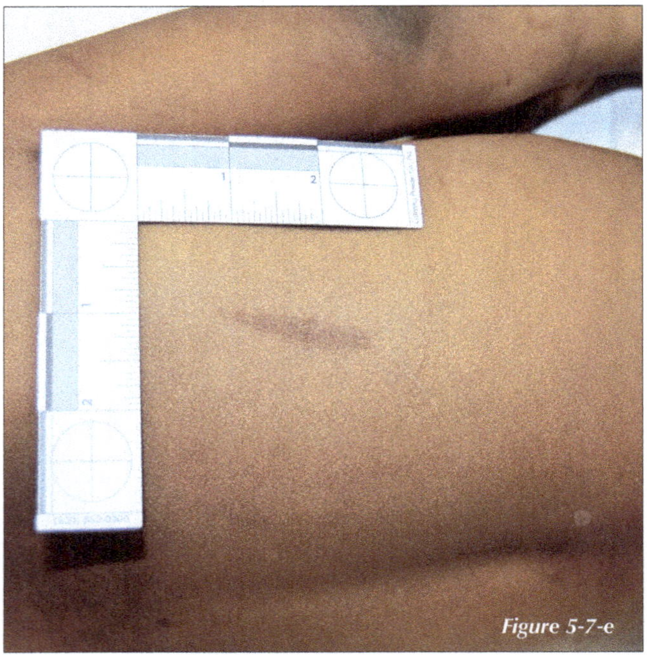

Figure 5-7-e

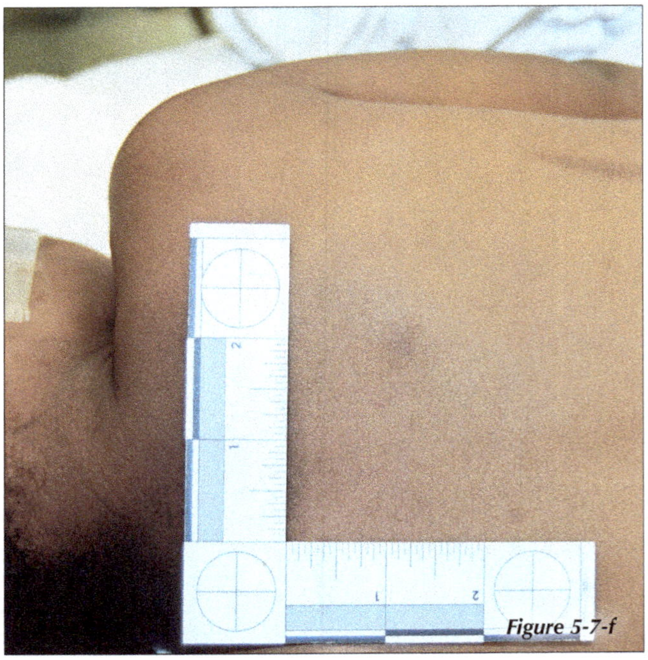

Figure 5-7-f

Abdominal Trauma Case Studies

Case Study 5-3

This 22-month-old boy's mother said that 2 days before taking her son to the hospital, he had a decreased appetite, and after work the next day, she found him lying in bed appearing unwell. She then took him to the ED. The child was found to have multiple bowel perforations and sepsis from injuries which appeared to be several days old. The child died after a few days in the hospital. There were prior department of family services (DFS) investigations of the family for lack of food, physical abuse, and a newborn crisis assessment. DFS subsequently removed all other children from the home. The child lived with his mother, his siblings, the mother's boyfriend, and 2 other adults. The boyfriend confessed to spanking the child, hitting him with a door, and punching him in the stomach. The boyfriend stated he had anger issues, and the mother said the boyfriend would become angry when he drank alcohol and used cocaine.

Cause of Death: Blunt abdominal trauma

Manner of Death: Homicide

Table 5-3-a. Autopsy Results

External Examination

— Vertical surgical incision in abdomen from which loops of small bowel were protruding and appeared hemorrhagic and swollen

— Scrotum and penis were swollen

Injuries

Head

Type	*Measurement*
Left forehead contusion	25 mm x 21 mm
Right cheek, preauricular area, scratch	10 mm x 1 mm
Right mid-cheek contusion	10 mm x 10 mm
Right upper lateral neck contusion	11 mm x 10 mm
Right parietal subgaleal hemorrhage	10 mm x 18 mm
Left frontal subgaleal hemorrhage	31 mm x 25 mm

Extremities

Left arm, petechial hemorrhages on antecubital fossa	70 mm x 40 mm area
Contusion, left wrist	25 mm x 5 mm
Left dorsal forearm contusion	45 mm x 12 mm
Left ventral forearm contusion	12 mm x 8 mm
Right thigh contusions	25 mm x 10 mm, , 30 mm x 15 mm
Right knee contusions	25 mm x 29 mm, 10 mm x 5 mm
Right leg contusion	9 mm x 8 mm
Right foot abrasion	10 mm x 10 mm
Right foot, linear punctate abrasions (4)	21 mm x 1 mm, 1 mm, 2 mm (2)
— With deep underlying hemorrhage in the soft tissue	
Abrasion on right big toe	4 mm x 1 mm
Left thigh contusion	10 mm x 18 mm
Left leg contusion	21 mm x 20 mm
Left foot abrasion	50 mm x 20 mm

Back

Area of hemorrhage within the right mid-back	
— Into soft tissues	10 mm
Mongolian spots on upper buttocks	
4 abrasions in a row, mid-back	
— Row length	48 mm
— Individual punctate abrasions with underlying hemorrhage in the soft tissue	4 mm (3), 5 mm

(continued)

Table 5-3-a. Autopsy Results *(continued)*

INJURIES

Abdominal Cavity

— Yellow purulent exudate on superior surface of the liver and under the diaphragm, forming a subdiaphragmatic abscess on both the right and left sides

— Fresh blood clot and liquid blood in right and left lower abdomen quadrants, 50 to 75 mL

— Jejunum enterotomies (2)

— Entire jejunum covered with purulent exudate with formation of early adhesions

— Early adhesions throughout entire small bowel

— Small and large bowel appeared dusky and necrotic

Lungs

— Poor crepitation and increased firmness

Spleen

— Mottled surface with flecks of exudate on cut section

Adrenals

— Associated with diaphragmatic abscesses

MICROSCOPIC EXAMINATION

— ***Lungs:*** Extensive and well-developed adult respiratory distress syndrome with prominent hyaline membranes; cuboidal cells lining alveoli and proteinaceous debris in alveoli

— ***Liver:*** Mixed acute and chronic inflammatory cells with fibrin

— ***Spleen:*** Congested, depleted of cells, and covered with an inflammatory exudate

— ***Small intestines:*** Serosal inflammation, acute and chronic with necrosis; extensive hemorrhage and necrosis of bowel wall

— ***Adrenals:*** Congestion with acute inflammation

— ***Right scalp:*** Acute hemorrhage

— ***Left frontal scalp:*** Acute hemorrhage

— ***Mesenteric fat:*** Acute hemorrhage, focal necrosis, and bacterial overgrowth

— ***Diaphragm:*** Necrotic inflammation with acute necrotizing inflammatory exudate in the abscess

— ***Back:*** Acute hemorrhage

— ***Right foot:*** Penetrating wound through epidermis

— ***Right thigh:*** Extensive acute hemorrhage

NEUROPATHOLOGY MICROSCOPIC EXAMINATION

— Multifocal axonal injury of hypoxic/ischemic pattern

Table 5-3-b. Diagnoses

Abdominal Blunt Trauma

— Status post resection of portion of duodenum following blunt trauma

— Acute suppurative peritonitis with subdiaphragmatic abscesses, right and left

— Hemoperitoneum, lower right and left abdomen, 50 to 75 mL

Other Blunt Trauma

— Subgaleal hemorrhage on right parietal, left frontal

— Contusions on left forehead, right cheek, right lateral upper neck

— Abrasions, right lateral cheek

— Contusions on left dorsal wrist, dorsal left forearm, ventral left forearm

— Contusions on right anterior thigh, right knee (2), right leg

— Abrasions, dorsum of right foot; linearly oriented punctate abrasions (4), dorsum of right foot

— Contusions on left lower thigh, anterior left leg

— Abrasion, dorsum of left foot

— Abrasions and linear punctate abrasions (4), midline mid-back

— Hemorrhage, right mid-back muscle

Figure 5-8-a. *Close-up of abrasions of midback.*

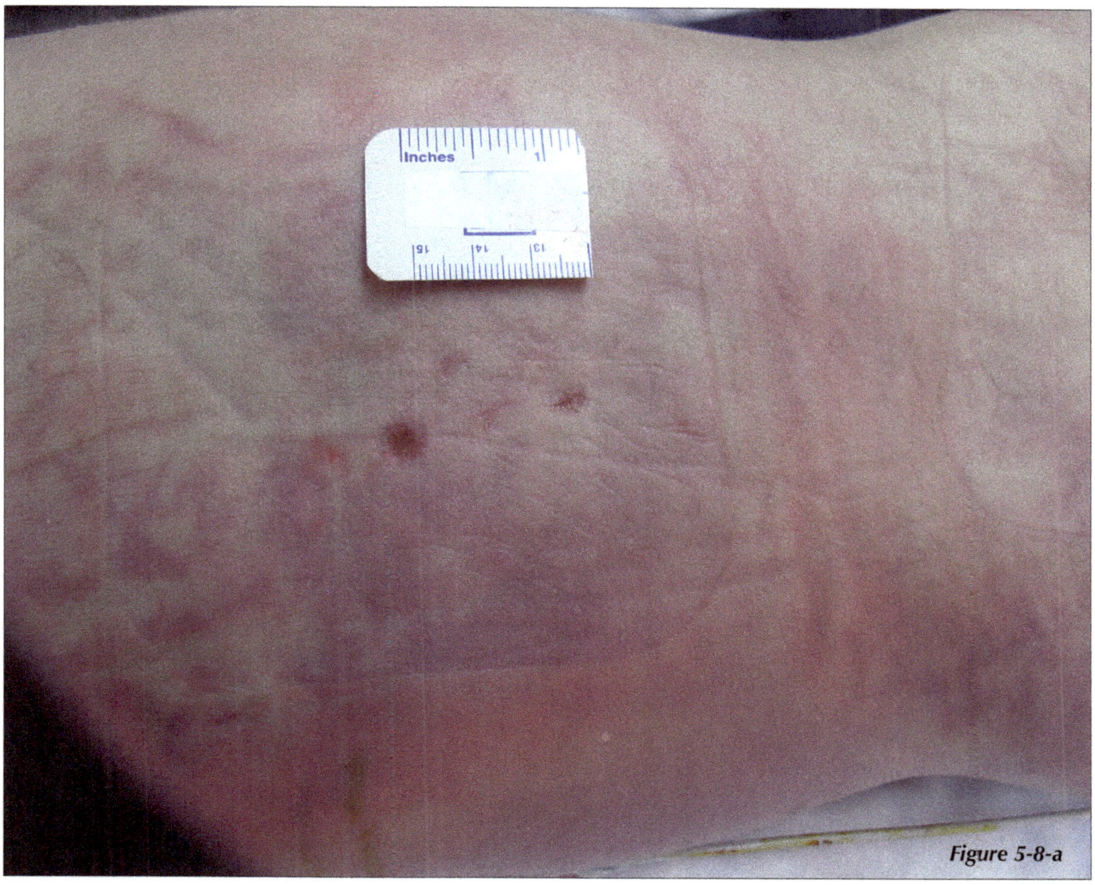

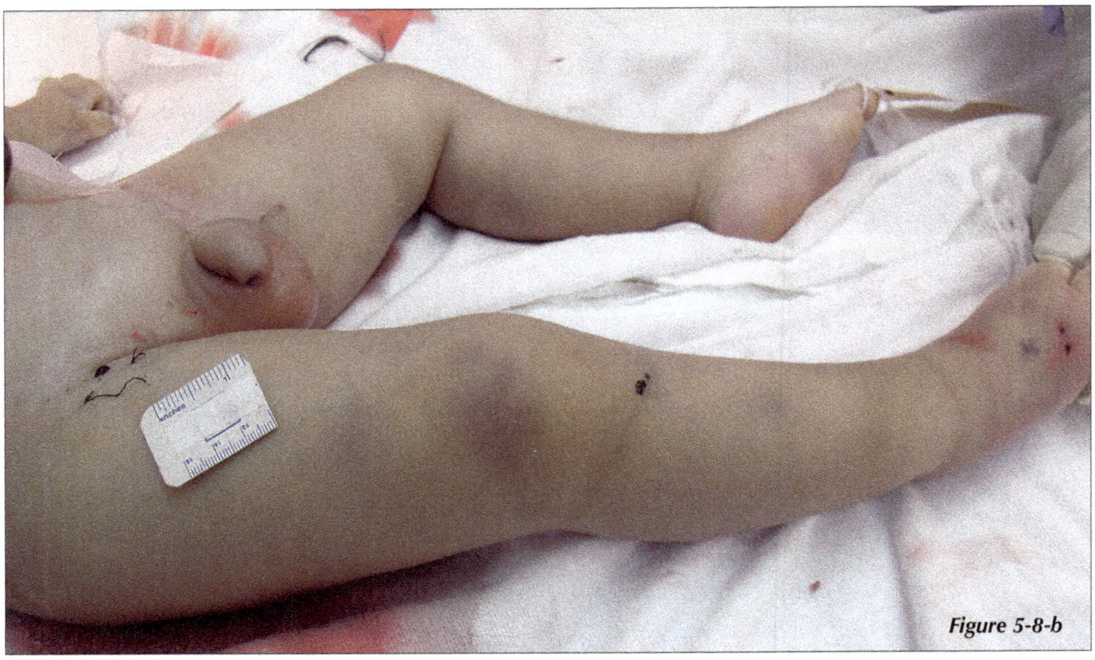

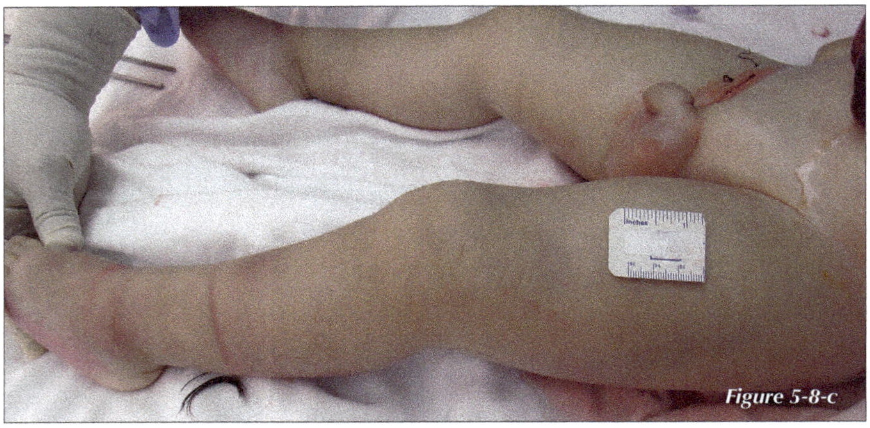

Figure 5-8-b and c. Contusions on thighs, knees, legs, and feet.

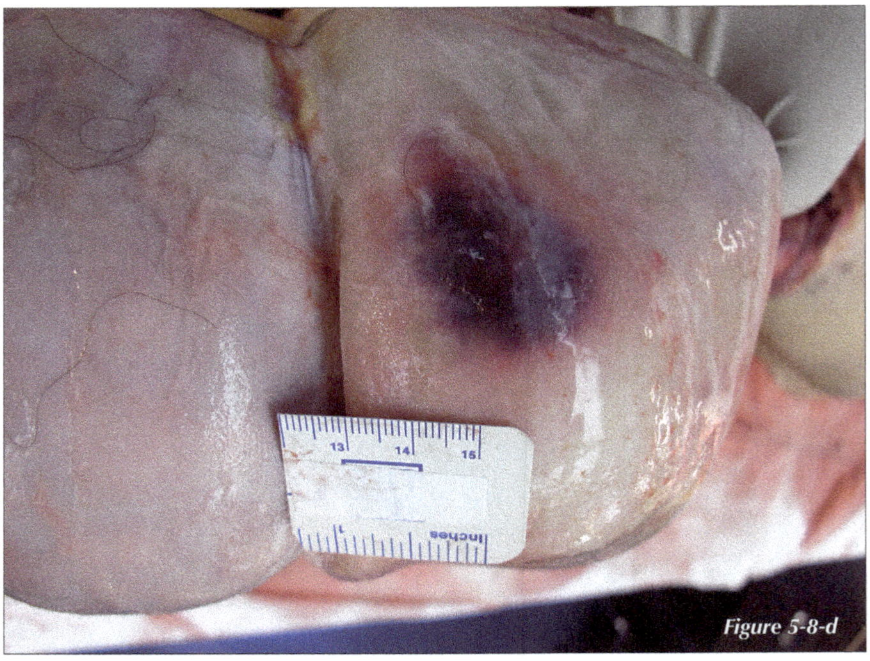

Figure 5-8-d. Scalp reflected to show subgaleal hemorrhage of right parietal.

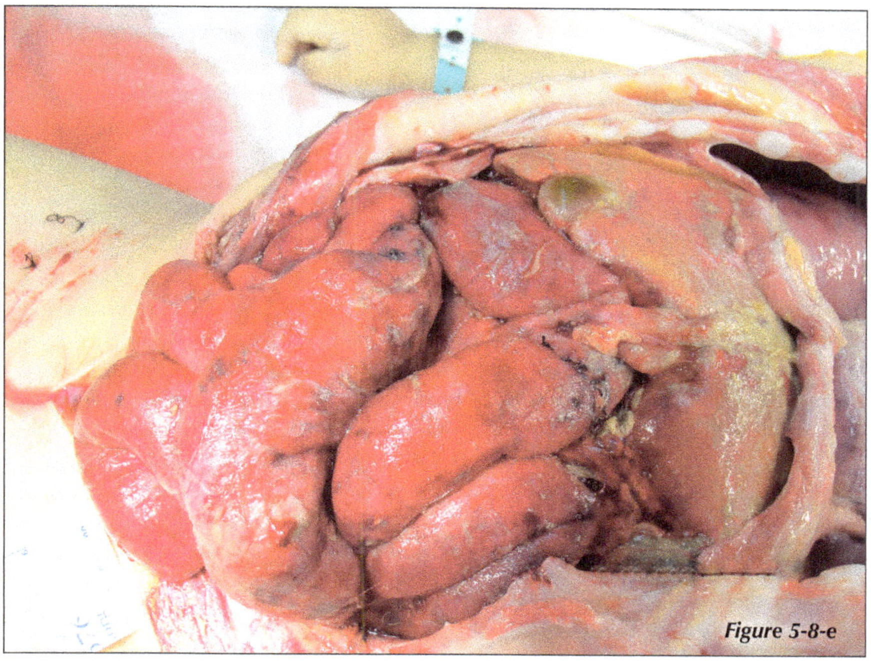

Figure 5-8-e

Figure 5-8-e. *Abdomen opened showing peritonitis with organizing purulent exudate over liver and loops of small bowel.*

Figure 5-8-f. *A posterior view of removed block of chest and abdominal organs to show organizing peritonitis.*

Figure 5-8-g. *Surface of liver with yellow purulent exudate.*

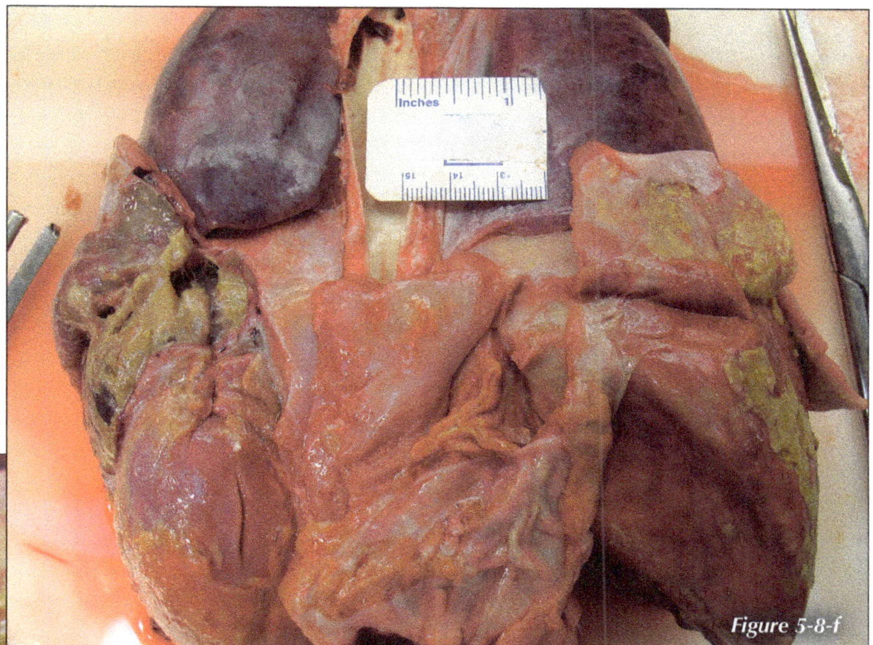

Figure 5-8-f

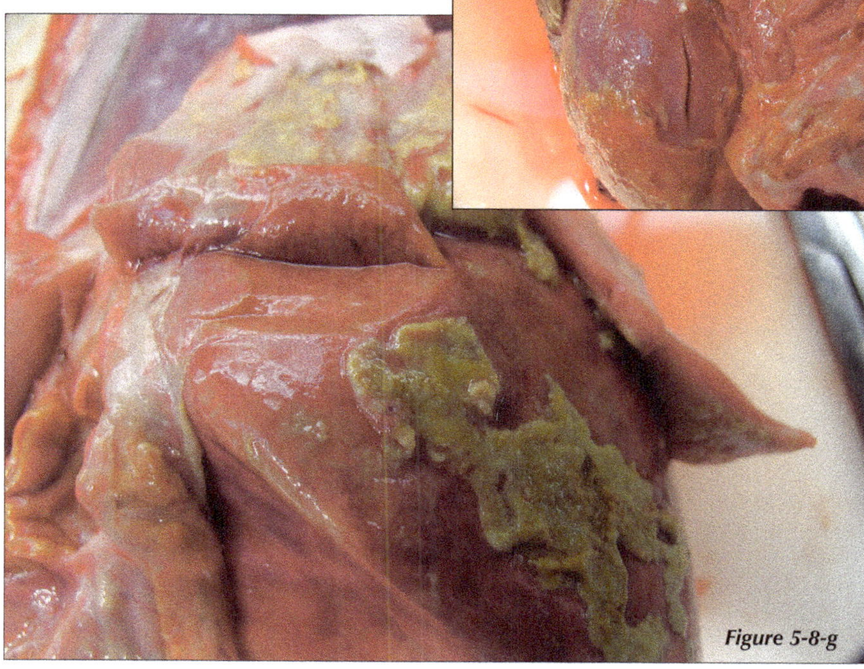

Figure 5-8-g

Abdominal Trauma Case Studies

Case Study 5-4

This 13-week-old girl was held underwater in a bathtub by her mother's boyfriend. The boyfriend said he did this because the infant would not stop crying. Initially, the boyfriend said he put her head underwater to rinse off shampoo, and the child went limp. He then took the child to the mother for help, and 911 was called. A neighbor performed CPR, and the child regained consciousness after coughing. However, when EMS arrived, the child was unconscious and was taken to the hospital where she was in arrest and died. DFS checked on a 2-year-old sibling who was found to have internal injuries and was also taken to the hospital. The mother eventually stated that she and her boyfriend were fighting about which chairs to sit in, and then the mother cut the cord to the TV set. After that, the boyfriend beat up the 2 children. The children were then bathed to clean them up from the beating.

Cause of Death: Blunt abdominal trauma

Manner of Death: Homicide

Table 5-4-a. Autopsy Results

Injuries

Type	*Measurement*
Lower left abdomen had an area of contusions with extensive hemorrhage into the subcutaneous fat	120 mm x 100 mm
Contusion of lower back and right flank	100 mm x 50 mm
Linear contusion, left lateral thorax	70 mm x 30 mm
Contusion, right scapula	25 mm
Abdomen was markedly distended with blood in the peritoneal cavity	200 mL
Multiple contusions over the occipital scalp	
Air within the small and large bowel	
Extensive laceration of the mesentery with intraperitoneal hemorrhage and some retroperitoneal hemorrhage	
Extensive perirenal and periadrenal hemorrhage on the left	
Complete avulsion of the pedicle of the left kidney from its vascular supply	
Renal artery and vein separated by abundant hemorrhage	
Callus of ribs 5 to 8 on both sides laterally	
Pancreas was surrounded by hemorrhage in the midportion	

Microscopic Examination

- ***Adrenals:*** Periadrenal hemorrhage on the left
- ***Kidney:*** Left kidney revealed focal areas of hemorrhage into the adipose tissue

Table 5-4-b. Diagnoses

Multiple Trauma

- Contusions
  - Lower abdomen
  - Back, multiple
  - Posterior scalp
- Intra-abdominal injury
  - Multiple lacerations of small and large bowel mesentery
  - Complete traumatic separation of left renal artery and renal vein
  - Hemoperitoneum, 200 mL
- Healed fractures, ribs 5 to 8, bilaterally

Abdominal Trauma Case Studies

Case Study 5-5

This 11-month-old girl lived with her mother, father, and 2 siblings who were aged 8 years and 2 years. The 8-year-old took a bath and refilled the tub once finished. Then, the mother placed the 2 younger children in the tub, leaving the 8-year-old to supervise them while she went to clean the dishes. About 5 minutes later, the 8-year-old told the mother that the child had fallen asleep in the tub. The mother found the child seated and bent forward in the tub with her face in 5 to 6 inches of water. The mother removed the child from the bathtub and did CPR. The child was unresponsive at the scene and was transported to a local hospital, where she was intubated. She was then transferred to a children's hospital, where she remained until she was pronounced dead 2 days later with hypoxic encephalopathy. The family had a disturbing history involving the father, who, 5 years earlier, caused fatal inflicted head trauma to a sibling and had been incarcerated and then released. Initially, the mother stated he was not in the home when this event occurred, but it was later ascertained that he was present. There were also several prior DFS reports concerning physical abuse, indifference to educational needs, lack of supervision, and verbal abuse.

Cause of Death: Acute purulent peritonitis complicating blunt trauma of abdomen with contusion of small bowel

Manner of Death: Homicide

Table 5-5-a. Autopsy Results

Injuries

— Right thigh had been damaged by an intraosseous vascular catheter that infiltrated, so it appeared swollen and deep purple from mid-thigh down the entire leg, sparing a portion of the posterior aspect and sharply demarcated at the edges with blisters at the margin and skin slippage. On cut section, the underlying fat was discolored reddish pink.

— 60 mL of yellow/orange purulent fluid in abdominal cavity

— Early adhesions forming between loops of bowel, between liver and diaphragm, and between loops of bowel and the lower abdominal peritoneal wall

— From the mid-ileum to the ascending colon and most marked in the distal ileum, the bowel was slightly thickened and reddish yellow with purulent material over the serosal surface

Microscopic Examination

— Lungs showed widespread atelectasis, many alveoli contained thick hyaline membranes lining alveoli, and some alveoli contained collections of neutrophils and some hemorrhage

— Sections of right thigh showed only edema of subcutaneous tissues

— Distal ileum showed extensive serosal layer of inflammatory cell collection of neutrophils and mononuclear cells with infiltration into the muscularis, and many vessels showed early thrombosis

— Other sections of ileum showed similar inflammatory changes with some actual necrosis

— Diaphragm showed a thick layer of purulent exudate on the subdiaphragmatic surface

— Small bowel mesentery showed a layer of purulent exudate and infiltration of the fat by inflammatory cells

Neuropathology

— The brain grossly was slightly softened in consistency

— The right eye had a small number of retinal hemorrhages in the posterior pole, and the left eye had a small number of retinal hemorrhage in the posterior pole and 1 hemorrhage at the ora serrata

— Neither eye had optic nerve sheath hemorrhage

— Beta-amyloid precursor protein (BAPP) staining demonstrated focal areas of hypoxic axonal injury in the posterior corpus callosum, midbrain, and pons

Table 5-5-b. Diagnoses

Blunt Abdominal Trauma

— Extensive contusion, small bowel

— Acute purulent peritonitis

Hypoxic Encephalopathy

— Respiratory Distress Syndrome with Pneumonia

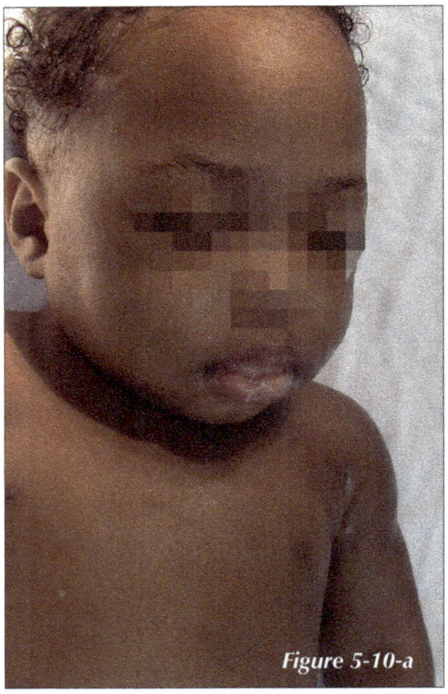

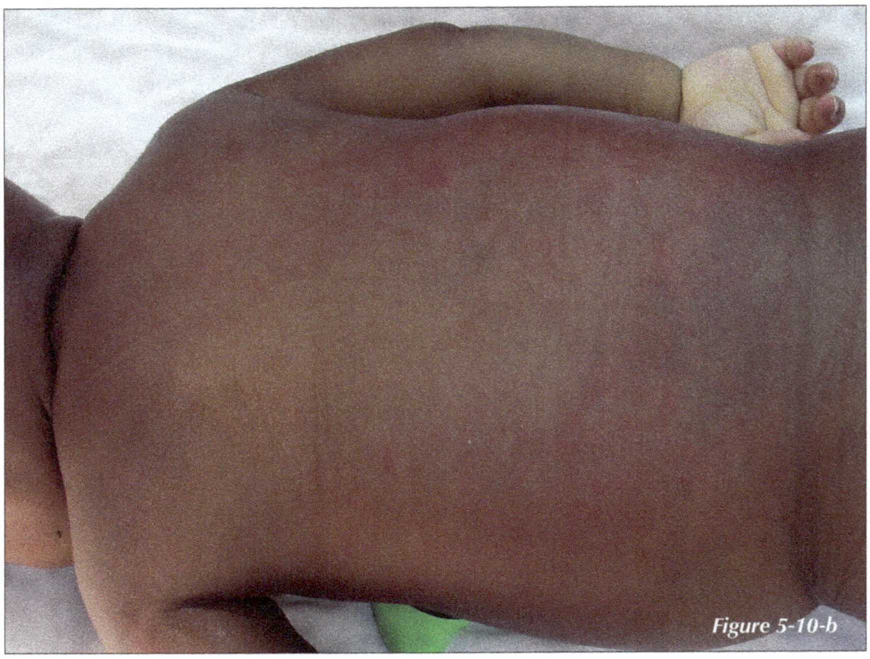

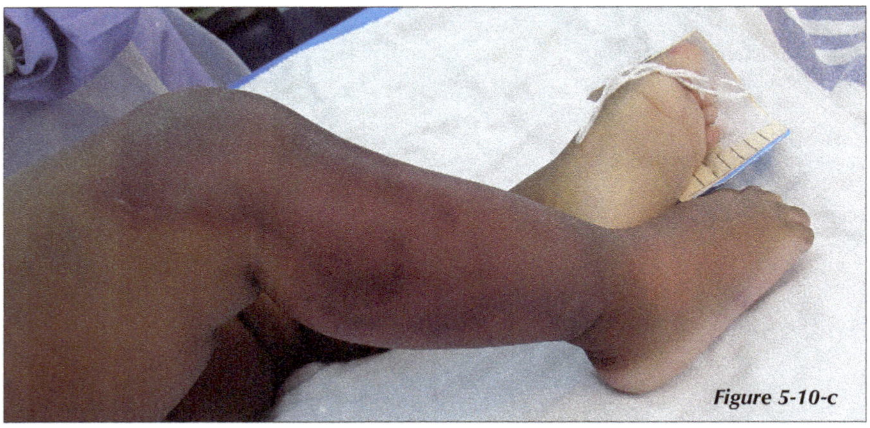

Figure 5-10-a. *Child at autopsy showing no injuries.*

Figure 5-10-b. *Back of body with no injuries.*

Figure 5-10-c. *Right lower extremity damaged by infiltrated vascular catheter with deep purple color.*

Figure 5-10-d. *Abdomen opened to show purulent exudate over bowel.*

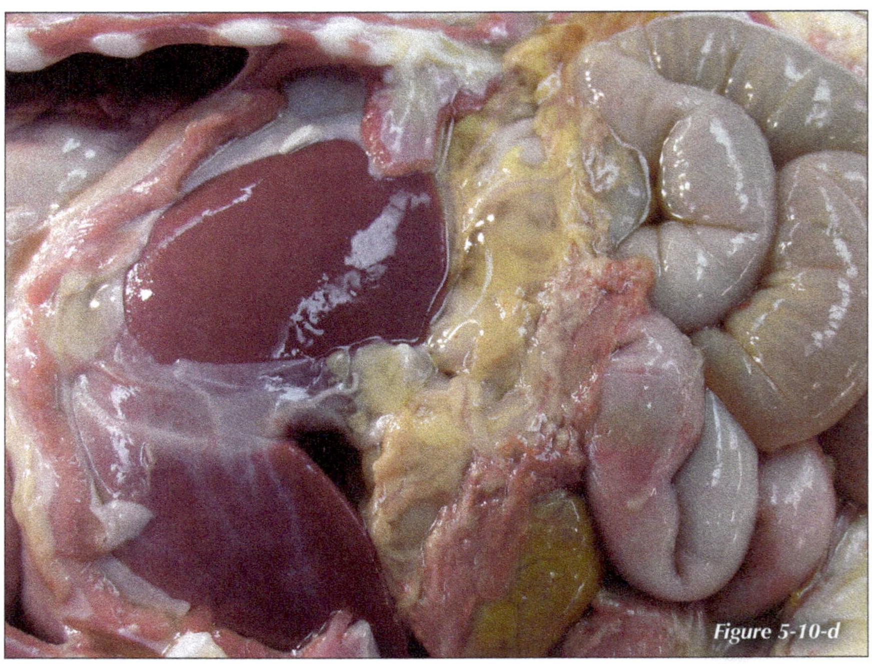

References

1. Lane WG, Dubowitz H, Langenberg P, Dischinger P. Epidemiology of abusive abdominal trauma hospitalizations in United States children. *Child Abuse Negl.* 2012;36(2):142-148.
2. Wood J, Rubin DM, Nance ML, Christian CW. Distinguishing inflicted versus accidental abdominal injuries in young children. *J Trauma.* 2005;59(5):1203-1208.
3. Kirks DR. Radiological evaluation of visceral injuries in the battered child syndrome. *Pediatr Ann.* 1983;12(12):888-893.
4. Ng CS, Hall CM, Shaw DG. The range of visceral manifestations of nonaccidental injury. *Arch Dis Child.* 1997;77(2):167-174.
5. Lane WG, Lotwin I, Dubowitz H, Langenberg P, Dischinger P. Outcomes for children hospitalized with abusive versus noninflicted abdominal trauma. *Pediatrics.* 2011;127(6):e1400-e1405.
6. Trokel M, Discala C, Terrin NC, Sege RD. Patient and injury characteristics in abusive abdominal injuries. *Pediatr Emerg Care.* 2006;22(10):700-704.
7. Roaten JB, Partrick DA, Bensard DD, et al. Visceral injuries in nonaccidental trauma: spectrum of injury and outcomes. *Am J Surg.* 2005;190(6):827-829.
8. Maguire SA, Upadhyaya M, Evans A, et al. A systematic review of abusive visceral injuries in childhood: their range and recognition. *Child Abuse Negl.* 2013;37(7):430-445.
9. Soames RW. Skeletal system: cranial characteristics at different ages. In: Williams PL, ed. *Gray's Anatomy.* 38th ed. Churchill Livingston; 1995:607-609.
10. Kleinman PK, Brill PW, Winchester P. Resolving duodenal-jejunal hematoma in abused children. *Radiology.* 1986;160(3):747-750.
11. Gaines BA, Shultz BS, Morrison K, Ford HR. Duodenal injuries in children: beware of child abuse. *J Pediatr Surg.* 2004;39(4):600-602.
12. Huntimer CM, Muret-Wagstaff S, Leland NL. Can falls on stairs result in small intestine perforations? *Pediatrics.* 2000;106(2 pt 1):301-305.
13. Wang MY, Kim KA, Griffith PM, et al. Injuries from falls in the pediatric population: an analysis of 729 cases. *J Pediatr Surg.* 2001;36(10):1528-1534.
14. Hilfer CL, Holgersen LO. Massive chylous ascites and transacted pancreas secondary to child abuse: successful non-surgical management. *Pediatr Radiol.* 1995;25(2):117-119.
15. Cooney DR, Crosfeld JL. Operative management of pancreatic pseudocysts in infants and children: a review of 75 cases. *Ann Surg.* 1975;182(5):590-596.
16. Ziegler DW, Long JA, Philippart AI, Klein MD. Pancreatitis in childhood. Experience with 49 patients. *Ann Surg.* 1988;207(3):257-261.
17. Case ME, Nanduri R. Laceration of the stomach by blunt trauma in a child: a case of child abuse. *J Forensic Sci.* 1983;28(2):496-501.
18. Meron G, Kurkciyan I, Sterz F, et al. Cardiopulmonary resuscitation-associated major liver injury. *Resuscitation.* 2007;75(3):445-453.
19. Bush CM, Jones JS, Cohle SD, Johnson H. Pediatric injuries from cardiopulmonary resuscitation. *Ann Emerg Med.* 1996;28(1):40-44.
20. Price EA, Rush LR, Perper JA, Bell MD. Cardiopulmonary resuscitation-related injuries and homicidal blunt abdominal trauma in children. *Am J Forensic Med Pathol.* 2000;21(4):307-310.

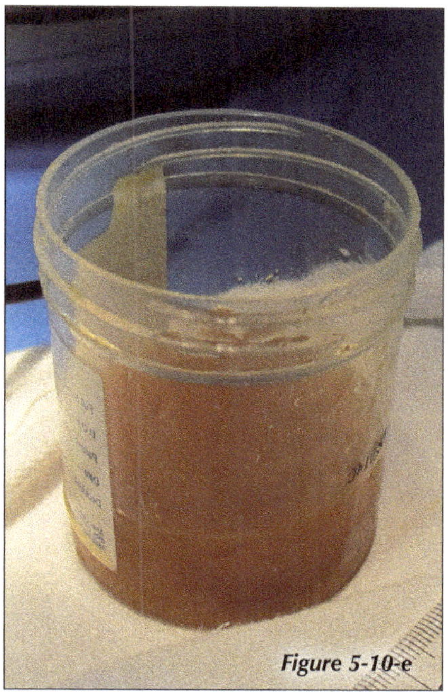
Figure 5-10-e

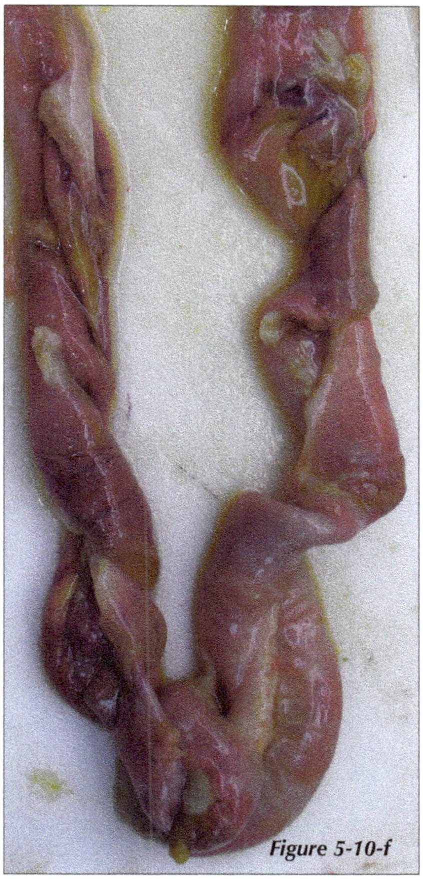
Figure 5-10-f

Figure 5-10-e. *Orange-yellow purulent fluid from peritoneal cavity.*

Figure 5-10-f. *Bowel showing purulent exudate over serosal surfaces.*

Chapter 6

Blunt Soft Tissue Trauma

Objectives

After reviewing this chapter, the reader will be able to:

1. *Recognize blunt soft tissue trauma as a rare form of lethal child abuse and list its potential mechanisms of death.*
2. *Describe the ways in which blunt soft tissue trauma can lead to heart lesions known as stress cardiomyopathy.*
3. *Identify expected autopsy findings of children who died from blunt soft tissue trauma.*

Blunt Soft Tissue Trauma

Blunt soft tissue trauma is a rare form of lethal child abuse with external evidence of beating but an absence of injury to the internal viscera. The lethal mechanism in these cases is not always certain and may be due to the large volume of blood shed into the soft tissue; the fat embolism released by the crushed fat of the soft tissues; or the effects of the stress associated with pain, fear, and traumatic shock.[1-3] Adults, in rare cases, have died with extensive external trauma without internal injury. In some of these cases, as well as in some children with these injuries, lesions in the heart can be found and have been termed ***stress cardiomyopathy***, which are believed to be related to catecholamine release from stress, causing damage to the heart.

The lesions in the heart are microscopic changes of myofibrillar degeneration and contraction band necrosis. Pavin[4] described 2 cases of reversible left ventricular dysfunction precipitated by acute emotional stress, which may be a similar mechanism. Autopsies on children who died from blunt soft tissue trauma demonstrate extensive contusions, abrasions, and patterned injuries of the extremities, chest, back, and buttocks. Incisions into the soft tissues of the extremities, back, and buttock reveal the large amounts of soft tissue hemorrhaging. These children should undergo thorough microscopic examination of the organs to exclude other causes of death and to determine whether there are catecholamine effects in the heart. In addition, the vitreous fluid should be analyzed for electrolytes, glucose, urea nitrogen, and creatinine to determine whether there is a dehydration pattern as well.

Blunt Soft Tissue Trauma Case Studies

Case Study 6-1

This 5-year-old girl came home from school early, and as a punishment, her father beat her with a variety of objects including: a belt, hair brush, fan belt, and paddle. At autopsy, the child had extensive abrasions and contusions on the surfaces of the torso and extremities. Incision into the soft tissue demonstrated extensive soft tissue hemorrhaging. There was no injury to the intracranial, intrathoracic, or intra-abdominal compartments.

Cause of Death: Blunt soft tissue trauma

Manner of Death: Homicide

Table 6-1. Diagnoses
Blunt soft tissue trauma with extensive abrasion and contusion of torso and extremities

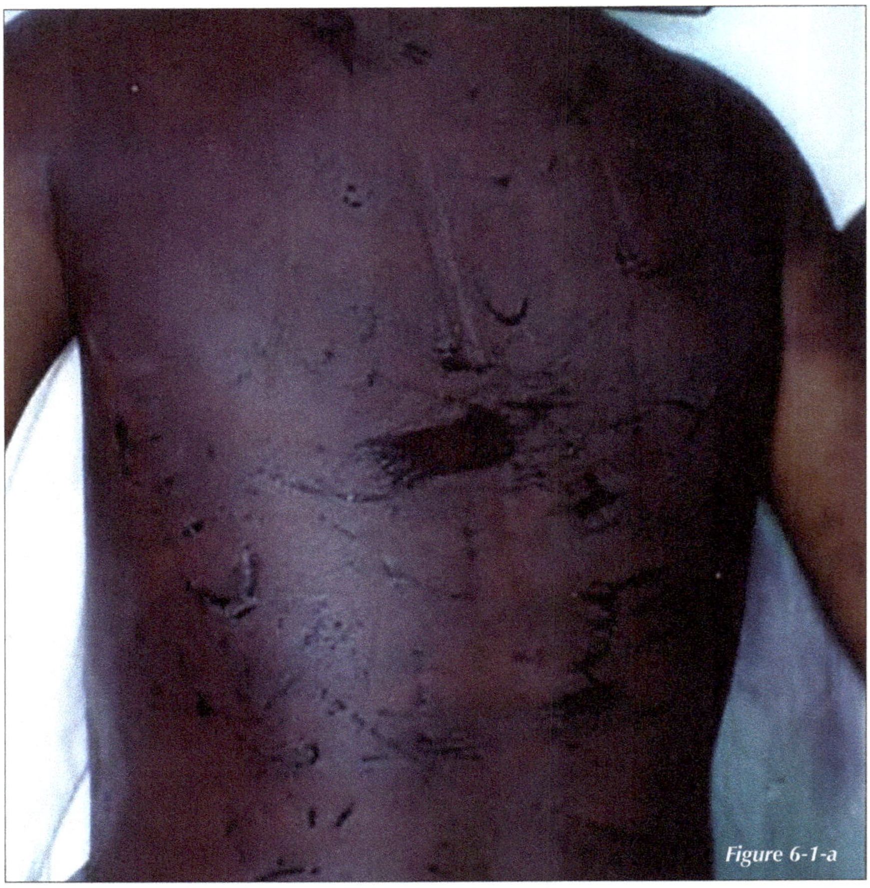

Figure 6-1-a

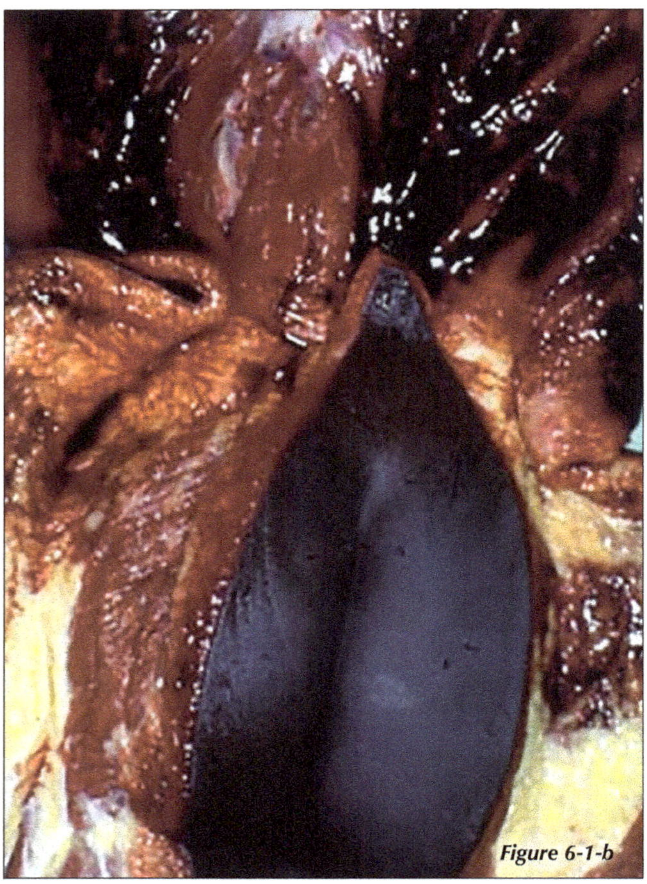

Figure 6-1-b

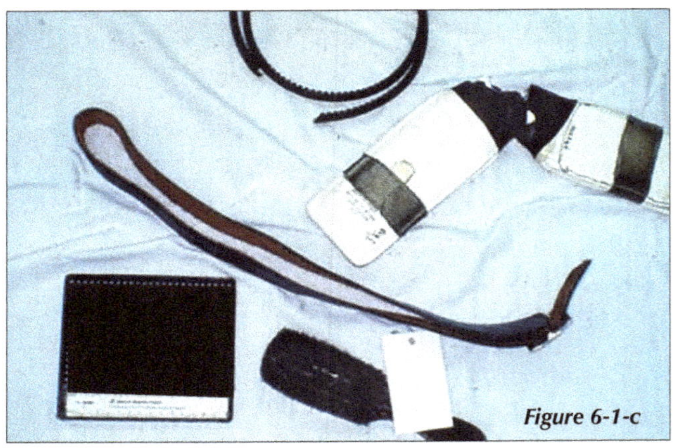

Figure 6-1-c

Figure 6-1-a. *Back of child showing abrasions and contusions with some of the abrasions demonstrating patterns of injury from inflicting objects.*

Figure 6-1-b. *Incisions into the soft tissue of the back and buttocks to demonstrate extensive underlying soft tissue hemorrhage.*

Figure 6-1-c. *Several of the objects used to inflict injury to the child, including a paddle, belt, and fan belt.*

Case Study 6-2

The mother of this 26-month-old girl rented a small basement room from a couple. The mother and child were upstairs in the owners' quarters. Between 4:00 AM and 4:30 AM, they reportedly drank a glass of milk. A short time later, the child became ill and said she needed to vomit. After vomiting, the child appeared very weak, and her eyes rolled back in her head. 911 was called. She was pronounced dead in the emergency department of a local hospital. The reporting physician stated that the child had been dead longer than the time the family reported because the body temperature would not reach above 90°F.

Cause of Death: Multiple blunt soft tissue traumas

Manner of Death: Homicide

Table 6-2. Autopsy Results

External Examination

— Child was 19 pounds and 32 inches tall

Injuries

Type	*Measurement*
Multiple injuries about the head and face, most notably a rectangular area of contusion involving the neck posterior and extending from right to left postauricular areas involving both neck and scalp regions and associated with considerable subcutaneous hemorrhage and edema	100 mm × 50 mm
Contusion on right forehead from eyebrow to hairline	55 mm × 45 mm
Pink contusion, superior midline forehead	30 mm × 20 mm
Contusion, left forehead extending from hairline to eyebrow	50 mm × 60 mm
Contusion, left malar eminence, upper cheek, and temporal areas	50 mm × 45 mm
At the inferior margin of that lateral contusion on the cheek were 2 crescentic, slightly curved abrasions	4 mm, 8 mm
Circumferential area of interrupted small abrasions on right cheek that resembled a bite mark	33 mm in diameter
White scar on right mandibular ridge, which was surrounded by an area of hyperpigmentation	6 mm
Gray scar below right nares	12 mm
Purplish-pink contusion on bridge of nose	15 mm × 15 mm
Chronically torn upper frenulum with recent injury	15 mm
Vertically oriented laceration of upper lip, right of midline	7 mm
Contusion and focal laceration on left lower gum adjacent to molar and incisor	15 mm
Denuded area of scalp at vertex with healing abrasion	18 mm × 15 mm
Linear fracture of left parietal bone above level of ear	50 mm
— Which had an inner aspect that extended downward	20 mm
Contusion extending from xiphoid down to umbilicus with considerable underlying subcutaneous hemorrhage	100 mm × 120 mm area
Contusion on left shoulder, superior and anterior	50 mm × 45 mm
Extensive contusion on left forearm and onto the dorsal surface that also involved the dorsal surface of the hand	180 mm in length; circumferential
Contusion, right anterior upper arm	5 mm
Contusion, right antecubital fossa	6 mm × 3 mm
Linear scar, medial aspect of right forearm	25 mm
Contusion, right forearm distal half, and involved right hand	160 mm in length; circumferential
Multiple scars, posterior right thigh and lower back; many had a J pattern or loop-type pattern	
Considerable underlying subgaleal hemorrhage	
Multiple areas of subgaleal/subscapular hemorrhage throughout scalp, both right and left but more on the left	

(continued)

Table 6-2. Autopsy Results *(continued)*

Injuries *(continued)*

Type	*Measurement*
Purplish-blue contusion on right lower leg proximally	70 mm × 45 mm
Extensive contusion, dorsum right foot	60 mm × 50 mm
Scar, medial left thigh	5 mm
Extensive contusion, anterior distal two-thirds of left thigh down upper left leg; the upper margin of that area had multiple linear parallel scars	170 mm × 160 mm
Contusion on lateral left thigh	30 mm × 1 mm
Bluish-purple contusion, left popliteal fossa superior	35 mm × 10 mm
Contusion on mid-left calf	10 mm
Examination of the brain demonstrated a contusion of the left frontal gyrus in the posterior one-third	15 mm
Multiple extensive scars on both buttocks with several J and loop patterns; these are seen on the presacral area and lower flank especially of the left	
Incision into the soft tissues of the body revealed corresponding involvement to the contusions with severe extensive subcutaneous hemorrhage and edema, especially of the forearms, thighs, and lower legs, but also the abdomen and buttocks	
Multiple scars on distal left anterior thigh; 1 has loop pattern	
Abrasion on left great toe	
Multiple abrasions on toes and partially avulsed skin on the tip of the third toe	
Extensive irregular scars, anterior right thigh; several have a J or loop pattern	
J-shaped scar and linear scar on distal medial right lower leg	
Extensive bluish-purple contusion on right knee and upper aspect of lower leg and thigh: anterior, laterally, and medially	
Multiple scars of distal medial right thigh	

Figure 6-2-a. *Several loop-shaped scars on lower leg.*

Figure 6-2-b. *Scalp reflected showing subgaleal hemorrhage over vertex.*

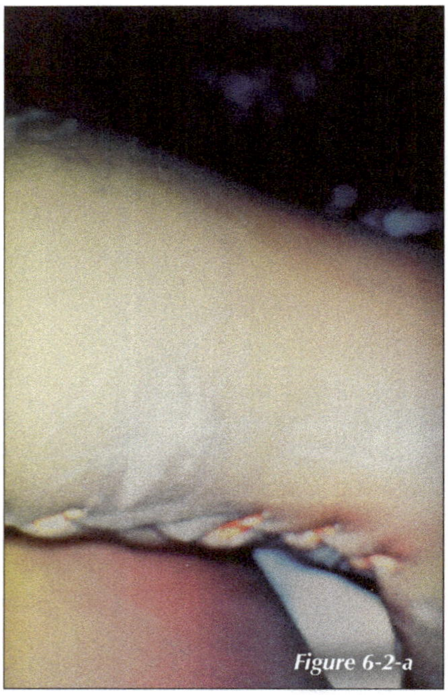

Figure 6-2-a

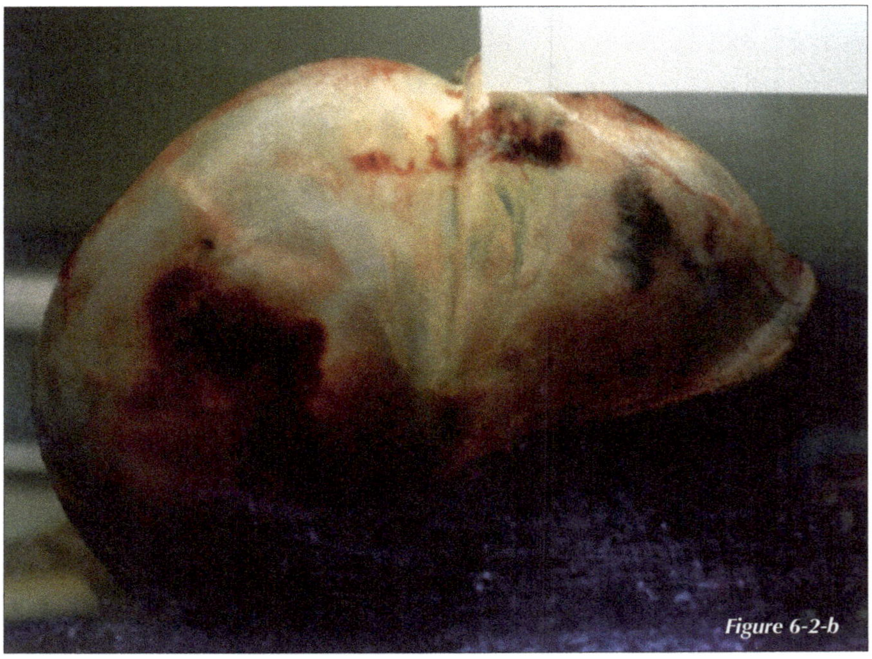

Figure 6-2-b

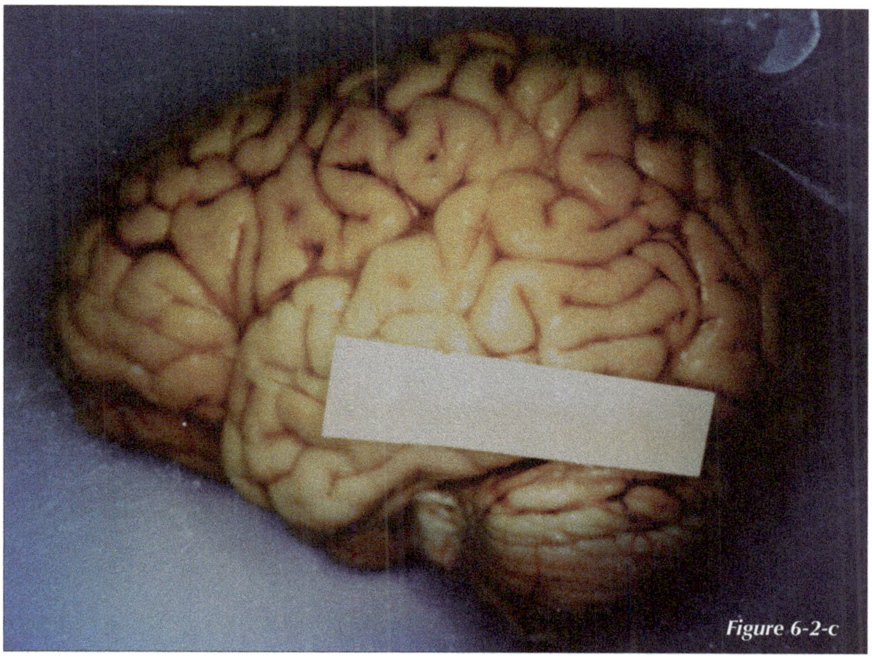

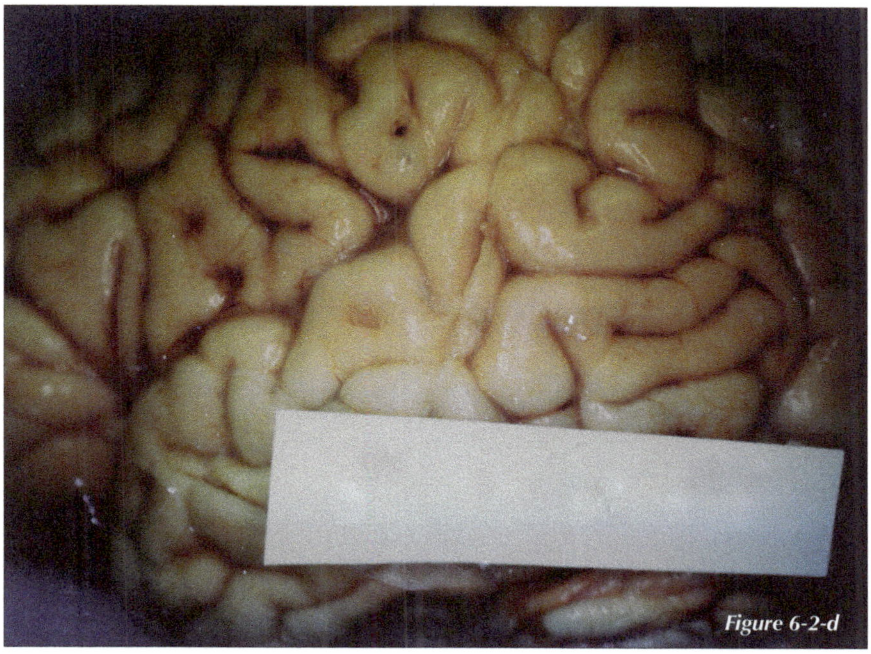

Figure 6-2-c. *Faint area of fracture contusion of left inferior frontal gyrus in posterior third.*

Figure 6-2-d. *Closer view of fracture contusion of left inferior frontal gyrus.*

References

1. Zumwalt RE, Hirsch CS. Subtle fatal child abuse. *Hum Pathol.* 1980;11(2):167-174.
2. Cebelin MS, Hirsch CS. Human stress cardiomyopathy. Myocardial lesions in victims of homicidal assualts without internal injuries. *Hum Pathol.* 1980;11(2):123-132.
3. Petty CS. Soft tisssues injuries: an overview. *J Trauma.* 1970;10(3):201-219.
4. Pavin D, Le Breton H, Daubert C. Human stress cardiomyopathy mimicking acute myocardial syndrome. *Heart.* 1997;78(5):509-511.

Chapter 7

Burns

Objectives

After reviewing this chapter, the reader will be able to:

1. *List the types of inflicted burn injuries and identify the most common lethal type.*
2. *Describe the pattern burns associated with both scalding and contact burns.*
3. *Distinguish between homicidal and accidental lethal burn injuries.*

Burns in Child Fatality Cases

There are many types of inflicted burn injury, including scalding, contact, chemical, and flame burns. Of these, the most commonly inflicted lethal burns are scalding burns. ***Scalding burns*** are produced by holding a child under hot water or submerging a child in a tub or sink of hot water. In young children, lethal inflicted hot water burns are often related to anger at toileting issues (ie, potty training) or in an attempt to discipline a child for soiling diapers or clothing.[1] When evaluating scalding burns, the relationship between the water temperature and the time it takes to produce full thickness burning of the skin needs to be taken into consideration. At 126°F, full thickness burning takes 120 seconds, but as the temperature goes up toward 140°F to 150°F, the time drops from less than 10 seconds for full thickness burning to 2 to 3 seconds.[2]

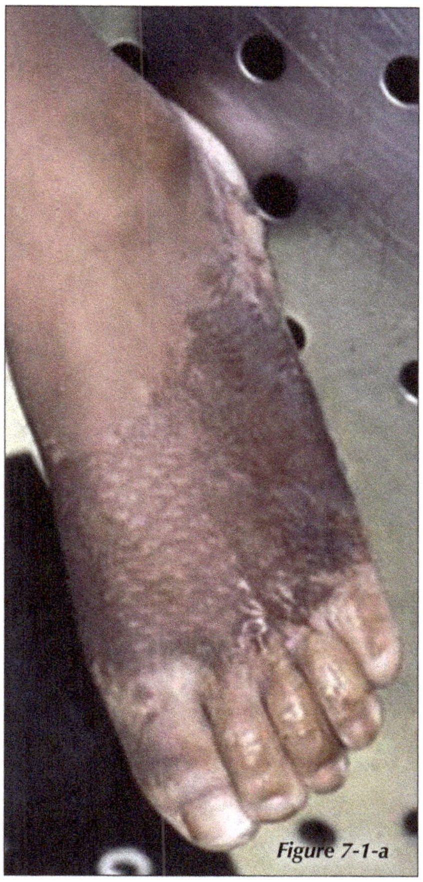

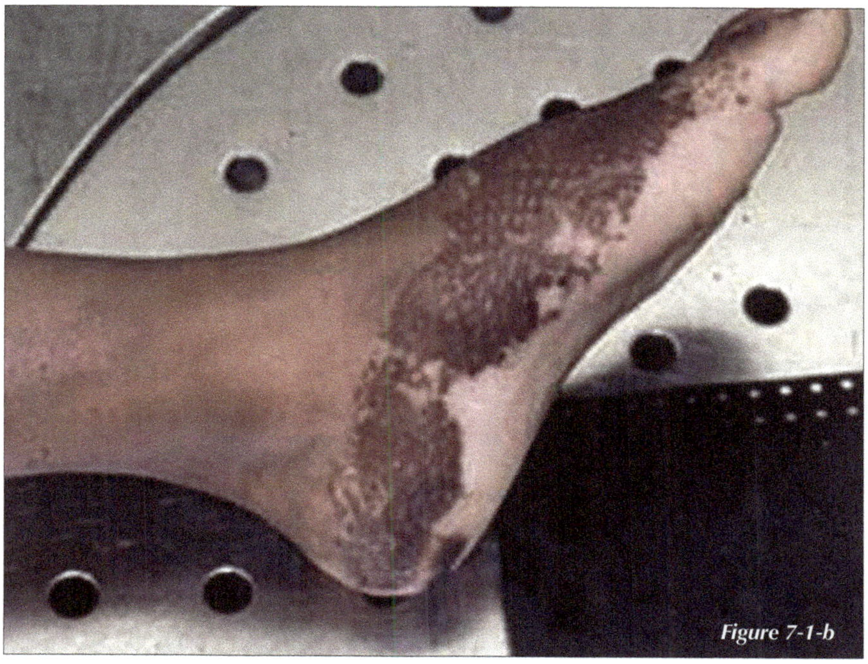

Figure 7-1-a. *Foot of a 24-month-old boy who died from blunt abdominal trauma with a lacerated spleen. He has scarring of the left foot from skin grafting for an old dipping-pattern scald burn.*

Figure 7-1-b. *Lateral view of foot with grafted burn scar.*

Recognizing the pattern of the burns is helpful in determining how the burning occurred. Inflicted burns tend to have large areas of solid burn with a "tide mark," which is a sharp line of distinction between the burned and unburned areas, rather than the tapering off and lessening of the degree of burning that is more commonly seen in accidental scalding injuries (**Figure 7-1-a** and **b**).[2] When a child is submerged into hot water, the child instinctually reacts by resisting and drawing their limbs upward or inward away from the water. Flexing the extremities while immersed results in a sparing of the inguinal, popliteal, and antecubital areas. If a child is submerged in a ceramic tub and held with a portion of their body, such as the buttocks or heels, against the floor of the tub, those areas may be spared from burn injury (**Figure 7-2-a** and **b**).

Accidental scalds in the home are unlikely to be lethal, so any death from scalding needs to be closely examined. The scene of the death needs to be examined for the temperature of the water at the site of injury, at the water heater, and during the recreation. Scene recreation is particularly helpful in evaluating scalding injuries. In recreating a described scenario, it may become evident that it would not be possible for the child's burn to have happened in the manner described by the caretaker. For example, when a scenario involves placing a child into a tub of hot water, the scene investigators need to consider that hot water will appear hot because of the heat radiating from the surface as one gets near it, indicating that the caretaker would have physically noticed the hot water, and by the child's reaction to the water, indicating that the water burns. It should not require several minutes, or even many seconds, of the child being submerged for someone to know to remove the child; therefore, if the child remained submerged, it may indicate lethal intent.

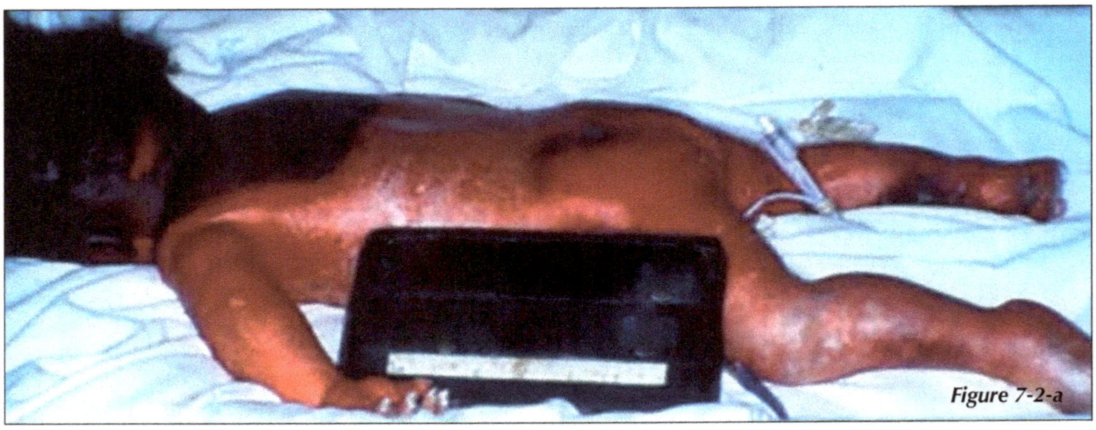

Figure 7-2-a

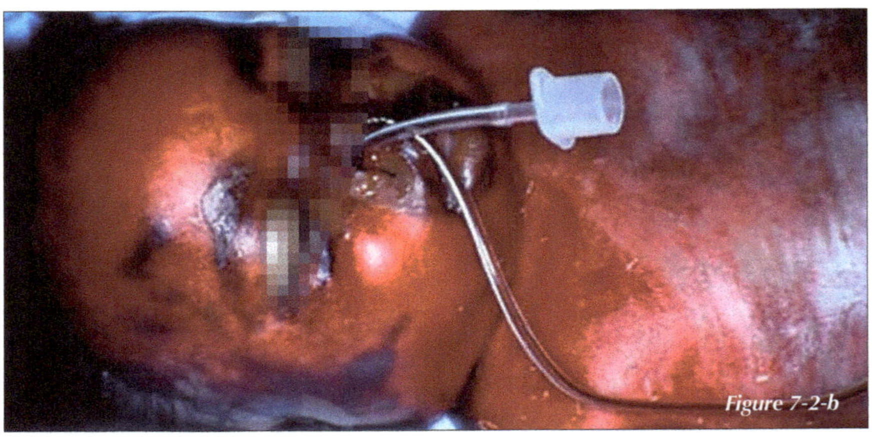

Figure 7-2-b

Figure 7-2-a. *A 10-month-old boy with extensive full-thickness scald burns from being placed into a tub of very hot water face down.*

Figure 7-2-b. *Face of child demonstrating sparing of the parts of the face in contact with the bottom of the tub.*

Contact burns are often seen by the medical examiner in children who died from other abusive injuries (eg, the child from **Figure 7-1-a** and **b** who had scalding burn scars on their foot, but who died from blunt abdominal trauma). Additionally, contact burns may have patterns that are recognizable, such as curling irons, heat grids, cigarettes, irons, or heater grates (**Figures 7-3** through **7-4**).[3] Sustaining a contact burn requires direct contact with the hot object for several seconds, thus creating a full thickness burn. Most hot objects that a child would come into accidental contact with, such as an object falling onto the child, would not cause a full thickness burn because the object would not be in contact with the child's skin for the necessary amount of time (eg, the hot object bounces off or the child touches the object and lets it go); therefore, if a contact burn occurs, it is typically a result of purposeful intent.

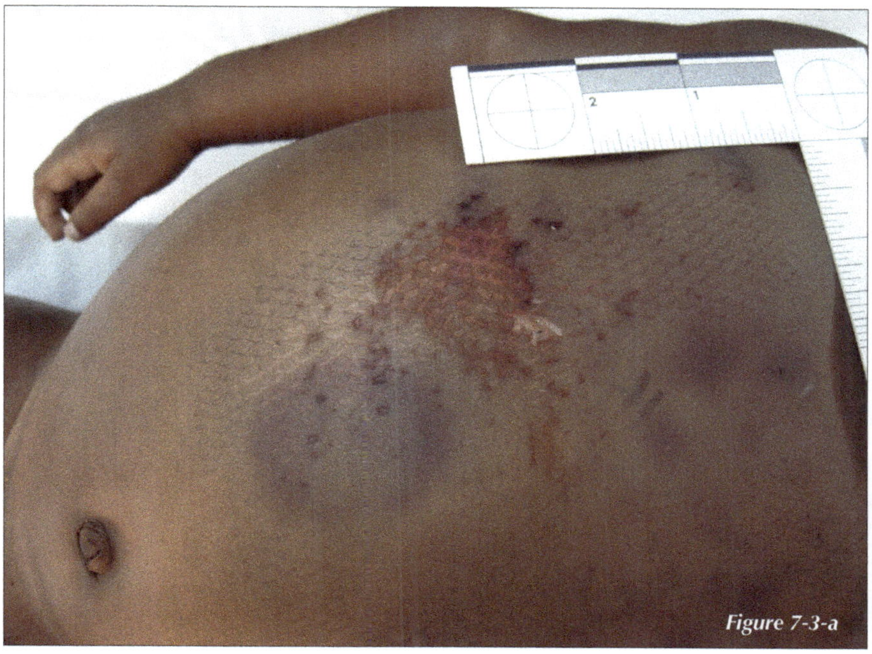

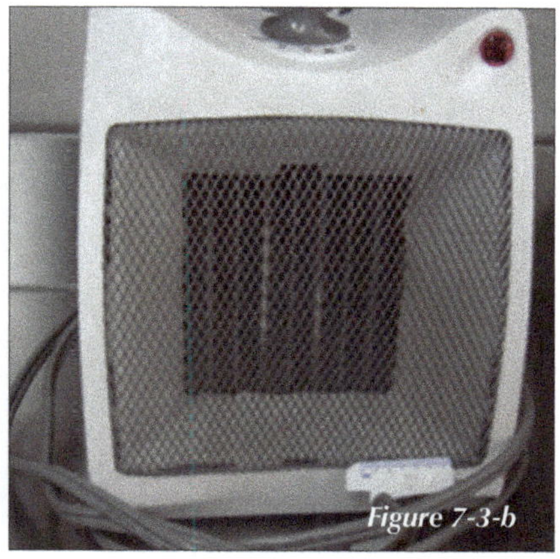

Figure 7-3-a. *A 13-month-old girl who died from head and abdominal trauma showing contact burns from a space heater on chest and abdomen.*

Figure 7-3-b. *Space heater that burned the child.*

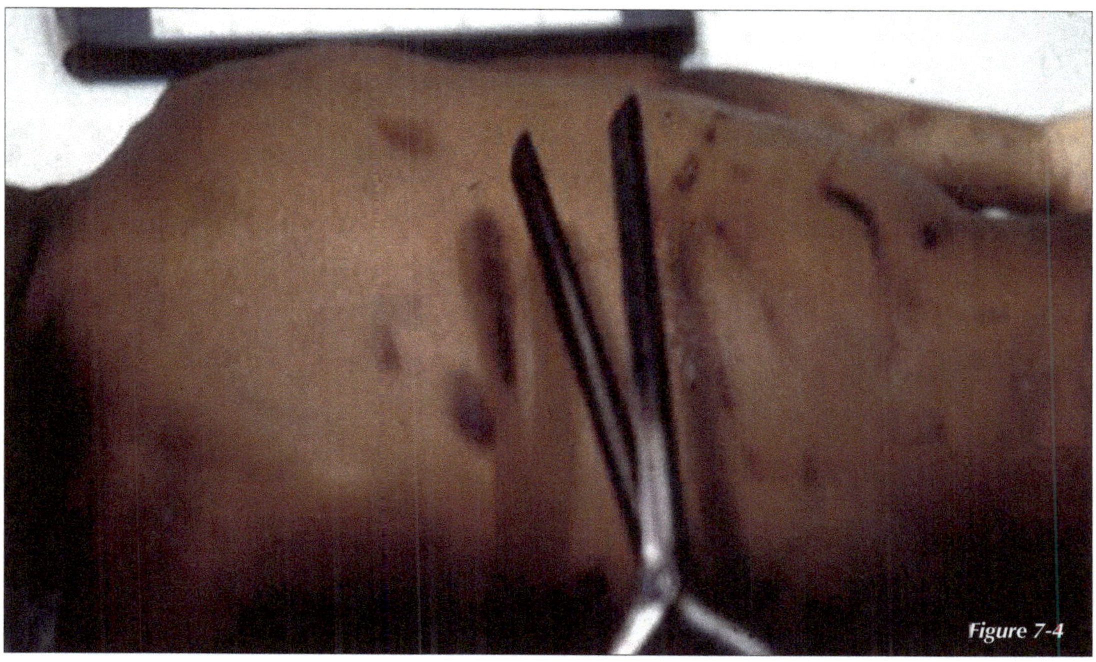

Figure 7-4. *A 14-month-old boy with curling iron-pattern contact burns on chest.*

Burn Case Studies

Case Study 7-1

According to the mother, this 13-week-old girl was sleeping with her mother in bed. The child rolled off the bed onto a heat register. The mother did not awaken at that time but later found the child and put cocoa butter on the burns. She did not take the child to the hospital for more than 12 hours after the injury occurred. The child was only taken to the hospital after she began gasping for breath. Further investigation found that the child had fallen face first into an open oven that was set to 500°F. The mother did not want to take the child to the hospital because of other department of family services investigations involving child neglect. The child was unresponsive in the emergency department (ED) and died after being admitted to the hospital.

Cause of Death: Complications of thermal injury after inordinate delay in seeking proper medical treatment; burn from oven; neglect

Manner of Death: Homicide

Table 7-1-a. Autopsy Results

Injuries

Type	*Measurement*
Eyes were swollen from edema	
Third-degree burns of the right side of face	120 mm × 120 mm
Third-degree thermal injury left cheek	70 mm
Second-degree thermal injury of the anterior chest wall	200 mm
Third-degree thermal injury right anterior chest wall	70 mm × 40 mm
Second-degree thermal injury of anterior abdominal wall surrounding the umbilicus	200 mm
Third-degree thermal injury inferior to the costophrenic junction	200 mm × 50 mm
Third-degree thermal injury of fingers	100 mm × 40 mm
Third-degree thermal injury overlying both patella	20 mm
Thermal injury covered approximately 20% of the total body surface	

Table 7-1-b. Diagnoses

Thermal Injuries

- Second- and third-degree burns over 20% of the body surface (including face, trunk, and all 4 extremities anteriorly)
- Metabolic acidosis
- Acute renal failure
- Pulmonary edema
- Bilateral pleural effusion
- Ascites
- Cerebral edema and brain death
- Sepsis

Case Study 7-2

This 17-month-old child was placed in contact with scalding hot water by the mother's boyfriend. The boyfriend admitted to causing the burns. The child was unresponsive in the ED and died after being admitted to the hospital.

Cause of Death: Complication of scald burns

Manner of Death: Homicide

Table 7-2-a. Autopsy Results

Injuries

- Extensive second- and third-degree burns involving the anterior aspect of the right foot, lower leg, and thigh and the anterior aspect of the left thigh, extending over the hip area and onto the lateral aspect of the left chest
- Burn area was contiguous with involvement of the left mid and lower back, with the burn continuing on to involve the posterior aspect of the left thigh, both buttocks, and the posterior aspect of the right thigh and leg
- Anterior half of right arm burned with extension of the same burn area to involve the lateral aspect of the right chest and posterior right shoulder and back

Lungs

- Parenchymal areas of adhesions to the thoracic wall
- These areas showed cavity formation; largest was 25 mm and contained some yellow semi-solid material

Cranial Cavity

- Sulci narrowed and gyri flattened

Microscopic Examination

- ***Lungs:*** Alveolar walls were thickened and lined with hyaline membranes; neutrophils present within and around bronchioles and alveoli
- ***Brain:*** Neurons darkly stained; perivascular and perineuronal clear spaces and disruption of neutrophils present

Table 7-2-b. Diagnoses

- Second- and third-degree body burns involving portions of torso and extremities
- Adult respiratory distress syndrome with superimposed bronchopneumonia
- Cerebral edema, mild

Case Study 7-3

According to the history, this 2-year-old boy fell into a pot of hot water. The grandmother went to the store and left a 12-year-old child in charge. There was a 14-quart pot of boiling water on a hotplate on the floor. The water was being heated to wash the kitchen floor. The 12-year-old said she accidentally kicked the child into the pot while she was getting something out of the deep freezer. She had been severely depressed since the incident and was threatening to kill herself. He was unresponsive at the scene and in the ED. The boy died after being admitted to the hospital with burns covering 70% of his total body surface area.

Cause of Death: Complications of hot-water scalding burns

Manner of Death: Homicide

Table 7-3-a. Autopsy Results

Injuries

— Extensive full-thickness burns, including 90 mm × 50 mm irregular area of scalding burns on right face and upper neck

— Similar burn on base of neck and right shoulder

— Burning on anterior deltoid areas and proximal medial arms

— Anterior chest and abdomen diffusely burned

— Burning on the dorsum of the penis

— Anterior, medial, lateral, and posterior surfaces of right thigh burned

— Left thigh diffusely burned

— 10 mm excoriated area at the right corner of the mouth

— Blisters, 3 to 30 mm, with clear fluid on the dorsal surface of the right foot

— ***Body cavities:*** 1000 mL fluid in peritoneal cavity

Neck Organs

— Upper airway contained frothy material

Lungs

— Increased firmness, edema; air passages contained frothy fluid

Liver

— Somewhat soft in consistency

Microscopic Examination

— ***Lungs:*** Diffuse alveolar damage

— ***Kidneys:*** Tubules dilated and lined by flattened epithelium with focal tubular epithelial necrosis present

— ***Skin:*** Resolving scald burns

Table 7-3-b. Diagnoses

— ***Thermal injuries:*** Skin, extensive resolving scald burns

— Diffuse alveolar damage syndrome (ARDS)

— Liver centrilobular necrosis

— Kidneys, focal tubular epithelial necrosis

— Ascites

Case Study 7-4

The family of this 2-year-old girl had just moved into a new home. An air conditioner unit and plug were removed from the home, but live wires were left behind. There were caps over the ends of the wires, which were hidden behind a curtain where the parents thought the child would not find them, because the parents were aware that this was a hazard. An electrician was coming soon and was going to "fix" the wires. The child found the wires and put them in her mouth (the wire caps were in the child's mouth when her mother found her). The child lived with her parents and her 5-year-old sibling. The father was out of the house to go deer hunting, and the child was home with the mother and sibling. The mother had gone downstairs quickly to do laundry. The 5-year-old came downstairs and told the mother that the child "was sleeping." The mother said the child could not be sleeping because she had just woken up from a nap. The mother rushed upstairs, and the child was lying on the floor with the wire caps in her mouth. The child was in full arrest when she arrived at the ED.

Cause of Death: Electrocution

Manner of Death: Accident

Table 7-4. Autopsy Results

External Examination	
— Many electrical marks and burns were present	
Injuries	
Type	*Measurement*
Raised burn on the mid-upper lip	5 mm × 5 mm
Raised burn on the right lower lip	5 mm × 3 mm
Linear scratch mark present on the right side of the mouth onto the right cheek	5 cm × 0.3 cm
Oval burn on the mid-lower neck with a wrinkled center	1 cm × 0.7 cm
Several electrical burns on the palmar surface of the left hand:	sizes varied from 5 mm to 2 cm × 5 mm
— 2 on the thumb	
— 2 on the hypothenar eminence	
— 5 on the adjoining surfaces of the second and third fingers	
Scratch on the lower right cheek	
Internal Examination	
Lungs	
— Aspirated gastric contents	
Nervous System	
— Gyri flattened, sulci narrowed, and ventricles compressed	

Figure 7-5-a. *Toddler-age child who chewed on an electric cord and 0sustained burns on lips and right cheek.*

Figure 7-5-b. *Electric burns on hand of child who chewed on electrical cord.*

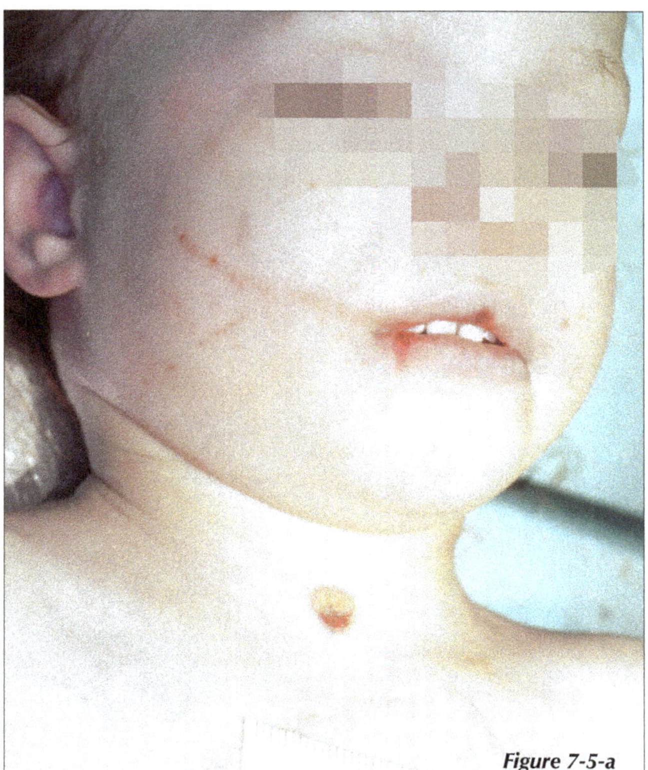

Figure 7-5-a

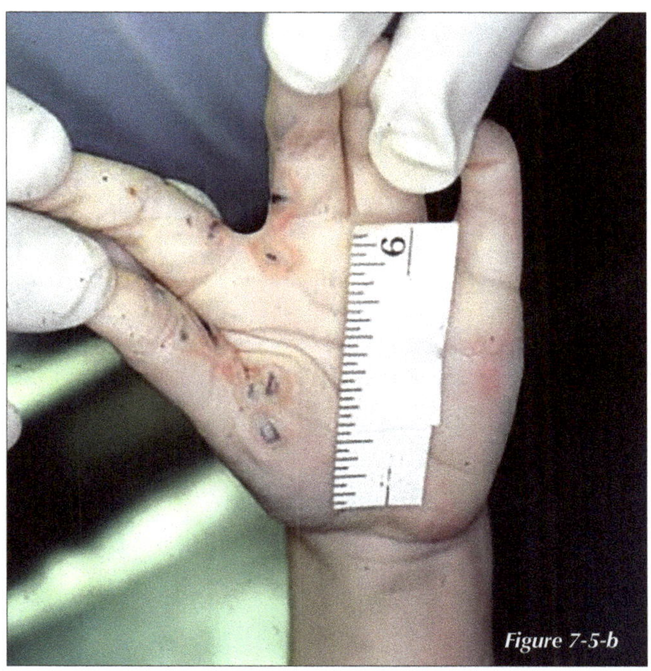

Figure 7-5-b

References

1. Peck MD, Priolo-Kapel D. Child abuse by burning: a review of the literature and an algorithm for medical investigations. *J Trauma.* 2002;53(5):1013-22.
2. Mortiz AR, Henriques FC. Studies of thermal injury: II. The relative importance of time and surface temperature in the causation of cutaneous burns. *Am J Pathol.* 1947;23(5):695-720.
3. Brent K. Scald burns should raise the clinician's suspicion for abuse. *Emerg Med News.* 2004;26(11):15-16.
4. Johnson CF, French G. Bruises and burns in child maltreatment. In: Giardino A, Alexander RC, eds. *Child Maltreatment: A Clinical Guide and Reference.* 3rd ed. GW Medical; 2005:63-82.

Editor's note: All references were used in the creation of the original work, *Forensic Pathology of Child Death,* but may not be cited directly in this chapter.

Chapter 8

Subtle Lethal Abusive Injury

Objectives

After reviewing this chapter, the reader will be able to:

1. *Differentiate between the various types of asphyxiation including suffocation, strangulation, and chemical asphyxia.*
2. *Identify the requirements to determine drowning as the cause of death in children.*
3. *Describe the role of an individual's history and crime scene investigation in identifying both the cause and manner of death in cases of lethal neglect and medical child abuse.*

Introduction

In addition to the more overt forms of child maltreatment, there are a number of subtle forms of child abuse that may be lethal. Included in this category of deaths are drownings; poisonings; asphyxia; and neglect of medical care, safety, or nutrition.[1] Establishing the fatal pathophysiologic mechanism of death may be the first step in understanding the cause of a child's death, along with consideration of the surrounding circumstances from scene investigation and police and other agency reports.

Deciding the manner of death may be a difficult choice, particularly in cases of subtle lethal deaths. All the cases discussed in this chapter were investigated by the medical examiner's office and underwent extensive police investigation. In addition, in cases after 1991, there were extensive child fatality reviews carried out. Despite these extensive reviews, in some cases there was not clear evidence for manner of death determination, and the manner was certified as ***undetermined***. The manner of death is the opinion of the forensic pathologist who performed the evaluation, often in conjunction with the chief medical examiner, but it is an opinion and is reflective of local traditions, as well as how an individual forensic pathologist was trained. In some cases, the manner of death being ruled an accident might also be questioned. The manners of death noted in these cases are not intended to represent what others might or should do but to illustrate how the cases were certified in a medical examiner's office.

It should be noted that prosecuting attorneys are not bound to adhere to the manner of death certified by the medical examiner. If they believe there is evidence to pursue a death from neglect or action on another's part, they are free to do so.

Drownings

Drowning, in all cases at all ages, is a diagnosis of exclusion. For the forensic pathologist to make a diagnosis of drowning, other causes of death must be excluded from a case in which an individual is seen to become submerged or is found in the water. There are no absolute pathologic changes that diagnose drowning, and homicidal drownings are difficult to distinguish from an accidental drowning. Gillenwater[2] reported 205 submersions in children younger than age 19, either drowning or near drowning, and found 16 (8%) were inflicted. The inflicted drowning victims were younger, with a median age of 2.1 years, and the bathtub was the most common site for the drowning. Nixon and Pearn[3,4] described several features that they believed helped to distinguish between accidental and deliberate immersion of a child. These features included: (1) the nonaccidental drowning took place in the bathtub, (2) the drowning took place at an unusual time of day for the child to be bathing, and (3) the child was alone in the bathtub. Griest and Zumwalt[5] described 6 childhood homicidal drownings and pointed out the importance of cooperation between the investigation by the medical examiner and the police. Their cases had a history of previous abusive actions by the parents in 3 cases and drug or alcohol abuse by the parents in 1 case. The wet state of the body or clothing were important clues in 2 cases, and in 4 of the cases, there was a delay between the event and the call for help.

Drowning Case Studies

Case Study 8-1

This 9-month-old boy was staying with the mother at an extended stay motel. The mother stated that she turned on the water in the bathtub and put the child in the tub. The mother then left the bathroom and was lying on the bed, talking on the phone. She eventually went back to check on the child, and he was floating in the water. She pulled him out and called 911. Investigation found that it would take about 9 minutes for the tub to fill up to 2 inches from the top of the bathtub, which is the level that the mother indicated the water was at when she found the child floating. He was pronounced dead in the emergency department (ED).

Cause of Death: Drowning

Manner of Death: Homicide; neglect of safety

Table 8-1. Autopsy Results

External Examination

— 30 mm x 10 mm area of hyperpigmentation left of the midline of the lower abdomen

— 15 mm x 5 mm abrasion on the right thigh

— 20 mm x 4 mm abrasion on the left thigh

Injuries

Type	*Measurement*
Petechial hemorrhages on right and left cheeks, lateral to right eye, right side of chin, and below lower lip	
Abrasion, right nose	10 mm x 3 mm
Right forehead contusions with underlying focal soft tissue hemorrhage	4 mm
Left forehead contusion with underlying soft tissue hemorrhage	8 mm x 8 mm
— Contusion with soft tissue hemorrhage	8 mm x 6 mm

Lungs

— Congestion and edema

Brain

— Edema with flattening of gyri and narrowing of sulci

Microscopic Examination

— ***Lungs:*** Congestion

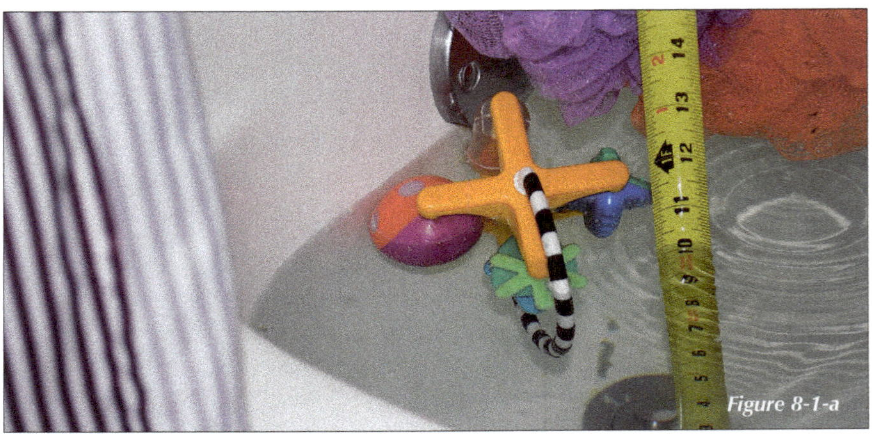

Figure 8-1-a. *Bathtub filled with water and many objects.*

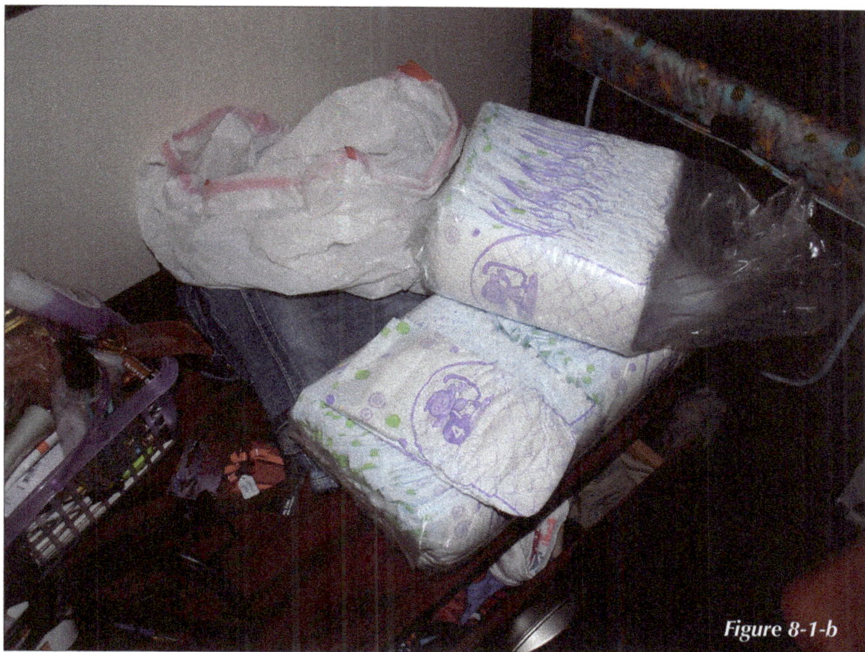

Figure 8-1-b

Figure 8-1-b. *Objects found in motel room.*

Figure 8-1-c. *Trash room near motel room.*

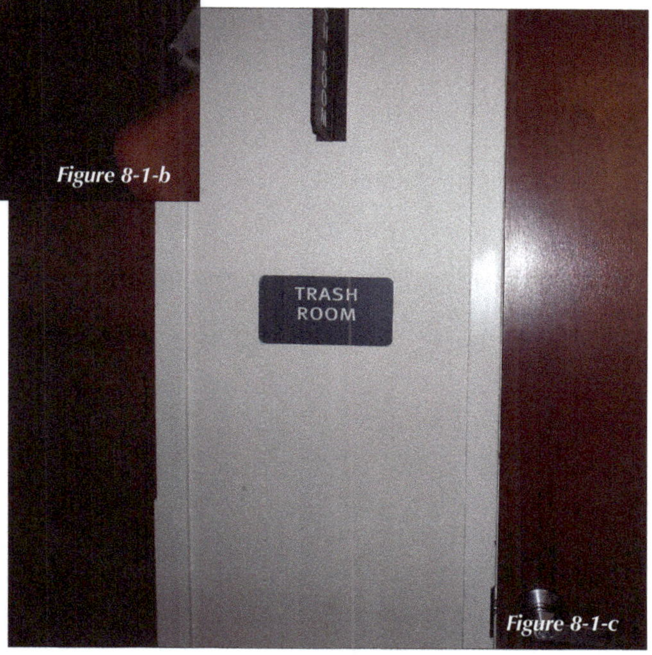

Figure 8-1-c

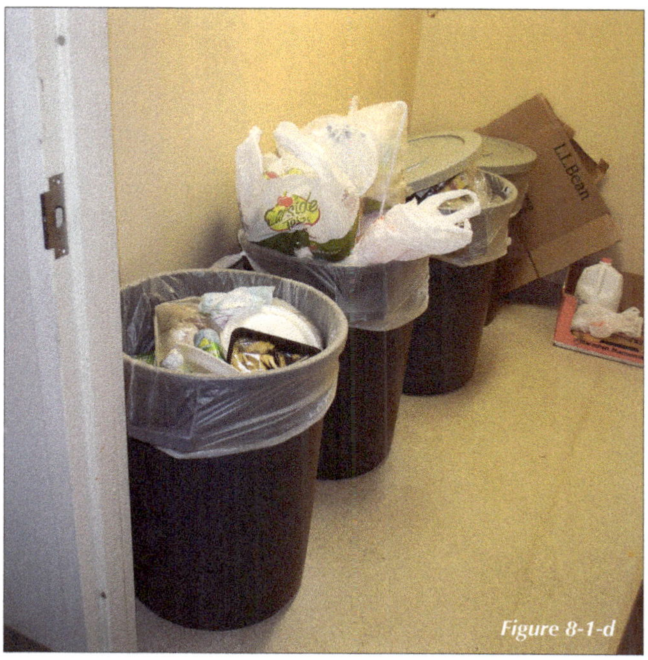

Figure 8-1-d

Figure 8-1-d and e. *Objects in trash room removed from motel room after child died.*

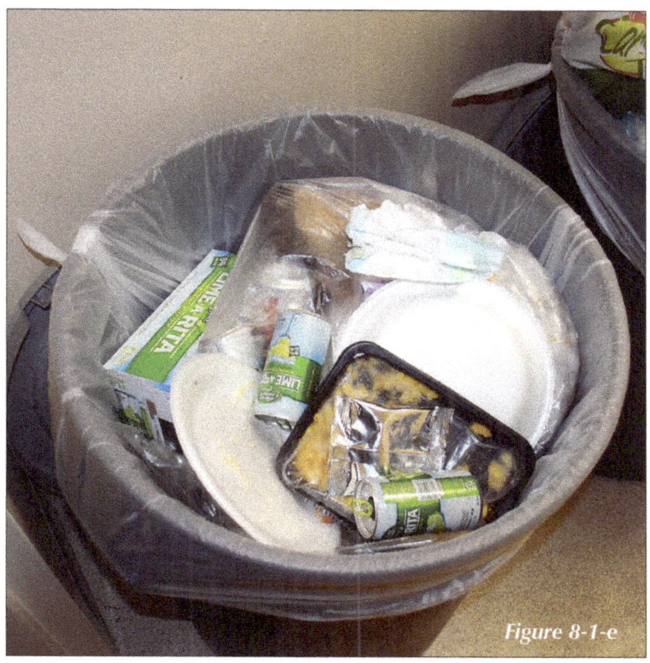

Figure 8-1-e

Case Study 8-2

This 8-month-old boy was found by his mother, unresponsive and floating on his back in 6 inches of water in the bathtub. The child was left in the bathtub with a 3-year-old to play in the hot water, not for a bath. The mother left to start the dryer and the dishwasher. When she did not hear the children in the tub, she ran upstairs to check on them and found the child with his face under the water. The police felt the mother was appropriately distraught. The mother was educationally challenged and had only completed the seventh grade. The child was in full arrest in the ED.

Cause of Death: Drowning

Manner of Death: Accident

Figure 8-2-a. *X-rays of child before autopsy showing no fractures.*

Figure 8-2-b. *Front surface of body showing small contusion on right forehead above medial edge of brow; moderate diaper rash.*

Table 8-2. Autopsy Results

External Examination

— 7 mm well-healed scar on chest lateral to nipple

— Moderate degree of diaper rash was present

Injuries

Type	*Measurement*
Circular contusion on right forehead above medial extent of the eyebrow	4 mm

Internal Examination

Neck

— Trachea contained a small amount of watery liquid

Lungs

— Tracheobronchial tree exuded frothy edema fluid

— Lobes on both sides showed splotchy areas of dark discoloration that exuded frothy edema fluid

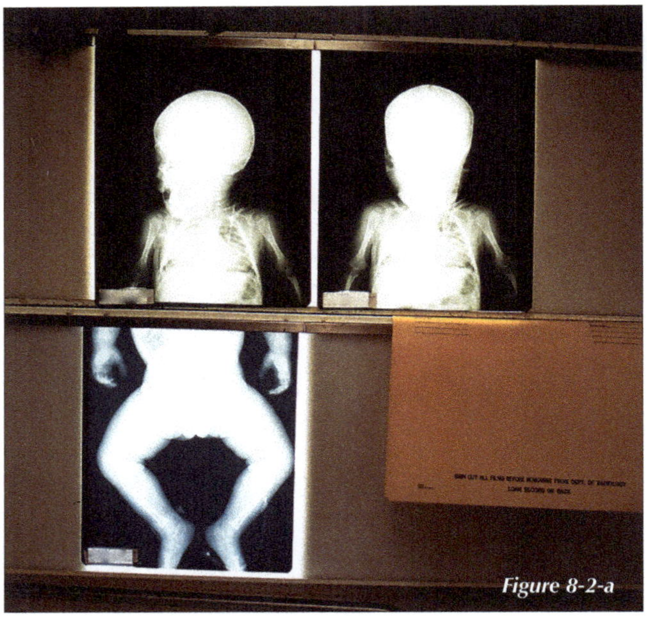

Figure 8-2-a

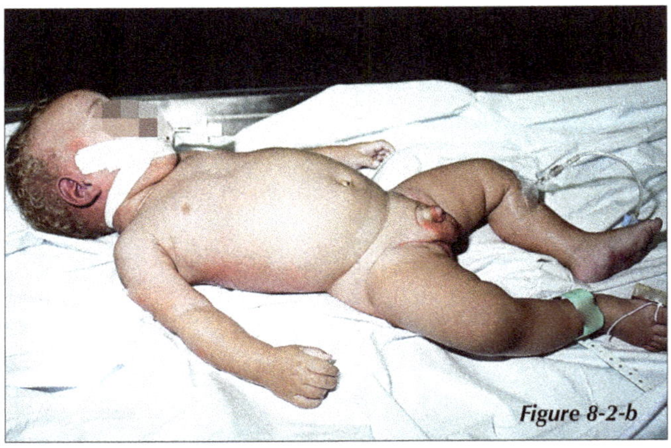

Figure 8-2-b

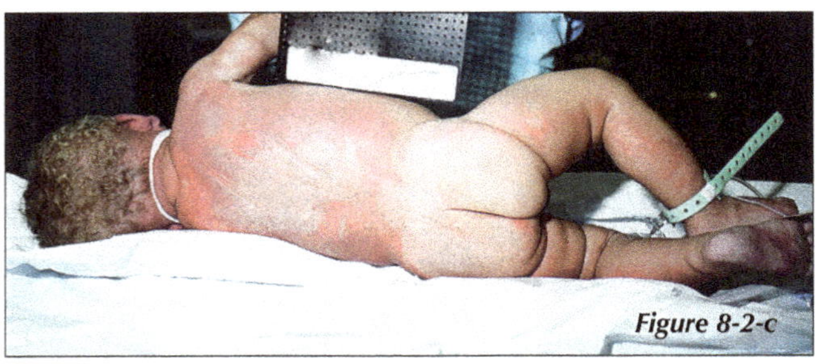

Figure 8-2-c

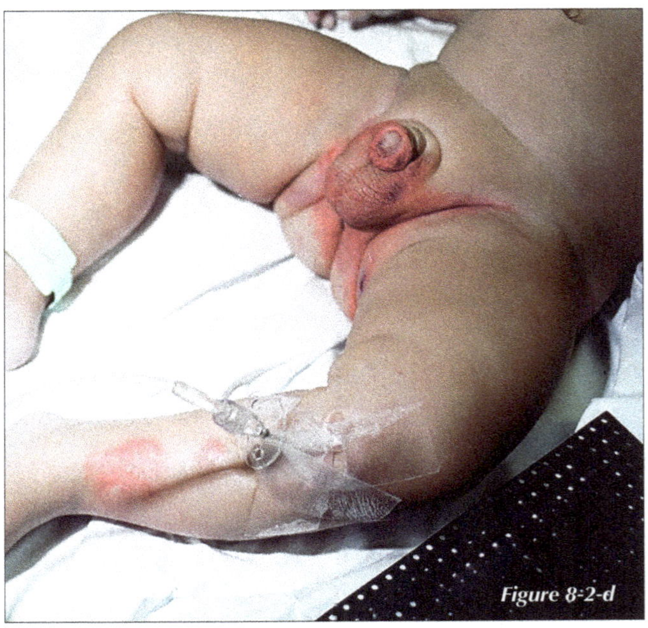

Figure 8-2-d

Figure 8-2-c. *Posterior surface of body with no injury; fixed lividity.*

Figure 8-2-d. *Child at autopsy with moderate diaper rash.*

Poisoning and Chemical Assault

Children may be poisoned by a variety of substances, including medications, alcohol, drugs, and even salt or water (**Figure 8-3**). Forensic autopsies should always include a complete toxicological analysis for determinations of such substances. The National Association of Medical Examiners maintains a registry for toxicological findings in children called PedTox for the purpose of assisting medical examiners in the interpretation of levels of various medications and drugs. In young children, the lethal or toxic levels of certain medications and drugs are unknown. PedTox is designed for forensic pathologists to register the findings in cases that have involved substances that may be related to the death of a child.

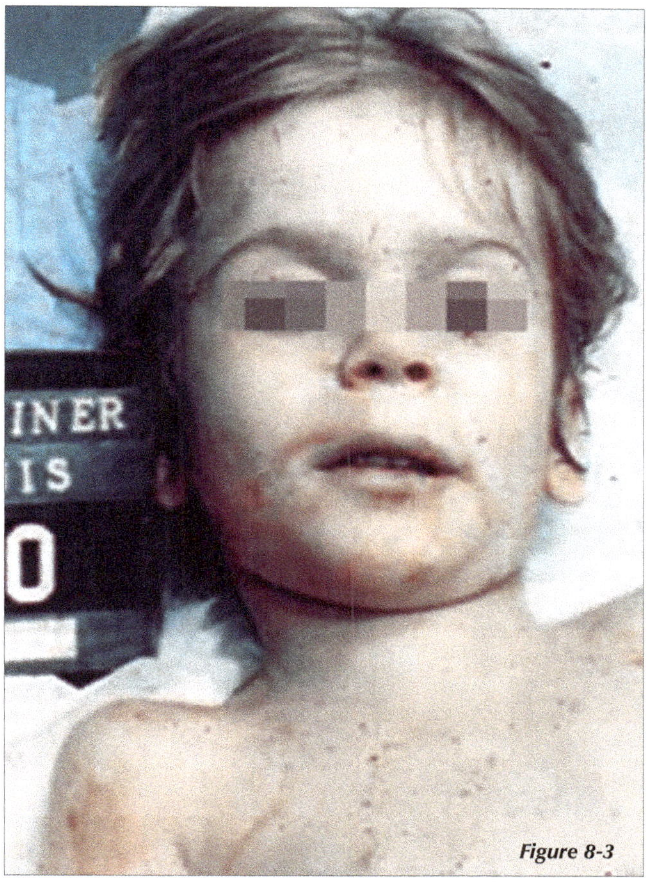

Figure 8-3

Figure 8-3. *A 4-year-old boy who died from intoxication with aspirin and alcohol from cologne. The parents did not seek medical care after the child was unconscious and waited many hours after the child died to report the death.*

Poisoning Case Studies

Case Study 8-3

This 22-month-old boy was put to bed on an air mattress by his mother. When she woke up, she found him unresponsive and called 911. When CPR was started, it was noted that "brown throw up stuff" was coming from the child's nose and mouth. The mother admitted to taking morphine, methamphetamine, Xanax, and Trazodone in the last 72 hours. Initially, the mother stated that she found the child with an open bottle of Xanax that had been filled with Trazodone, but she did not believe he took any so she did nothing about it. The mother reported that the child later had labored breathing. She allowed the child to nurse even though she was on narcotics and had taken 10 morphine pills that day. The mother also admitted to giving the child melatonin and "maybe some ibuprofen" to help him sleep. The father of the child was a registered sex offender for crimes involving minors and children.

Cause of Death: Morphine intoxication

Manner of Death: Homicide

Table 8-3. Autopsy Results

Internal Examination

Lungs

— Mild acute congestion on cut surface

Stomach

— 50 mL of opaque, dark green, well-digested material with suggestion of gray-white fragments

Cranial Cavity

— Cerebral edema with effacement of some sulci

Microscopic Examination

— ***Lungs:*** Extensive bronchopneumonia

Toxicology

— Urine positive for amphetamines and opiates

— Individual drug quantitation:

— 0.11mcg/mL methamphetamine

— 0.11 mcg/mL hydromorphone, > 4 mcg/mL morphine

— ***Blood:*** Free morphine 0.46 mcg/mL, total morphine 1.2 mcg/mL

Case Study 8-4

The mother gave this 9-month-old girl a bottle containing 5 Thorazine tablets to use as a rattle. The bottle had a childproof cap, so she thought it was safe. The mother said that she had done this before with similar bottles that had pennies inside, and the tops had never come off. The mother was watching television in the same room as the child when she noticed the container was open and the child was trying to eat the pills. The mother attempted to induce vomiting with no success. The child became lethargic and did not improve, so the mother took her to the hospital. The child was unresponsive in the ED and was admitted and died inpatient. Treatment included giving the child activated charcoal.

Cause of Death: Acute chlorpromazine (Thorazine) intoxication

Manner of Death: Accident

Comment: The question of whether a 9-month-old child could open a childproof bottle is a legitimate concern. The manner of death is the opinion of the forensic pathologist, but others might consider this an undetermined manner.

Table 8-4. Autopsy Results

External Examination

— Black carbonaceous material seen within and around oral cavity

Internal Examination

Lungs

— Black carbonaceous material surrounding airways

Digestive System

— Stomach contained 10 mL of black carbonaceous material

Nervous System

— Flattened gyri

Microscopic Examination

— ***Lung:*** Charcoal particles seen within airways with neutrophilic inflammatory infiltrate

— ***Liver:*** Scattered neutrophils within blood vessels

Toxicology

— ***Blood:*** Chlorpromazine 5.8 mcg/mL

— ***Bile:*** Phenothiazine

— ***Gastric:*** Positive for chlorpromazine

— ***Urine:*** Positive for phenothiazine

Chlorpromazine Levels

— ***Liver:*** 25.5 mcg/mL

— ***Kidney:*** 24.4 mcg/mL

— ***Brain:*** 47.0 mcg/mL

— ***Muscle:*** 7.5 mcg/mL

— ***Fat:*** 18.5 mcg/mL

Asphyxiation

Asphyxia is the failure of cells to receive or use oxygen.[6] Asphyxial deaths include suffocation, strangulation, and chemical asphyxia. Suffocation includes entrapment, smothering, choking, mechanical asphyxia, and suffocating gases.

Smothering is caused by occluding the nose and mouth and can be easily done to children and infants without always leaving evidence. In some cases, there are findings that demonstrate evidence of contact with obstructing materials (eg, hands, pillows) to the child's face (**Figure 8-4**). Abrasions or contusions of the nose, lips, and cheeks may be present, as well as contusion or laceration of the mucosal surfaces of the mouth (**Figure 8-5**). Smothering may cause some petechial hemorrhages, but not always.[7] Meadows[8] described 27 young children who were suffocated by their mothers.

Table 8-5. Meadows Findings

Case Study Group	
— 27 children suffocated by mothers	
No marks of external injury	52%
Previous apneic episode	90%
Previous unexplained disorder	44%
Older than 6 months of age	55%
Dead sibling	48%

It is not possible to determine how many children are suffocated, as it is difficult to detect. Some of the infants in the sudden infant death syndrome (SIDS) category are felt to be homicides, but the actual number is unknown.

Strangulation in infants and young children is also difficult to recognize in some cases. Ligatures are more likely to leave abrasions on the neck; however, manual strangulation in children as old as 6 years of age may not leave any external markings on the neck; nor petechial hemorrhages; nor any internal injury to the muscles, hyoid, or larynx. Strangulation in young children differs from strangulation later in life because the airway itself is soft and can be compressed with much less pressure. If the airway is actually compressed, the mechanism of asphyxia changes from vascular disturbance by lack of carotid flow and venous return to simply occlusion of the airway. Without the vascular disturbance, there may be no petechial hemorrhages. Because the airway is compressible, there may be no evidence of trauma to the neck. One of the methods forensic pathologists have used to learn what has happened to a child is through confessions by individuals who have killed children.

The author autopsied a child who presented with evidence of hypoxic encephalopathy of unknown origin, which subsequently was found to be because of asphyxia by neck compression. This child presented to the ED at age 4 months with seizures and was worked up at a children's hospital and thought to have possible encephalitis. At autopsy at age 7 months, there was hypoxic encephalopathy in a laminar distribution throughout much of the brain. The father of this child later killed a second child by shaking. During his confession of the shaking, he described holding the first infant so that his neck extended over the crib railing until the child convulsed. McIntosh[9] described a similar finding in an infant. Because of these experiences, any child found to have hypoxic encephalopathy of undetermined etiology must be thoroughly examined and evaluated for possible asphyxial events.

Asphyxial deaths may result from unusual practices to quiet a crying child. The author has seen homicidal cases in which an infant's chest was compressed in an effort to to make them stop crying. The author also noted 1 father who killed an infant at 3 months of age and a second infant at 4 months of age by placing them under several layers of folded blankets and pillows to muffle their crying. In a similar case, another father killed his 9-month-old son by wrapping him in a heavy comforter and placing him face down to muffle the crying. In all these cases, the autopsy did not demonstrate a cause of death. The death scene investigation revealed the details of what had been done to the child so that cause and manner of death could be determined as homicidal asphyxiations.

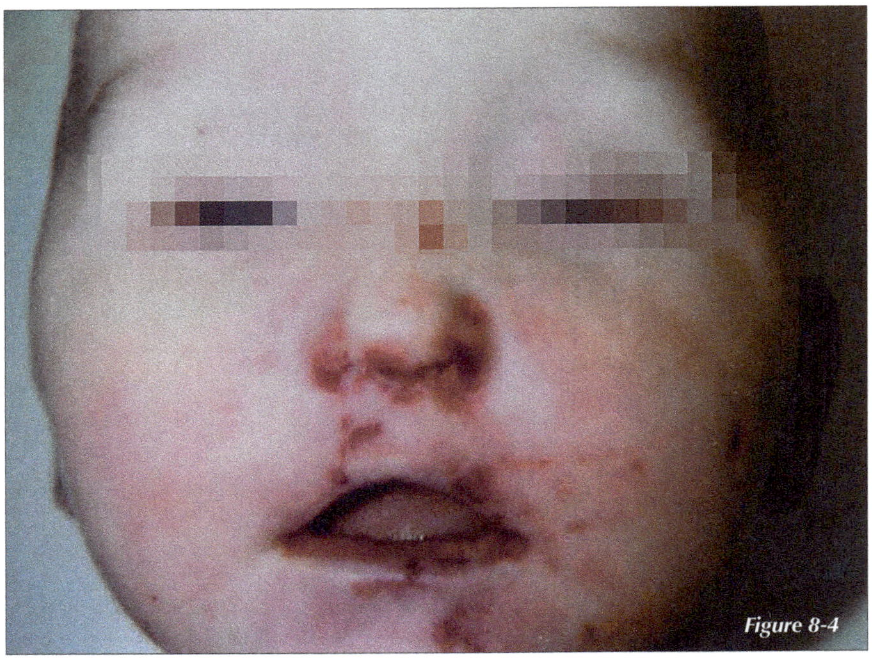

Figure 8-4. *A 3-month-old infant showing abrasions of nose and mouth from suffocation.*

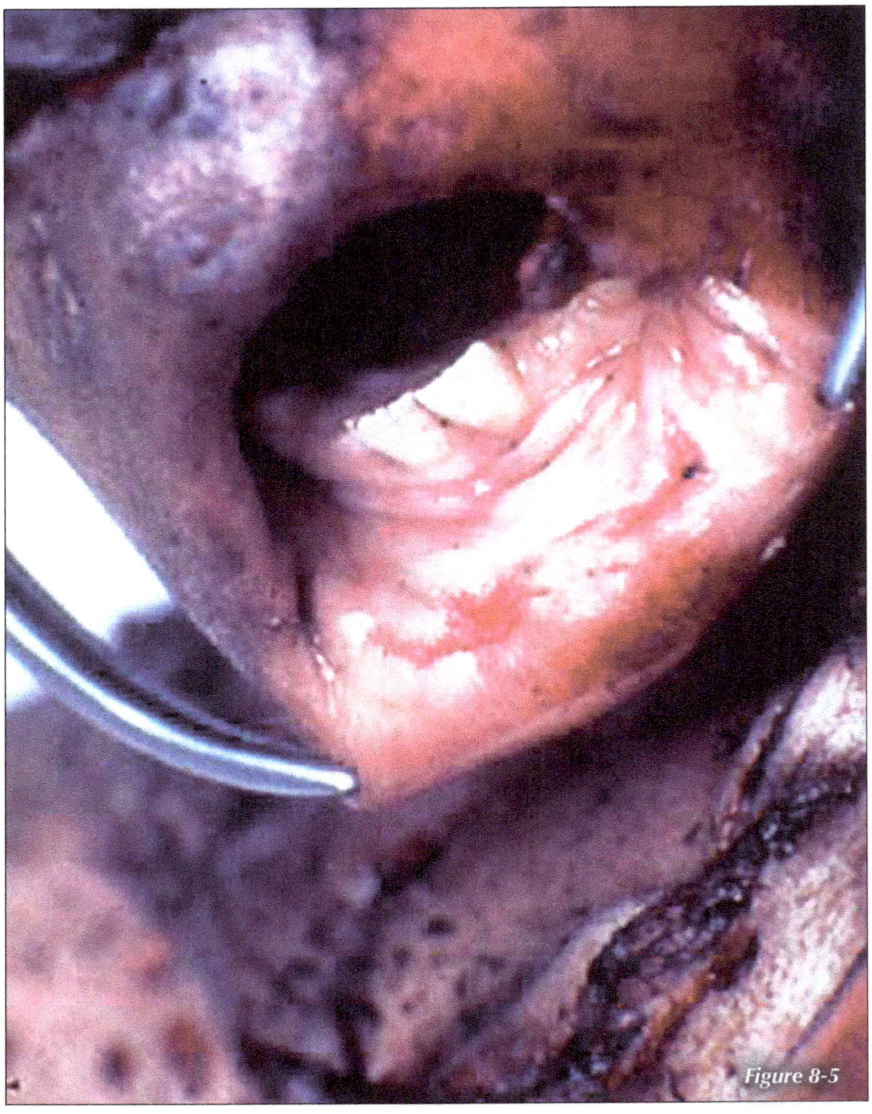

Figure 8-5. *A 5-year-old child who was suffocated by their mother showing lacerations of inner lower lip from pressure of a hand against the mouth. Child was burned to conceal the injuries. Autopsy did not show any soot in the airway or carbon monoxide in the blood.*

Asphyxiation Case Studies

Case Study 8-5

This 3-week-old girl had been placed on her back to sleep in bed with her mother and the mother's boyfriend. In the morning, she was found not breathing, unresponsive, and was positioned face down. When paramedics and police arrived at the scene, no one was performing CPR. The mother said the child had been rolling over on her own for about a week and that the laceration on the infant's head was from a cut during C-section at the child's birth. The mother had another child who was 3 years old and had been taken by the father. This child was conceived as a result of a criminal sexual assault, and the mother had not been certain about keeping the child. No police report had been made of this assault. The mother said she had been sexually assaulted at least 8 times. She also gave a history of being molested as a child by family members which caused her to leave home at age 16. The mother smoked cigarettes during the pregnancy.

Cause of Death: Chest compression with multiple rib fractures; asphyxiation

Manner of Death: Homicide

Table 8-6. Autopsy Results

Injuries

— Diffuse hemorrhage surrounding some of the ribs and in the intercostal spaces on both the right and left sides

— Multiple fractures of ribs

— Right ribs 1 through 6 laterally

— Right ribs 9, 10, and 11 posteriorly

— Left ribs 2 through 6 anteriorly

— Left ribs 7 through 10 posteriorly

— Contusions, soft tissue posterior to the left fifth rib and right sixth rib posteriorly

— Contusions on scalp in left parietal

Microscopic Examination

— Rib fractures were fresh with no evidence of healing

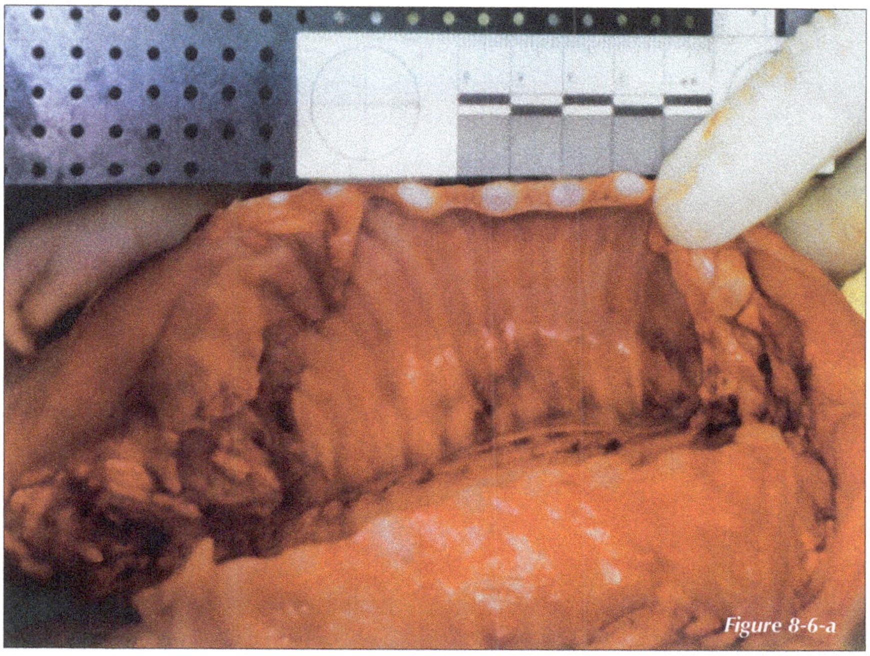

Figure 8-6-a

Figure 8-6-a. *Body opened and organs removed showing fractures of right ribs 1 through 6 laterally and 9, 10, and 11 posteriorly.*

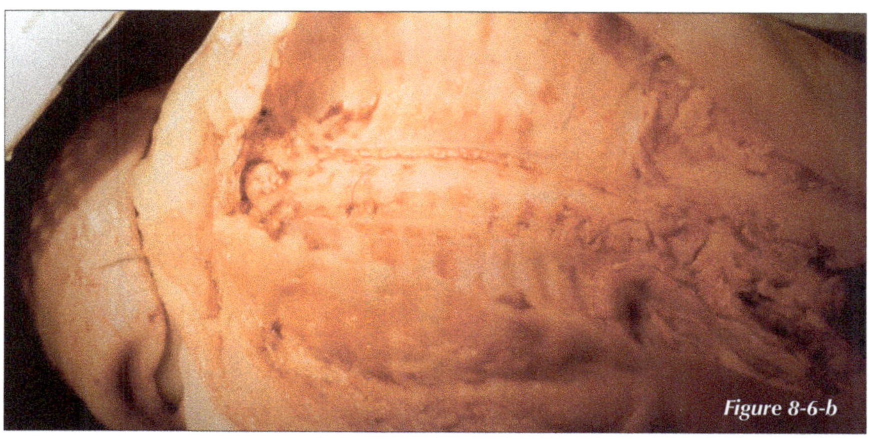

Figure 8-6-b

Figure 8-6-b. *Body opened and organs removed showing fractures of left ribs 2 through 6 anteriorly and 7 through 10 posteriorly.*

Case Study 8-6

This 4-year-old boy's mother worked as a cashier at a fast food hamburger restaurant and did not have a babysitter, so she brought the child and his 6-year-old brother to work and let them play alone on the indoor playground. The playground had a crawl tube that children could crawl through to different parts of the play structure. The child became wedged upside down next to the crawl tube and the padded metal exterior of the structure. He was positioned facing the crawl tube. His brother went to get his mother to help, thinking that the child was "just messing around." The child was unresponsive and had no vitals by the time paramedics arrived. In the ED, he was placed on a ventilator and transferred to the intensive care unit and died later that evening. Examination in the hospital noted a horizontal mark on the anterior region of the neck.

Cause of Death: Mechanical asphyxiation

Manner of Death: Accident

Table 8-7. Autopsy Results

EXTERNAL EXAMINATION

— Petechiae on both lower palpebral conjunctivae; many petechiae diffusely covering the orbital skin and cheeks as well as extending to the forehead

— A few petechiae on the maxillary and mandibular gingivae

— Healing 5 mm abrasion on the anterior right knee

— 25 mm scar on the posterior proximal left thigh

INJURIES

TYPE	*MEASUREMENT*
Red mark extending inferolaterally from the right corner of the mouth (could be from endotracheal tube)	15 mm x 10 mm
A few tiny abrasions on the upper lateral right neck	
Horizontal area of abrasion across the mid-lower anterior right neck	15 mm x 3 mm
— With an internal display of punctate abrasions	3 mm apart
Similar abrasion across the anterior left neck	5 mm x 3 mm
A few abrasions scattered over the back	each less than 2 mm
Abrasion on the lower left back	13 mm x 6 mm
2 faint abrasions on the lateral left hip	10 mm each
Contusion on the mid-distal right shin	20 mm

Figure 8-7-a. *Fast food restaurant indoor play area with crawl tubes. The crawl tube on the left side has a padded area where the child became wedged upside down.*

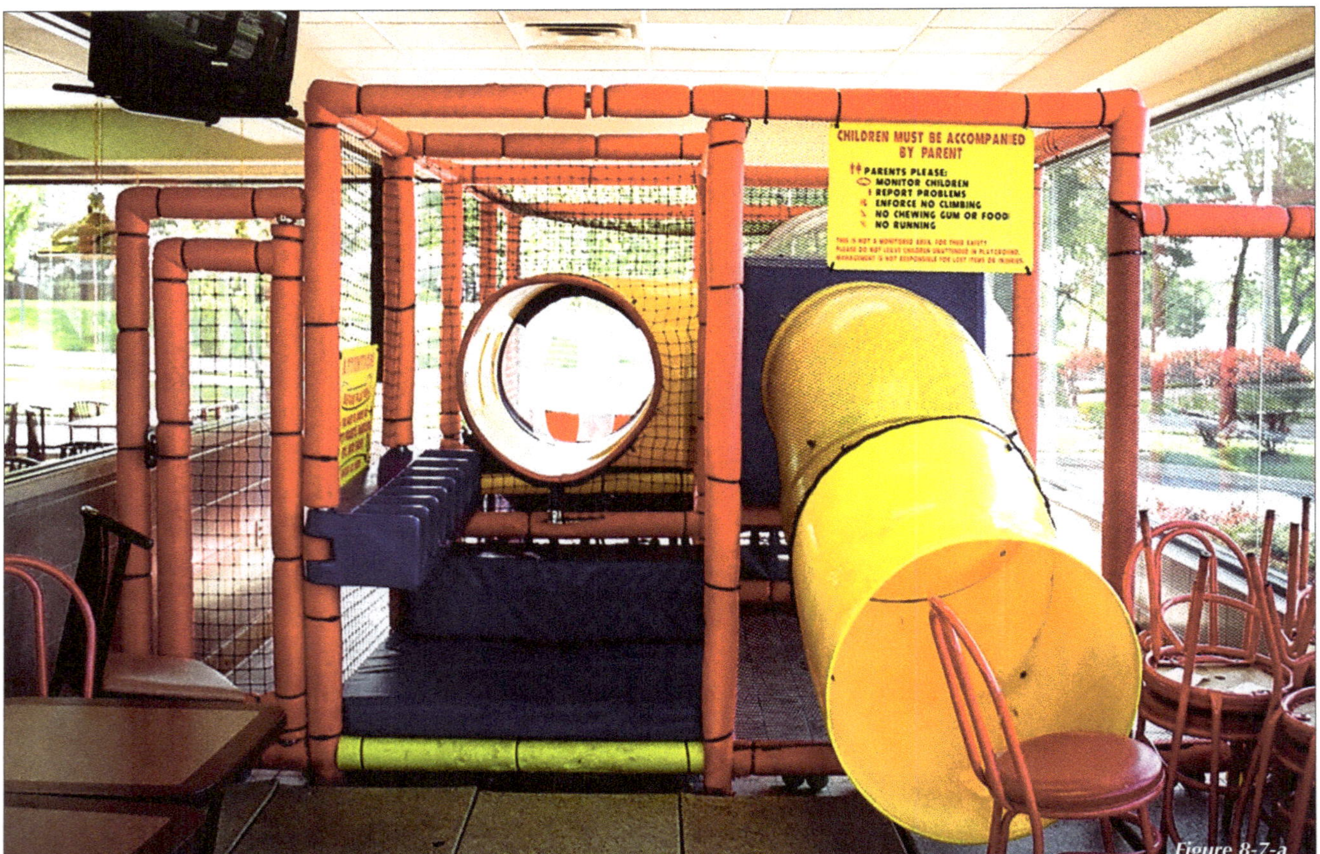
CHILDREN MUST BE ACCOMPANIED BY PARENT
PARENTS PLEASE:
MONITOR CHILDREN
REPORT PROBLEMS
ENFORCE NO CLIMBING
NO CHEWING GUM OR FOOD
NO RUNNING
Figure 8-7-a

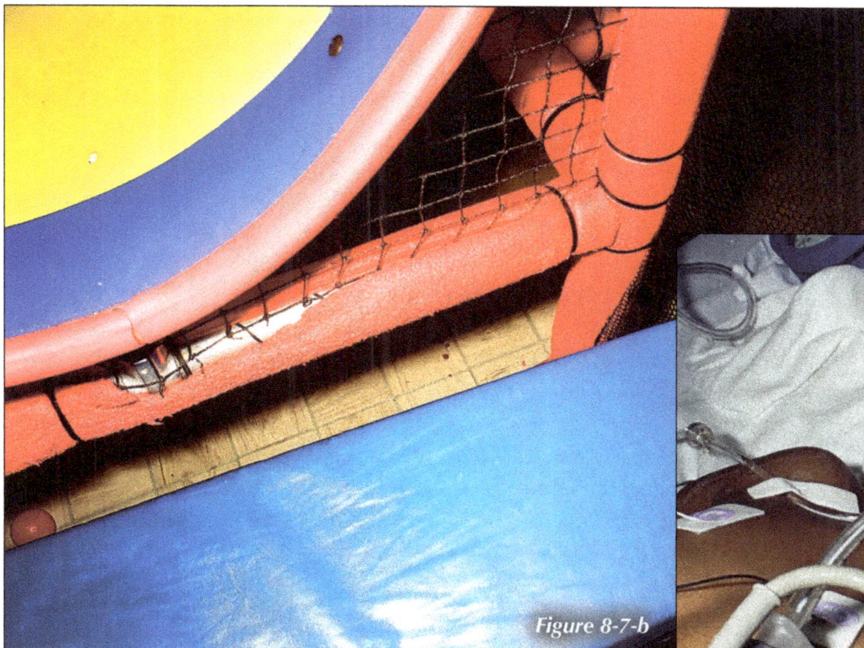

Figure 8-7-b. Below site of where child became wedged.

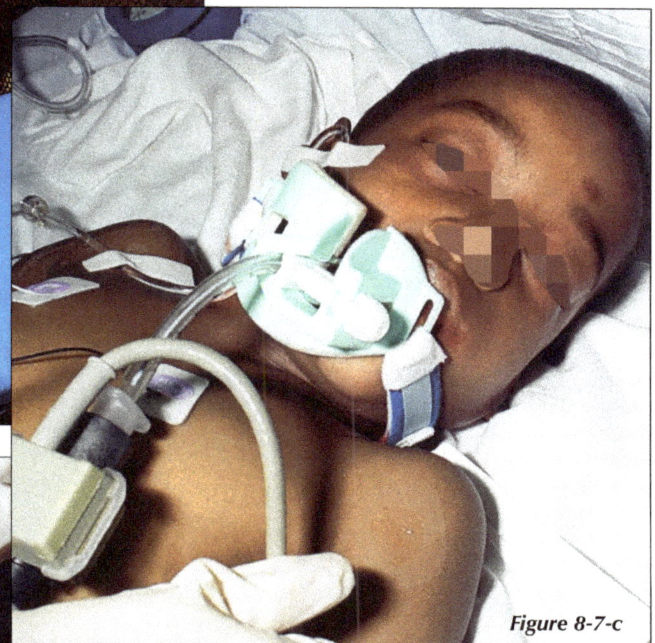

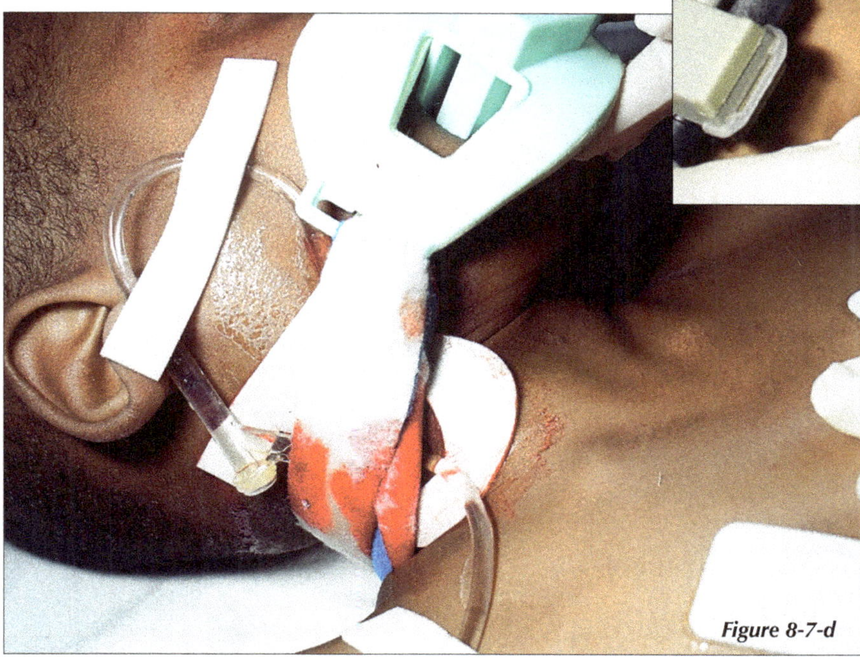

Figure 8-7-c. Petechial hemorrhages of orbital skin and cheeks.

Figure 8-7-d. Tiny abrasions on upper lateral right neck and horizontal abrasion across mid-lower anterior right neck.

Lethal Neglect

Parents or caretakers of children have a responsibility to those children to supply certain requirements that the children cannot obtain by themselves, including food, a safe environment, and medical care. Failure of the parent or caretaker to provide these essentials constitutes neglect. If a child dies from lack of these essentials, then the medical examiner may consider the death a homicide.

All of these cases require the medical examiner to complete an extensive examination of the family history and circumstances to understand how the child died. Many medical examiners take a less aggressive approach to calling these cases homicides. In the case of a child whose family practices a religion that forgoes medical treatment, if the child dies from a condition that would be treatable if taken to medical care (eg, onset of diabetes in a 12-year-old child who died in ketoacidosis after a period of coma that was evident to the parents), the author has certified the death as a homicide. This practice varies from medical examiner to medical examiner.

Starvation is an area where the pathology is not well-studied nor described. Gamble[10] demonstrated that consuming 100 grams of glucose per day in an otherwise starving adult who was allowed free access to water reduced the consumption of body protein by half and prevented ketosis. It is not known how much glucose or its equivalent is needed to produce a similar effect on an infant. There is no one degree of weight loss or starvation that is lethal. In adults, when the loss of weight reaches 40%, deaths begin to occur.[6] Infants and young children are in a stage of life when growth and weight gain should be occurring on a daily basis, so weight loss alone in a child is not the proper predictor of lethality. Comparing the child's height and weight to standard growth curves will provide information of where the child falls in comparison to age-mates and possibly will indicate how long the child had been deprived of nutrition.[11] At autopsy, the thickness of the subcutaneous layer of fat and muscle of the abdominal wall is noted, and in starvation cases the layer tends to be only skin. The extremities are atrophic and show loss of muscle. The skin may demonstrate other stigma of neglect such as skin infections or scars from infection or chronic diaper rash. Autopsy will usually demonstrate atrophy of the thymus, heart, liver, spleen, and kidneys. The stomach may show mucosal erosions, and the colon may have ulcerations of the mucosa.[12] Kellogg[13] described 12 prosecuted cases of infant and child starvation. These 12 cases ranged from children who were 2.25 months to 13 years of age. Half of the children died before or shortly after presentation to medical care or law enforcement. Survival was more common in the older children. At death, children dying from inanition, as it is termed on the death certificate, will often have some microscopic evidence of bronchopneumonia.

Lethal Neglect Case Studies

Case Study 8-7

This 7-month-old boy was born at 6 months gestation via emergency cesarean section because the mother had toxemia. At birth, the infant weighed 2 pounds. The infant remained in the hospital for 1 month. On the day of death, the mother stated the infant had recently had cold-like symptoms and had not been eating well. The mother said she fed the infant twice in the 12 hours before his death. She placed him on his back to go to sleep in a room with his 8-year-old sister, and she later found him face down on the floor next to his bed, unresponsive. She then called 911 and attempted CPR. The mother had 5 children living in the residence, including a 2-year-old, 5-year-old, 6-year-old, and 8-year-old in addition to the infant. When first responders arrived on the scene, the other children asked the police for food, so they left and bought hamburgers for the children. Investigation revealed that the children were frequently left in the care of the 8-year-old. The 5-year-old sibling was in charge of feeding the infant. The food that was provided to the infant consisted of adult leftovers, such as pizza.

Cause of Death: Malnutrition; inanition; failure to feed

Manner of Death: Homicide

Table 8-8. Autopsy Results

External Examination

- Very thin, poorly nourished infant, weighing 8 pounds and measuring 22 inches in length
- Appeared considerably younger than stated age; size was off the chart for age

Injuries

- Multiple scabbed-over 1 mm abrasions in the left upper frontal portion of the scalp, over forehead, and 1 on the nose
- Abdomen was scaphoid

Internal Examination

GI Tract

- Stomach was distended with air and contained a small volume of clear fluid
- Small bowel contained a scant amount of thin, bile-stained liquid
- Large bowel was filled with firm, pale-brown dried fecal material, which had the consistency of carpet fiber

Microscopic Examination

- One section of the lungs had a focal area of interstitial collections of neutrophils and mononuclear cells; they were also present in adjacent alveolar spaces
- Several nearby bronchioles also showed neutrophils within the lumen
- Vitreous electrolytes demonstrated urea nitrogen of 36 (H), creatinine of 0.2, chloride of 131 (H), sodium of 138

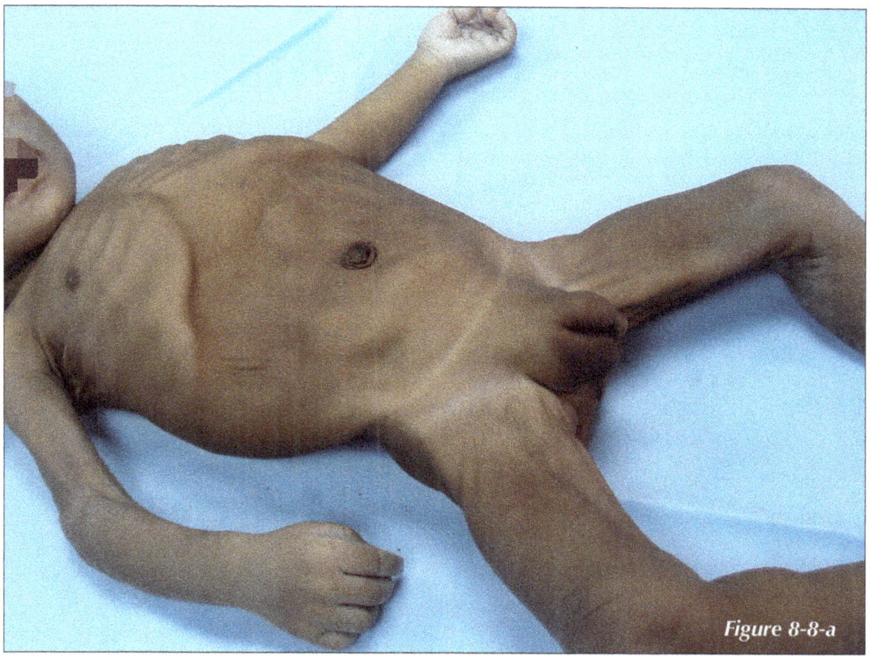

Figure 8-8-a

Figure 8-8-a. *Anterior view of child at autopsy showing small size with lack of subcutaneous fat and prominent ribs.*

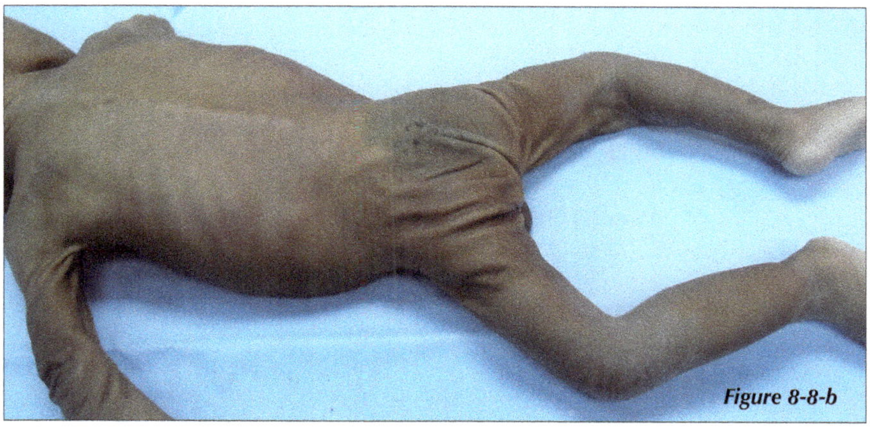

Figure 8-8-b

Figure 8-8-b. *Posterior view of body showing poorly nourished state.*

Figure 8-8-c. *Large bowel opened to show firm dried fecal material having the consistency of carpet fiber.*

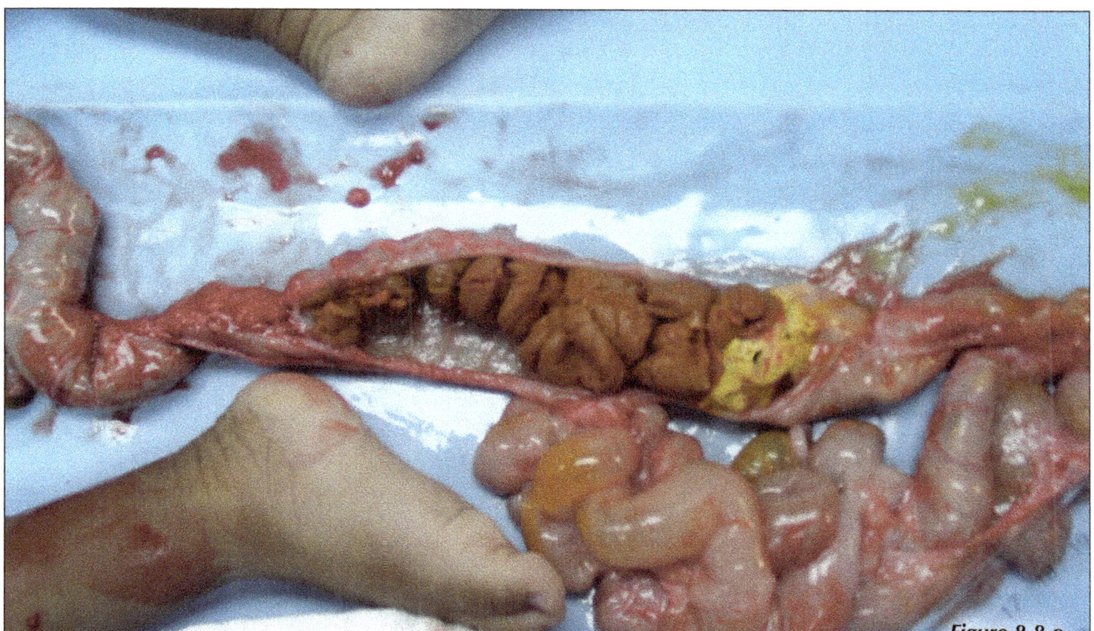

Figure 8-8-c

Medical Child Abuse

Medical child abuse (MCA) has replaced the previous entity of Munchausen syndrome by proxy and is defined as, "A child receiving unnecessary and harmful or potentially harmful medical care at the instigation of the caretaker."[15] It is a factitious disorder in which a parent, usually the mother, either feigns a disorder in a child or creates an illness by some harmful practice, such as dosing the child with adult blood pressure medication or injecting fecal material into the child.[16,17] The fictitious disorder then results in medical investigation with extensive testing and diagnostic procedures in an attempt to determine the source of the problem. This health care-seeking behavior may have devastating and even lethal effects on the child.

The most common type of MCA seen by the medical examiner is an infant who presents with multiple episodes of apnea, often with a history of resuscitation by the mother. One case seen by the author was a 3-month-old infant whose death was under review by the child fatality panel and was found to have had 17 hospitalizations because the child had "stopped breathing." Extensive workup in the hospital eventually resulted in a differential diagnosis that included seizure disorder, although no actual evidence of such was found. After an entire year of reviewing medical records by the fatality review panel, the case was finalized as MCA-induced apnea. By that point, the panel believed it was important to try to establish whether the mother might again be pregnant or if she might have delivered other infants. She was found to have another 3-month-old child. Further, the pattern of multiple hospital visits for apnea had begun with the second sibling. At this point, police were asked to again interview the mother, and on further questioning, the mother confessed to killing the first child. This case demonstrates the value of the fatality review system. The initial autopsy on this child was performed at a medical examiner system separate from where the fatality review was carried out. The autopsy found nothing to explain the death, and the pathologist used hospital records to provide a diagnosis of seizure disorder. The medical examiner who did the autopsy did not thoroughly review every hospitalization. Once every hospitalization was assessed in the fatality review, it became evident that this was MCA.

There is overlap of MCA with apnea in cases of multiple asphyxial deaths of children who have the same parent or caretaker. These are deaths that occur when the child is found dead with no history of previous episodes of apnea and autopsy can find no cause of death. Some of these cases in the past have been called SIDS deaths. If more than one death in similar circumstances occurs with the same caretaker, investigation of the case as a homicide should ensue. Although few medical examiners would make that conclusion from 2 deaths, they may do so with 3 deaths in the care of the same individual. The investigation and circumstances of previous deaths are crucial to the elucidation of these cases.

References

1. Zumwalt RE, Hirsch CS. Subtle fatal child abuse. *Hum Pathol.* 1980;11(2):167-174.
2. Gillenwater JM, Quan L, Feldman KW. Inflicted submersion in childhood. *Arch Pediatr Adolesc Med.* 1996;150(3):298-303.
3. Nixon J, Pearn J. Non-accidental immersion in bathwater: another aspect of child abuse. *Br Med J.* 1977;1(6056):271-272.
4. Pearn J, Nixon J. Bathtub immersion accidents involving children. *Med J Aust* 1977;1(7):211-213.
5. Griest KJ, Zumwalt RE. Child abuse by drowning. *Pediatrics.* 1989;83(1):41-46.
6. DiMaio V, DiMaio D. *Forensic Pathology.* 2nd ed. CRC Press; 2001.

7. Meadow R. Suffocation, recurrent apnea, and sudden infant death. *J Pediatr.* 1990;117(3):351-357.

8. Emery JL. Child abuse, sudden infant death syndrome, and unexpected infant death. *Am J Dis Child.* 1993;147(10):1097-1100.

9. McIntosh BJ, Shanks DE, Whitworth JM. Child abuse by suffocation presenting as hypoxic-ischemic encephalopathy. Report of a patient. *Clin Pediatr.* 1994;33(9):561-563.

10. Gamble JL. The Harvey Lectures, series XLIII, 1946-1947: physiological information gained from studies on the life raft ration. *Nutr Rev.* 1989;47(7):199-201.

11. Wehner F, Schieffer MC, Wehner HD. Percentile charts to determine the duration of child abuse by chronic malnutrition. *Forensic Sci Int.* 1999;102(2-3):173-180.

12. Zumwalt RE, Hirsch CS. Pathology of fatal child abuse and neglect. In: Helfer RE, Kempe RS, eds. *The Battered Child.* 4th ed. University of Chicago Press; 1987:247-260.

13. Winick M, ed. *Hunger Disease: Studies by the Jewish Physicians in the Warshaw Ghetto.* John Wiley & Sons; 1979.

14. Kellogg ND, Lukefahr JL. Criminally prosecuted cases of child starvation. *Pediatrics.* 2005;116(6):1309-1316.

15. Roesler TA. Medical child abuse. In: Jenny C, ed. *Child Abuse and Neglect.* Elsevier; 2011:586-591.

16. Fish E, Bromfield L, Higgins DJ. A new name for Munchausen Syndrome by Proxy: defining fabricated or induced illness by carers. *Child Abuse Prev Issues.* 2005;23:2-12.

17. Sanders MJ, Bursch B. Forensic assessment of illness falsification, Munchausen by proxy, and factitious disorder, NOS. *Child Maltreat.* 2002;7(2):112-124.

Editor's note: All references were used in the creation of the original work, *Forensic Pathology of Child Death,* but may not be cited directly in this chapter.

Chapter 9

Organ and Tissue Procurement

Objectives

After reviewing this chapter, the reader will be able to:

1. *Identify and understand the deaths and categories of deaths that medical examiner coroners (ME/Cs) have jurisdiction over.*
2. *Explain why the need for children's organs and tissues is acute.*
3. *Summarize the ME/C's decision making process for organ and tissue procurement of a child in relation to documentation and other bodily injuries.*

Introduction

Every state has statutes that create a ME/C jurisdiction over individuals who die suddenly, unexpectedly, or by possibly unnatural causes of death (eg, accidents, suicides, homicides) as well as many natural deaths due to age or circumstances of death. There are also certain categories of deaths that medical examiners will always have jurisdiction over: all children; those in the custody of law enforcement or who die during an interaction with law enforcement; deaths in the workplace; and deaths outside of medical care. The ME/C mandate is to determine the cause and manner of death, seize evidence from the body (eg, bullets, material for DNA, specimens for toxicology, clothing, hair, fibers), and document injuries and disease. The National Association of Medical Examiners has taken the position that ME/Cs should permit procurement of organs and tissues in cases under their jurisdiction, as well as have cooperative agreements with the organ and tissue procurement organizations (O/TPO) in order to enable these procurements while still fulfilling the ME/C mandate.[1]

Organ and Tissue Procurement

The success and 5-year survival rate for both solid organ and tissue transplantation is impressive; however, the perpetual shortage of them continues to increase. The need for organs and tissues for children is especially acute, and children are a special concern in organ and tissue procurement. Because children must receive size-matched organs and tissues, the scarcity of these are greater than for adults. Additionally, the transplant programs for children tend to be smaller and require special expertise. Children and adolescents cannot give antemortem permission for donations, as might be done with an adult driver's license, so the parents must make this decision during a time of great emotional stress.

Most of the candidates for tissue and organ procurement involve cases that fall into the jurisdiction of the ME/Cs, and before a case is released for donation, permission must be obtained from the ME/C after reviewing the case details. Forensic pathologists working in large medical examiner systems generally have extensive experience and interaction with the O/TPO in their community, so, in most cases, they are comfortable with allowing the donation of organs and tissues. However, in cases of homicide or sudden infant deaths, donation can be a difficult decision for the

ME/C. In many child abuse homicides, the victim dies in a children's hospital where there has been extensive examination by child protective services and social services. In these types of cases, most injuries have been documented; therefore, at the time of death, the pathologist can review the medical records and determine if organs and tissues that were not impacted by injury can be recovered. In addition, many pathologists will even attend the procurement procedure to assure that if any internal injury becomes apparent during the removal, the injury can be properly documented.

Infants and young children who are found dead outside of hospital care will often still be eligible for donation of certain organs and tissues without the fear of lost evidence. However, in the past, in smaller coroner communities, it was not unusual for the coroner to refuse any recovery of organs or tissues simply because they were unfamiliar with the procedures and protocols. In response to this attitude, many states have enacted laws that bar ME/Cs from forbidding procurement of organs and tissues.

Organ and Tissue Procurement Case Studies

Case Study 9-1

This 2-year-old girl lived with her mother and the mother's boyfriend in the boyfriend's parents' home. The boyfriend was home alone with the child when she became unresponsive. He admitted to being "ridiculously violent" to the child. There were previous injuries and bruises to the child. The boyfriend texted pictures of the bruises to the mother, and the mother noted that they could cover up the bruises with makeup. There were also videos of the child that showed her stumbling around and then becoming unconscious. The child was transported to a children's hospital where she remained for 2 days, unconscious. She was able to donate a beating heart, lungs, liver, kidney, pancreas, and intestines after an extensive workup of her injuries in the hospital. The O/TPO was instructed to take full-body photographs before organ procurement and to take photographs during the removal of organs if trauma was present.

Cause of death: Closed head trauma

Manner of death: Homicide

Comment: This case has multiple significant injuries that were able to be demonstrated, photographed, and documented, despite having organs donated.

Table 9-1-a. Autopsy Results

External Examination

- 2-year-old female, 37 inches and 38 pounds
- Sutured horseshoe-shaped incision, right fronto-parietal-temporal scalp, for evacuation of subdural blood
- Y-shaped sutured incision, chest, midline down abdomen

Injuries

Head

Type	*Measurement*
Swollen face	
Contusion, pinna of right ear	10 mm
Contusion, posterior right pinna	30 mm x 10 mm
7 to 8 contusions, right temporal scalp below surgical incision	5 to 12 mm each
Contusion, bridge of nose	3 mm
Contusion, midline upper lip	5 mm
Contusion, right forehead	30 mm
— With central abrasion	10 mm
Contusion, upper right forehead at hairline	5 mm
6 to 8 contusions, left forehead	5 to 10 mm each
2 contusions, left cheek	10 mm, 3 mm
2 contusions, inside left pinna	5 mm, 10 mm
Shower of red petechial hemorrhages below left pinna	15 mm area
2 contusions, right occipital scalp	5 mm, 10 mm
Subgaleal hemorrhage from midline right frontal through right temporo-parieto-occipital	20 mm x 30 mm area, up to 10 mm thick
Bone of right fronto-temporo-parietal craniotomy was removed and left out, and brain was herniating out of defect	
Acute subdural blood, thick layer, over cerebral convexities and anterior, middle, and posterior cranial fossae	
Heavy optic nerve sheath hemorrhage, bilateral	
Subdural blood over spinal cord	

(continued)

Table 9-1-a. Autopsy Results ***(continued)***

Other Blunt Trauma

Type	Measurement
Multiple contusions, 6 on the right shoulder and 3 on the left	5 to 20 mm
Shower of petechial hemorrhages, left upper chest	10 mm area (2)
Contusion, left upper chest	3 mm
2 contusions, left lower abdominal quadrant	5 mm each
Contusion, right lateral	10 mm x 15 mm
2 contusions, dorsal surface of right forearm	5 mm, 10 mm
Contusion, anterior right arm	5 mm
Contusion, medial right elbow	10 mm
Contusion, lateral right knee	6 mm
Contusion, right upper leg	5 mm
2 contusions, left arm lateral	10 mm each
Contusion, upper lateral left arm	5 mm
Contusion, lower lateral left arm	5 mm
3 contusions, anterior left arm	10 mm, 5 mm (2)
3 contusions, left elbow	5 mm each
Contusion, ventral surface of left wrist	30 mm
Contusion, anterior lower left thigh	20 mm x 10 mm
Contusion, lateral left thigh	30 mm x 10 mm
7 contusions, left upper back	5 to 10 mm
3 contusions, right upper back	5 mm each
4 contusions, right mid-back	5 mm each
Contusion, right upper buttock	15 mm
Contusion, left lower back	5 mm
Compression fractures of T4 and T5	

Dissection of soft tissue of back revealed extensive deep hemorrhage in the posterior right thigh in muscle and fat

Neuropathology Examination

— Acute subdural blood, cerebral convexities
— Early brain death
— Mixed pattern of traumatic and hypoxic axonal injury
— Bilateral retinal hemorrhages, too numerous to count, in all layers, out to ora serrata
— Bilateral optic nerve sheath hemorrhage

Microscopic Examination

— ***Right shoulder:*** Acute hemorrhage within subcutaneous and deep fat without inflammatory response
— ***Medial left knee:*** Minimal acute hemorrhage in deep fat without inflammatory response
— ***Left upper back:*** Minimal acute hemorrhage without inflammatory response
— ***Right buttock:*** Extensive acute hemorrhage in deep fat without inflammatory response
— ***Right frontal:*** Massive subgaleal hemorrhage without inflammatory response
— ***Right temporal:*** Massive subgaleal hemorrhage associated with minimal inflammatory response with neutrophils and mononuclear cells
— ***Right occipital:*** Massive subgaleal hemorrhage with minimal mixed neutrophil and mononuclear cell response
— ***Left radius and ulna:*** Acute fracture with disruption of bone and acute hemorrhage

Table 9-1-b. Diagnoses

Closed Head Trauma

- Contusions on pinna right ear (2), right mastoid (7 to 8), right occipital (2)
- Contusions on bridge of nose, upper lip, right forehead (2), left forehead (6 to 8), left cheek (2), left ear (2)
- Massive subgaleal hemorrhage, right fronto-temporo-parieto-occipital
- Status post right frontoparietal craniectomy for evacuation of subdural hemorrhage and pressure monitor left frontal
- Subdural hemorrhage, cerebral convexities and basilar
- Mixed pattern of traumatic and hypoxic axonal injury
- Early brain death
- Bilateral retinal hemorrhages, too numerous to count, extending out to ora serrata
- Bilateral optic nerve sheath hemorrhage

Blunt Trauma

- Contusions on right (6) and left (3) shoulders, left lower quadrant (2)
- Petechial hemorrhages on left upper chest (2 areas), below left pinna
- Contusions on right arm lateral, right elbow (2), dorsum right forearm (2), anterior right arm, medial right elbow, right thigh, right leg
- Contusions on left arm (7), left elbow (3), left thigh (4)
- Contusions on left upper back (7), right upper back (3), right mid-back (4), right upper buttock, left lower back
- Massive deep contusion, posterior right thigh
- Fractures, left ulna and radius
- Compression fractures, T4 and T5

Figure 9-1-a. *Thoracic spine after defleshing of the spine showing compression fractures of T4 and T5.*

Figure 9-1-b. *Lateral view of thoracic spine after defleshing of the spine showing compression fractures of T4 and T5.*

Figure 9-1-c. *Lateral radiograph of thoracic spine showing compression fractures of T4 and T5.*

Figure 9-1-d. *Anterior posterior radiograph of thoracic spine showing compression fractures of T4 and T5.*

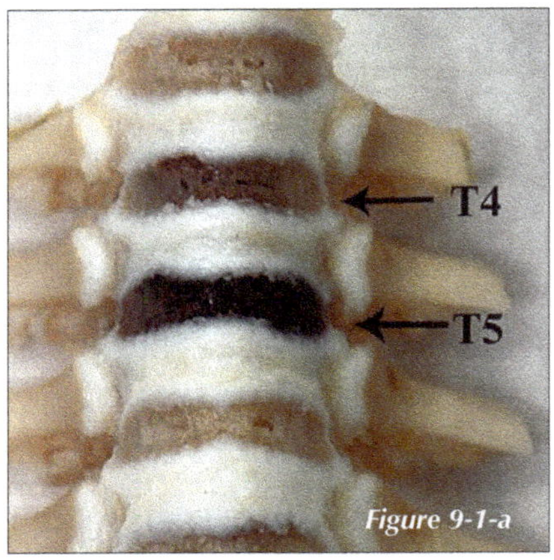

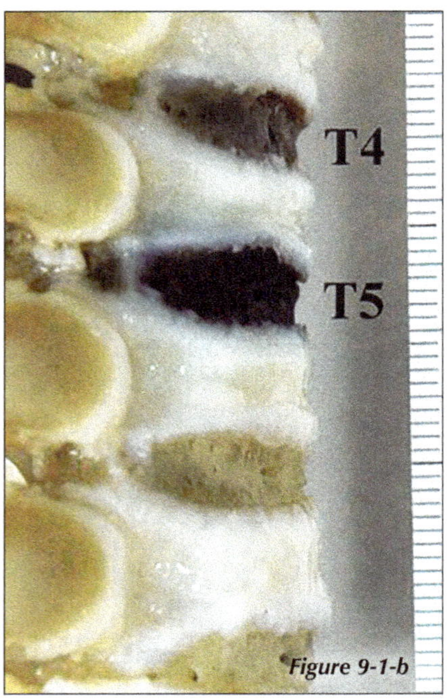

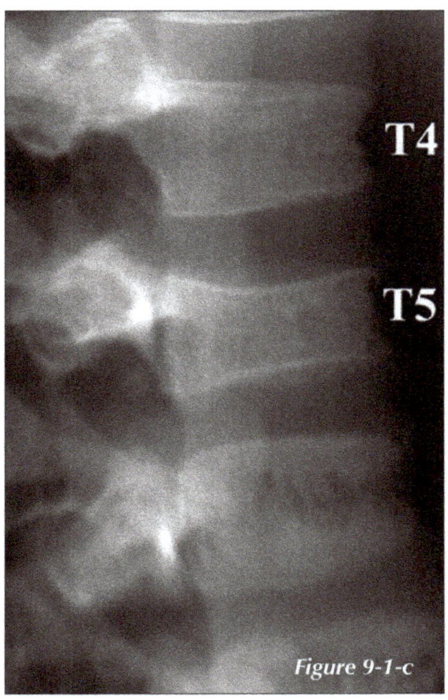

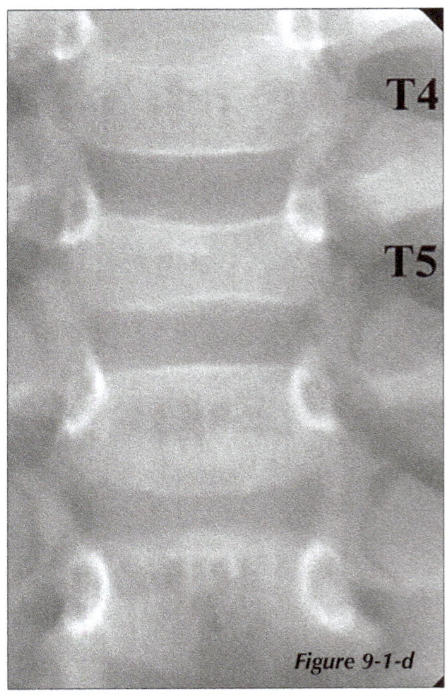

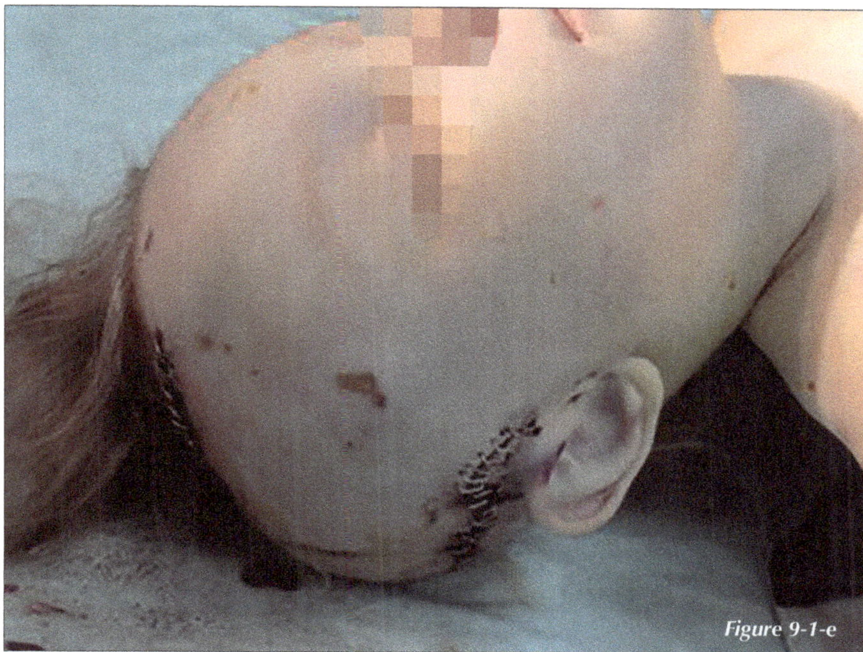

Figure 9-1-e

Figure 9-1-e. *Right side of face showing incision of the right frontotemporoparietal craniotomy, contusion of right ear, and 2 contusions of right forehead.*

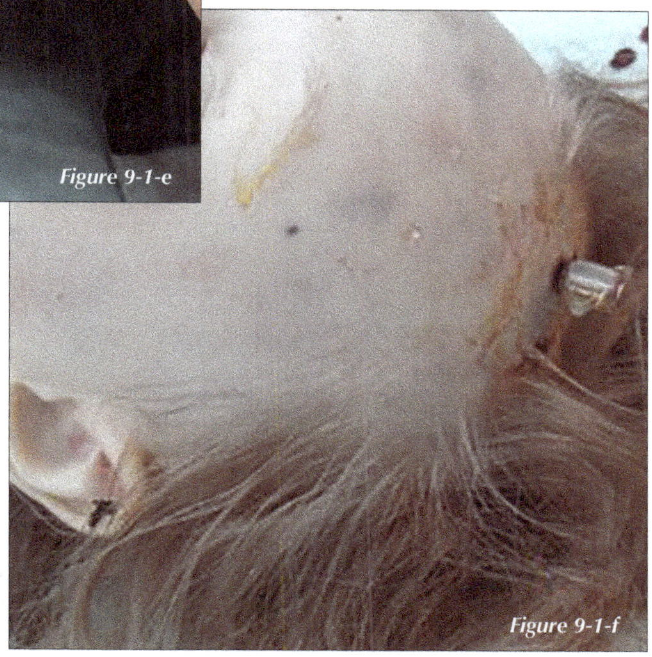

Figure 9-1-f

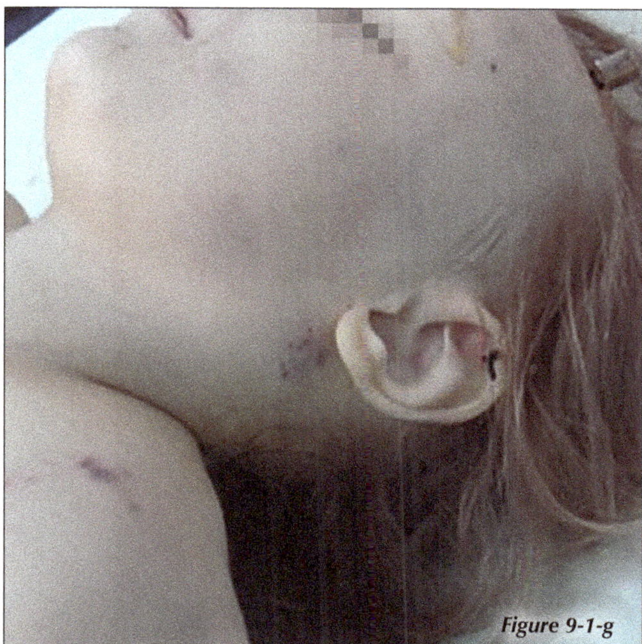

Figure 9-1-g

Figure 9-1-f. *Left side of face showing pressure monitor in left frontal and 6 to 8 contusions of left forehead.*

Figure 9-1-g. *Left side of face showing 2 contusions on left cheek, 2 contusions on pinna of left ear, and petechial hemorrhages below left ear.*

Figure 9-1-h. *Posterior aspect of head showing 2 contusions of right occipital scalp.*

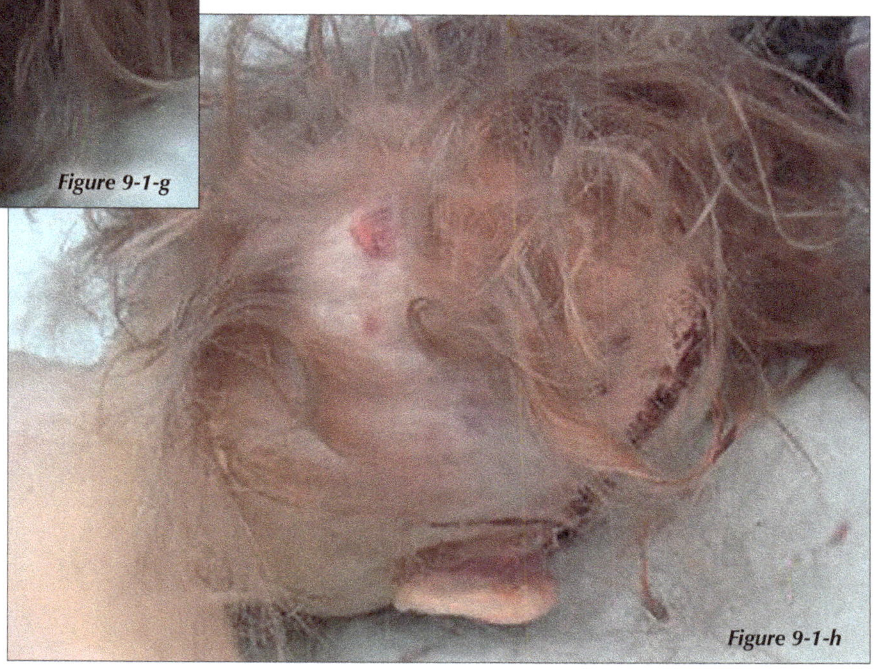

Figure 9-1-h

Figure 9-1-i. *Sutured incisions for harvesting chest and abdominal organs/tissues; multiple contusions right shoulder.*

Figure 9-1-j. *Right forearm showing 2 contusions on dorsal surface.*

Figure 9-1-k. *Right arm showing contusion elbow.*

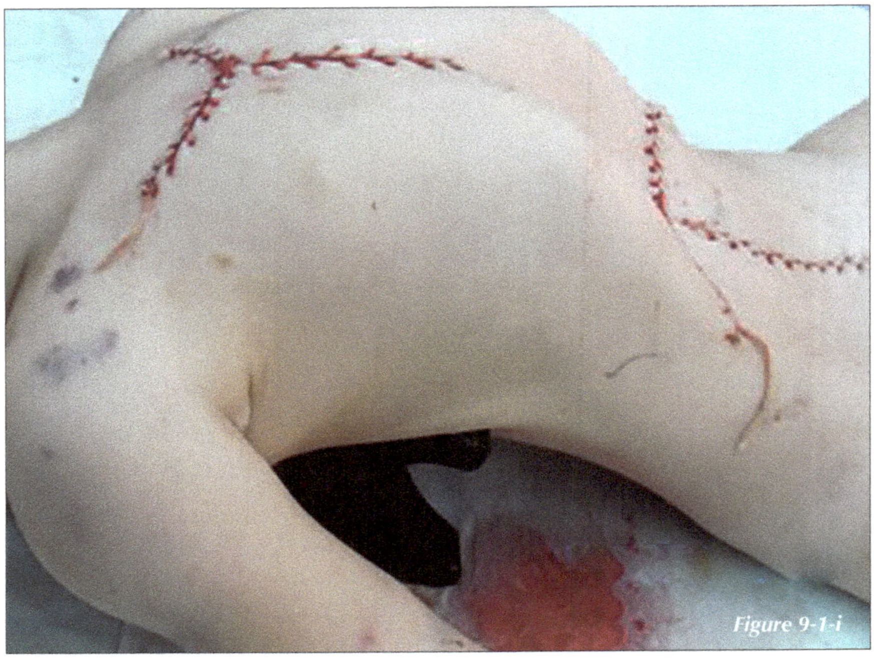

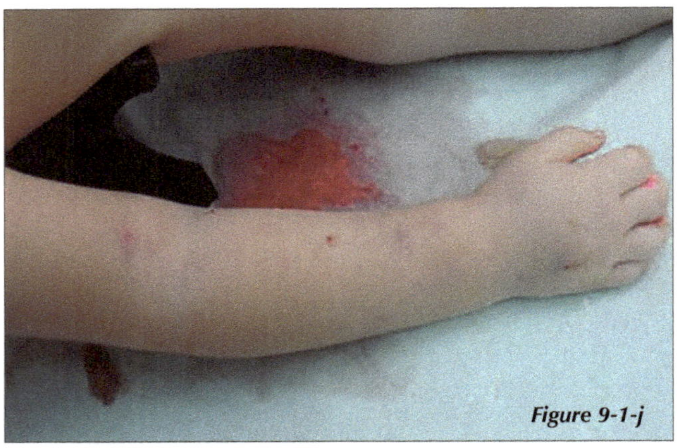

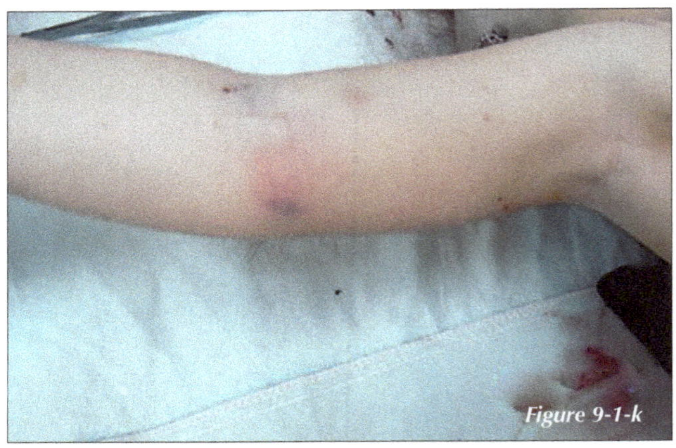

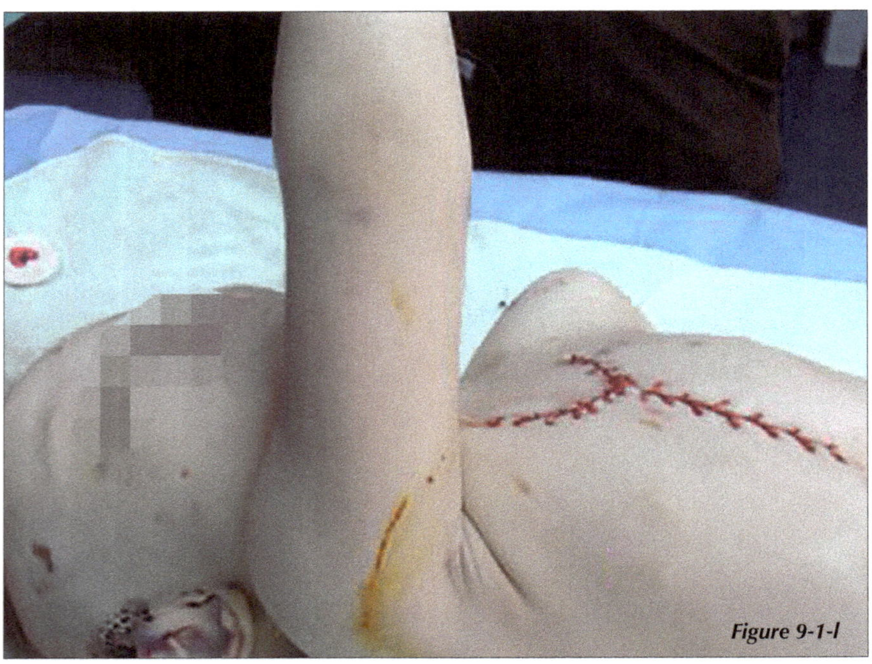

Figure 9-1-l. *Right arm showing contusion at elbow.*

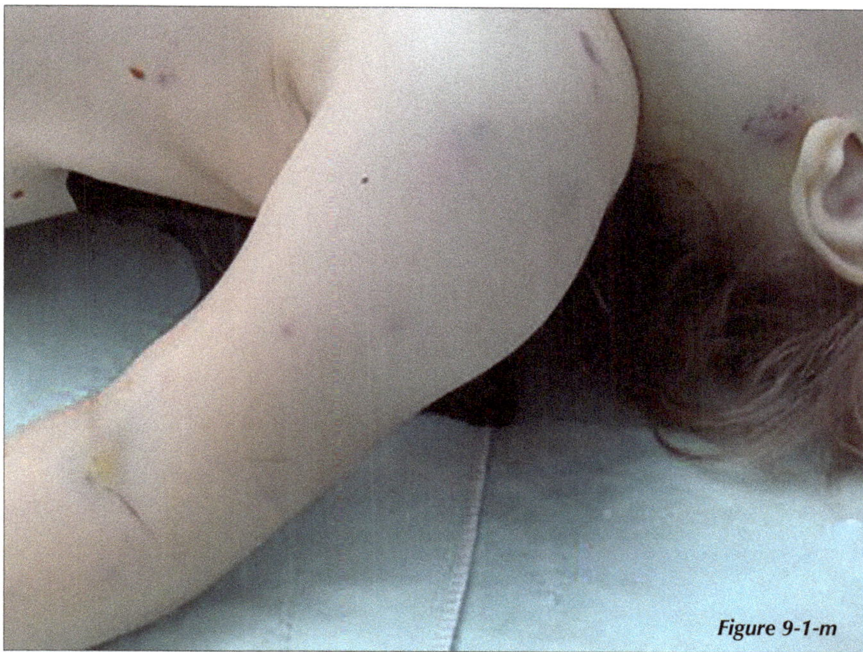

Figure 9-1-m

Figure 9-1-m. Left arm showing contusions on shoulder and lateral arm.

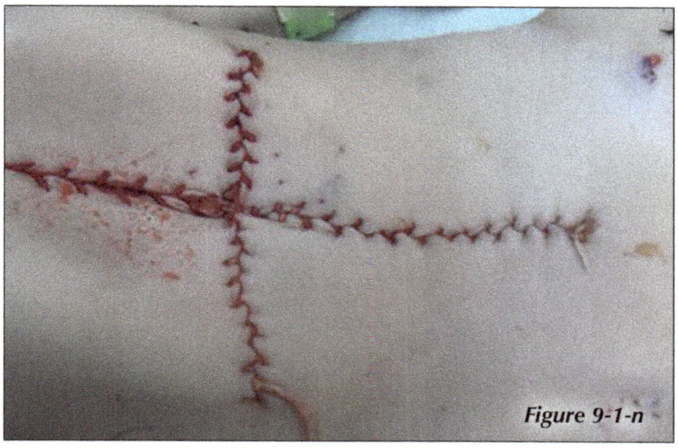

Figure 9-1-n

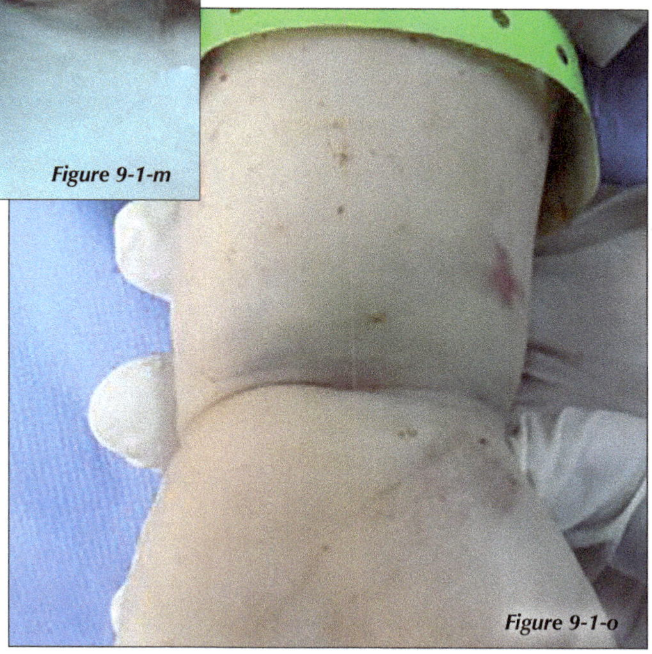

Figure 9-1-o

Figure 9-1-n. Abdomen with sutured incisions for organ harvesting and showing contusions on left lower quadrant.

Figure 9-1-o. Left wrist showing contusion on ventral surface.

Figure 9-1-p. Abdomen showing contusions on left lower quadrant.

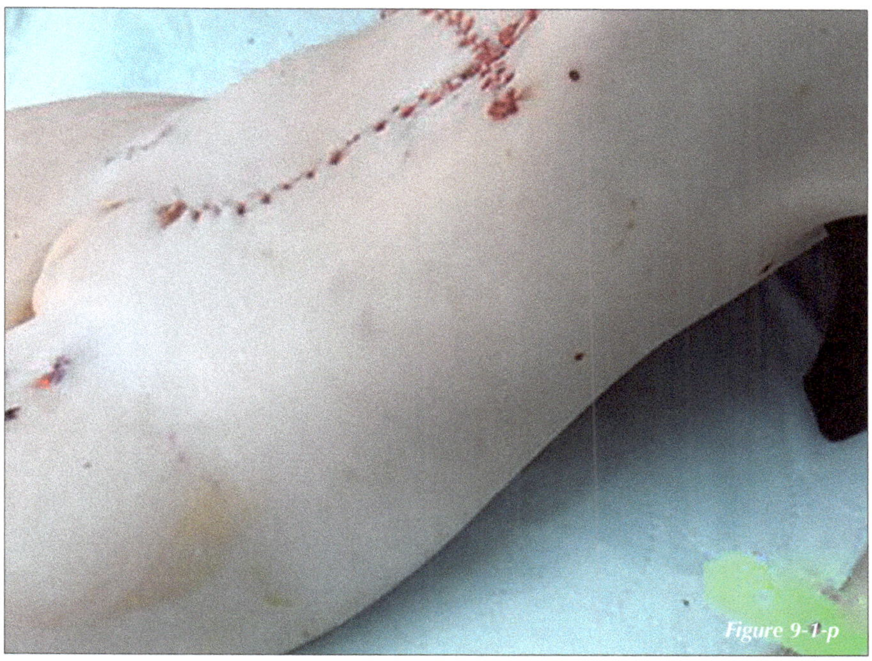

Figure 9-1-p

Figure 9-1-q. *Right shoulder with contusion and cassette to document identification of section taken from the contusion.*

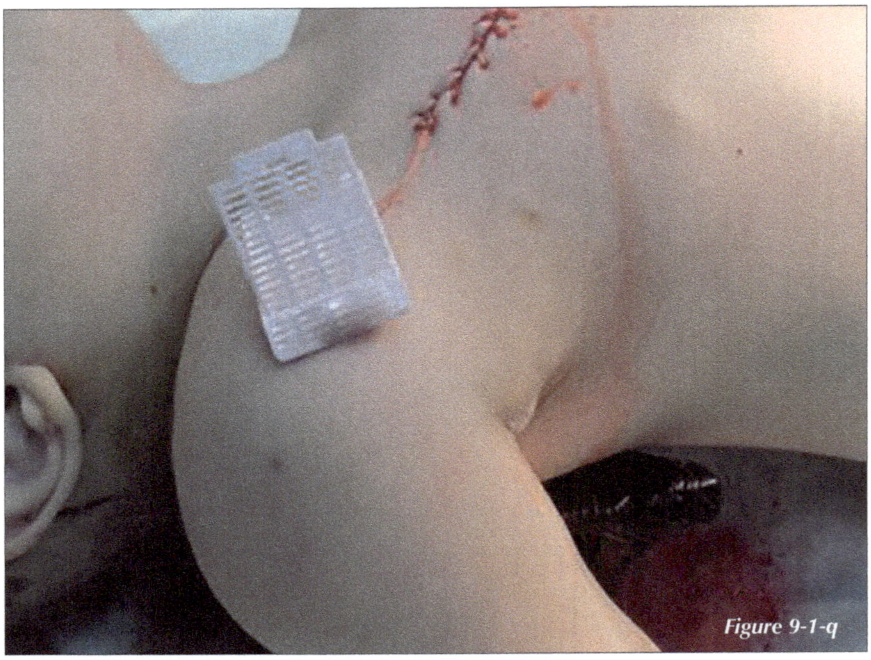

Figure 9-1-q

Figure 9-1-r. *Left shoulder with contusion and cassette to document identification of section taken from contusion.*

Figure 9-1-s. *Back of body showing 3 contusions of right upper back.*

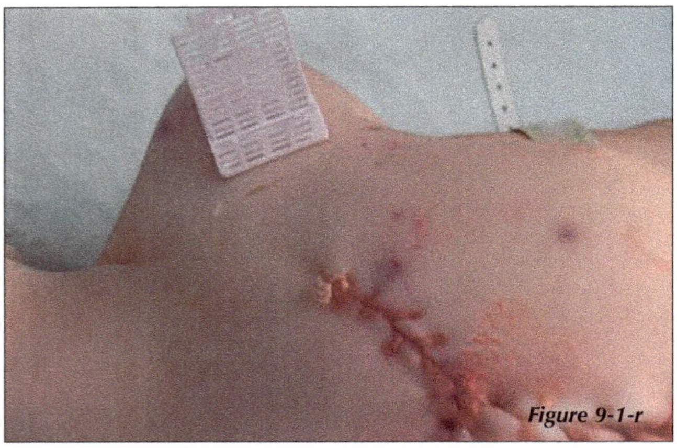

Figure 9-1-r

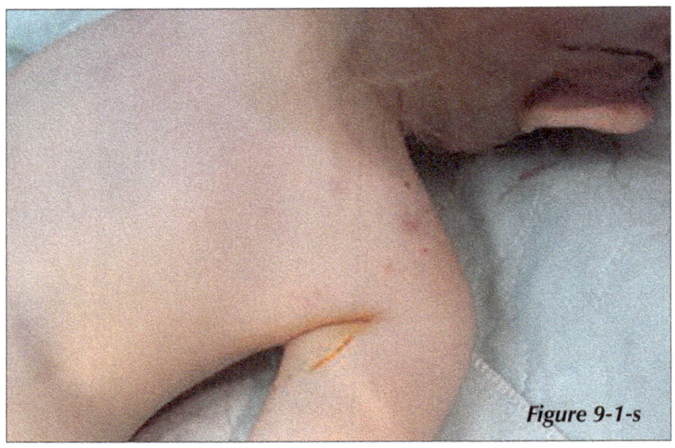

Figure 9-1-s

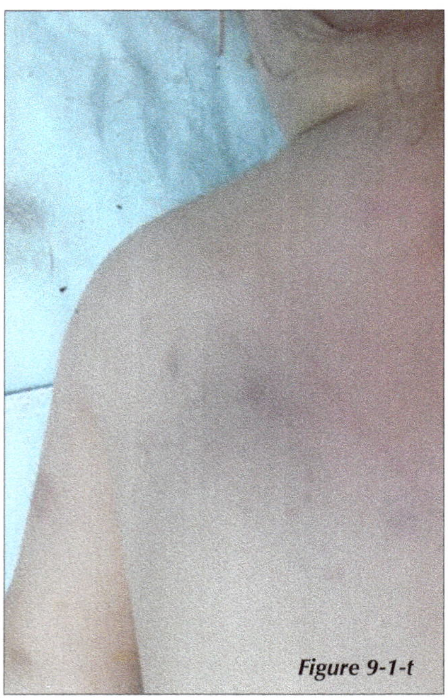

Figure 9-1-t

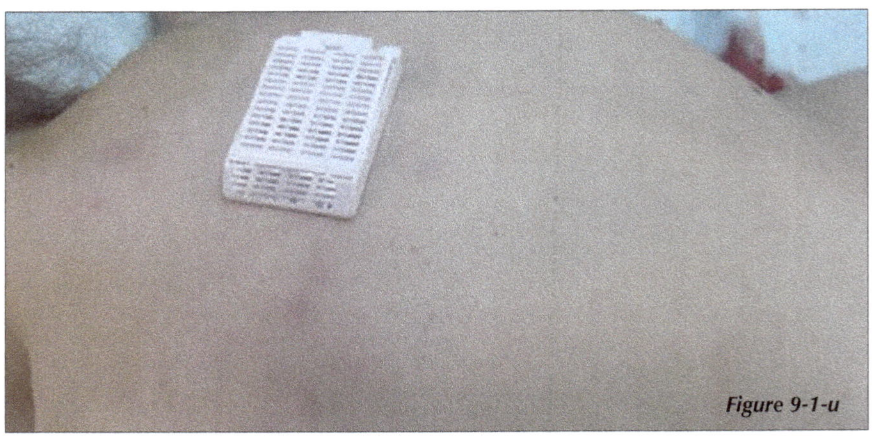

Figure 9-1-u

Figure 9-1-t. *Back of body showing 7 contusions of left upper back.*

Figure 9-1-u. *Back of body showing right upper back with cassette to document identification of section taken from contusion.*

Figure 9-1-v. Back of body showing contusion of right upper buttock.

Figure 9-1-w. Back of body showing cassette to document identification of section taken from contusion of right buttock.

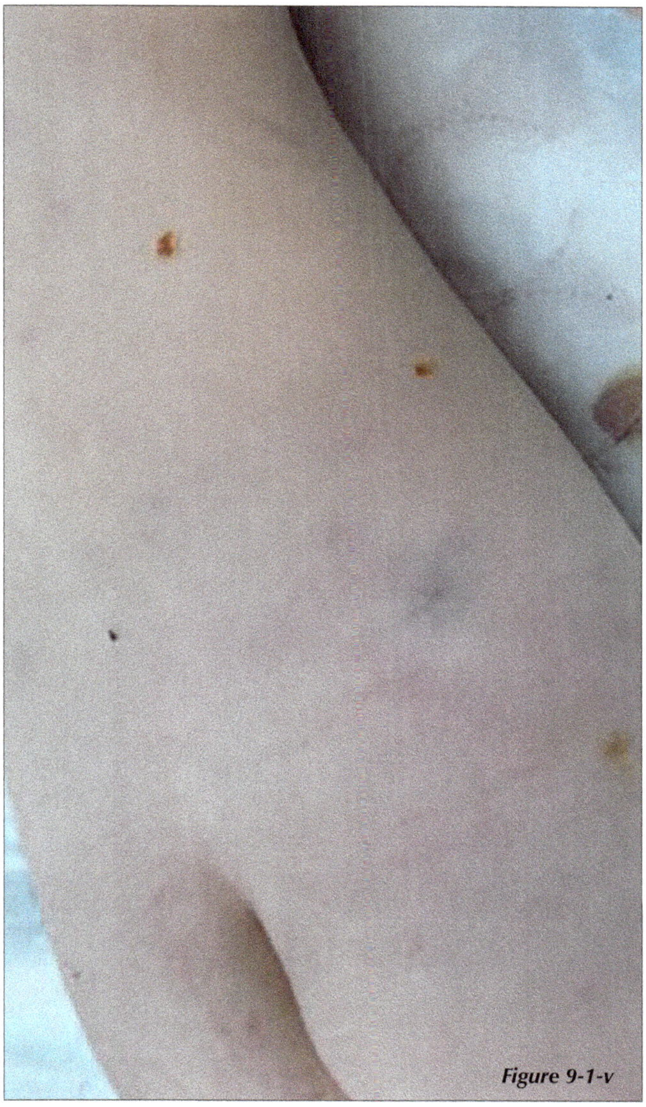

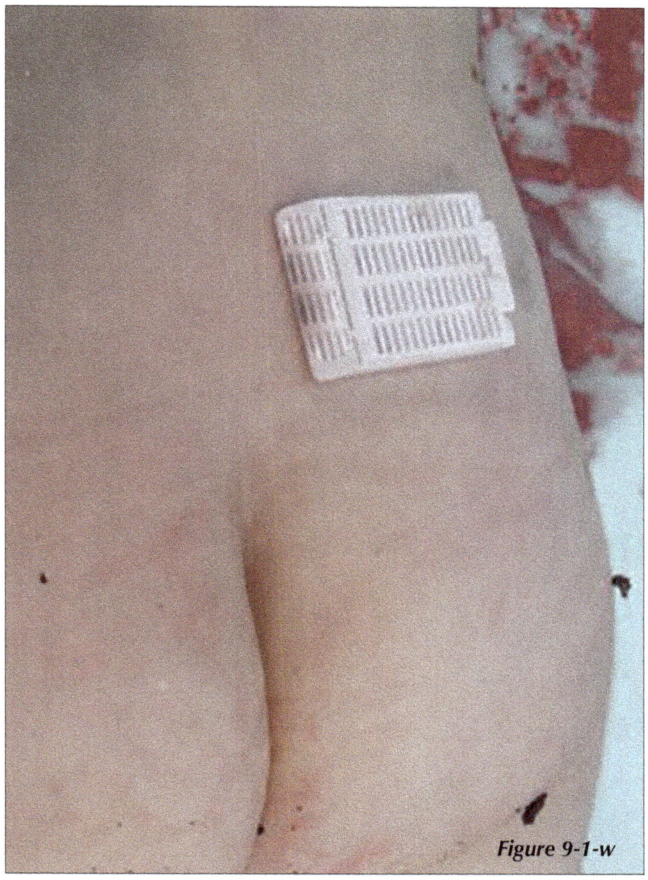

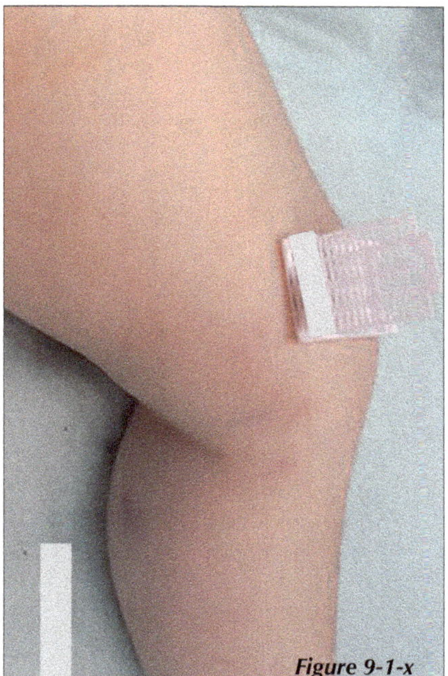

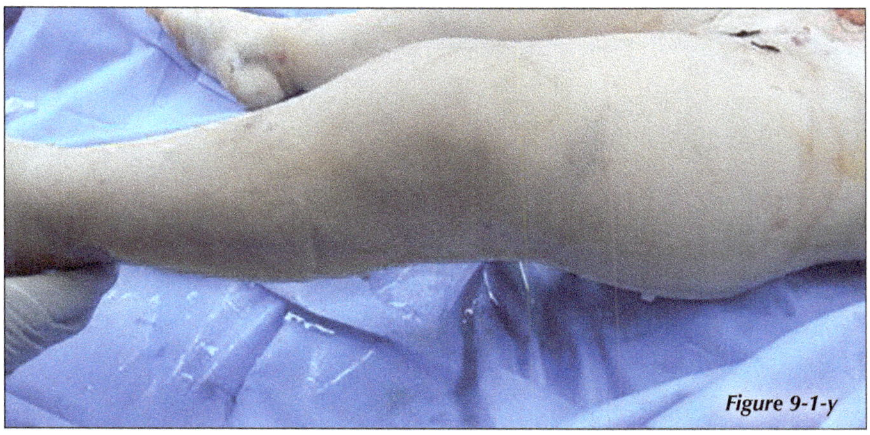

Figure 9-1-x. Right knee showing contusion of lateral knee.

Figure 9-1-y. Left lower extremity showing contusion, left anterior lower thigh.

Figure 9-1-z. Scalp opened and reflected to demonstrate subdural hemorrhage where the bone was removed from the craniotomy site.

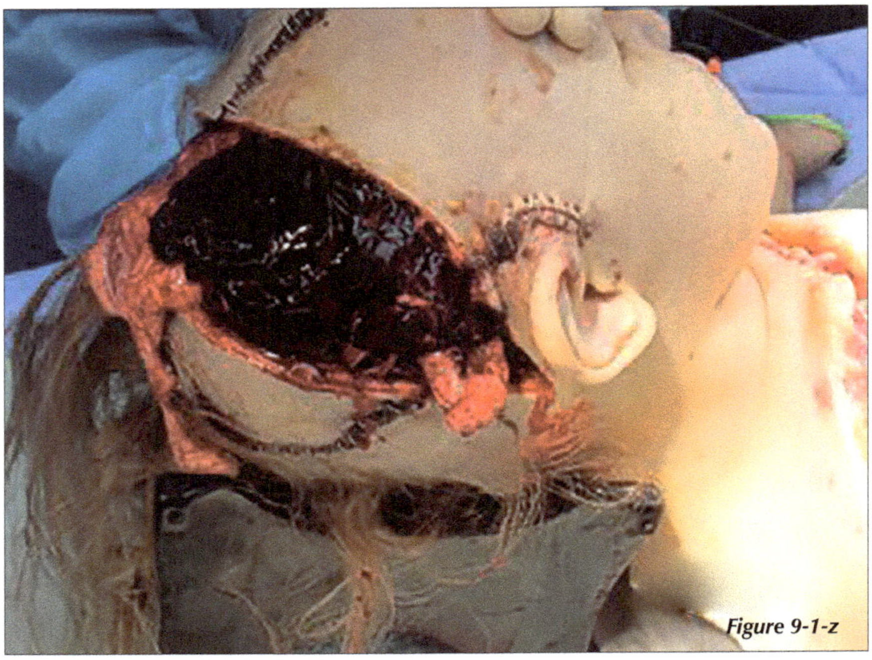

Figure 9-1-a.1. Reflected scalp showing subgaleal hemorrhage. As calvarium is removed, subdural hemorrhage over the cerebral convexities can be observed.

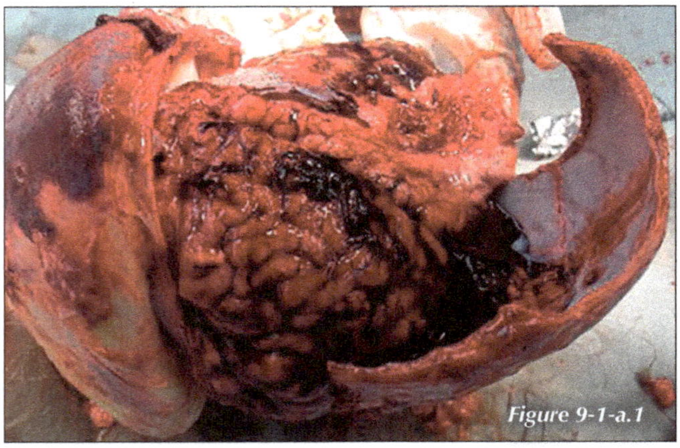

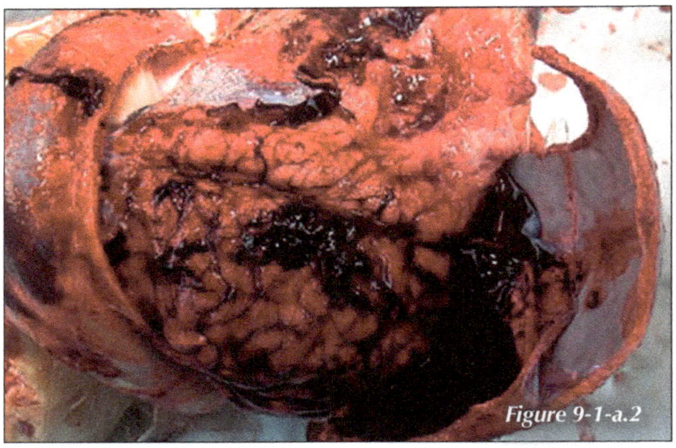

Figure 9-1-a.2. Removed calvarium showing residual subdural hemorrhage over cerebral convexities.

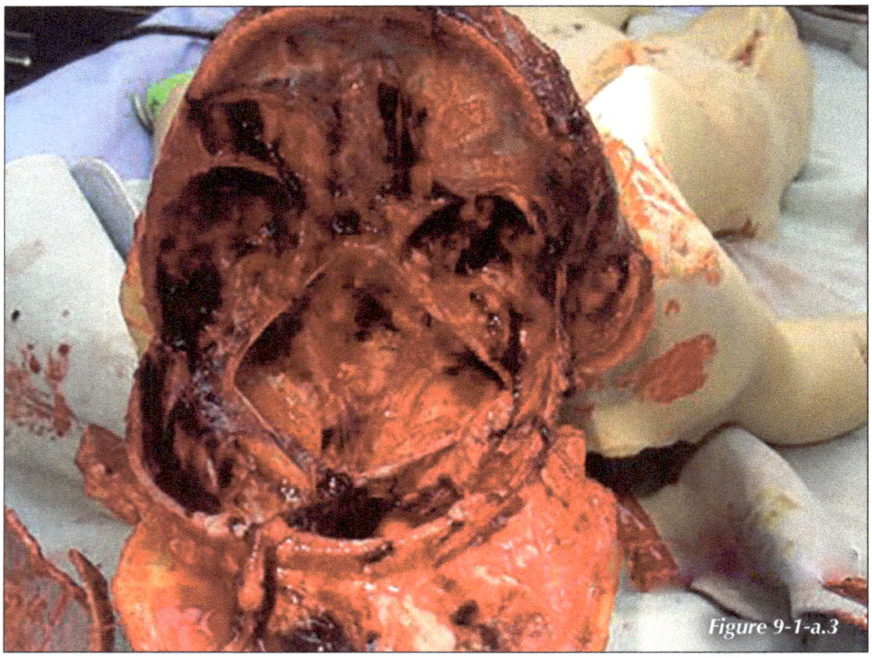

Figure 9-1-a.3. Calvarium and brain removed, showing subdural hemorrhage in anterior, middle, and posterior cranial fossae.

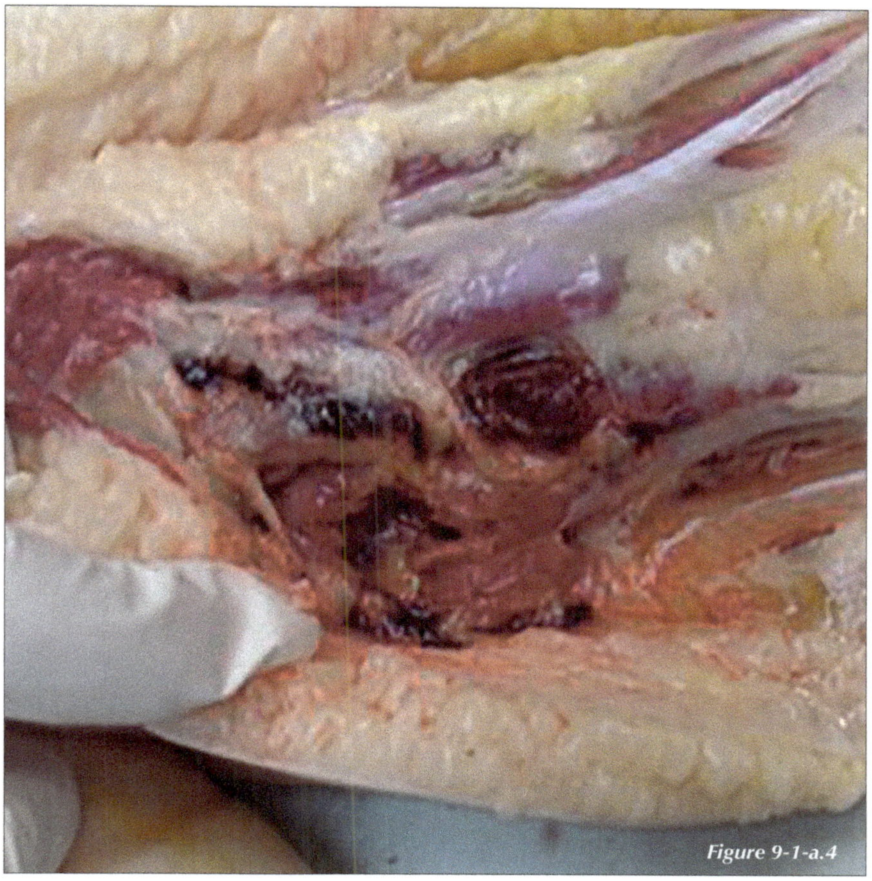

Figure 9-1-a.4. *Dissection of soft tissue, demonstrating extensive deep hemorrhage in posterior right thigh.*

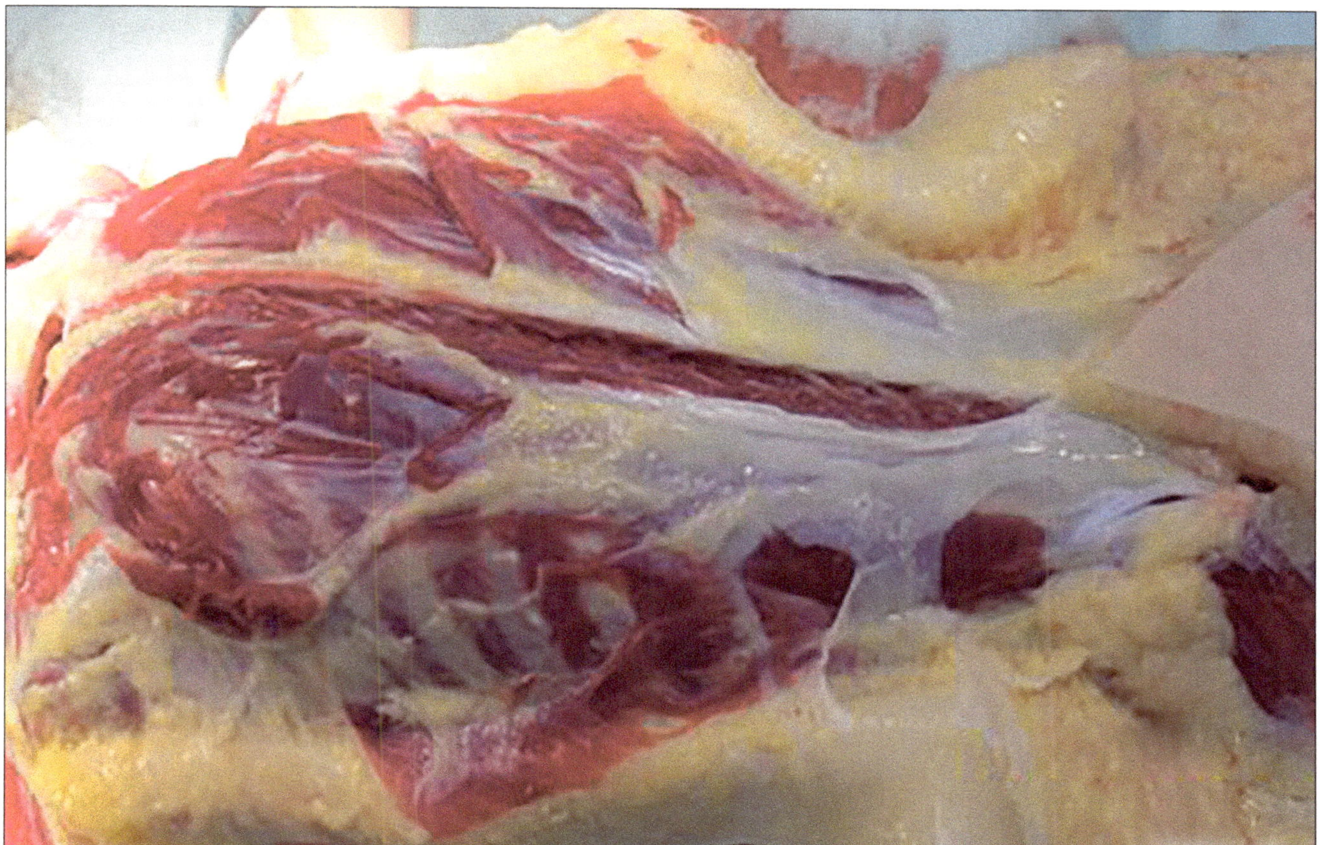

Figure 9-1-a.5. *Dissection of soft tissue of back.*

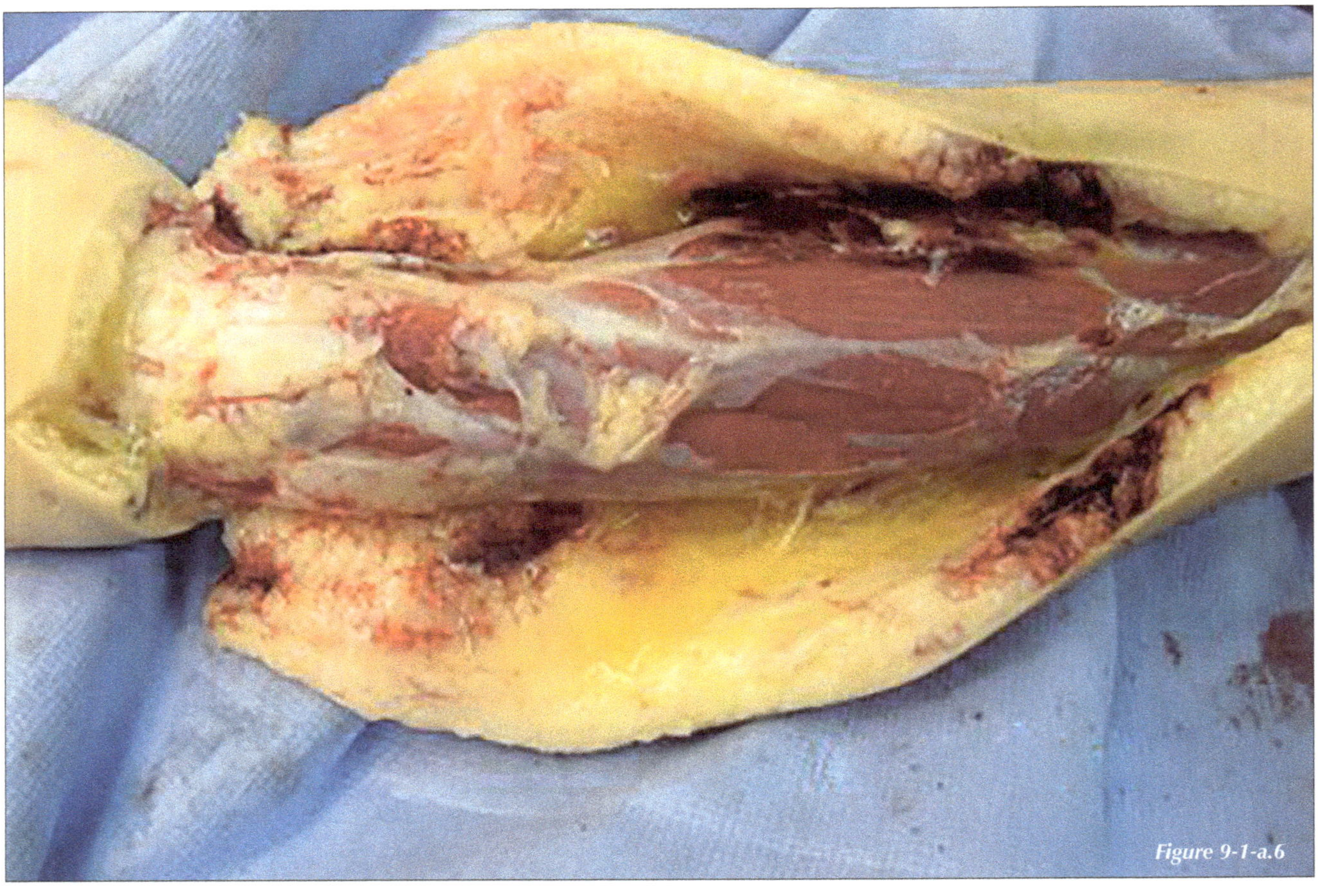

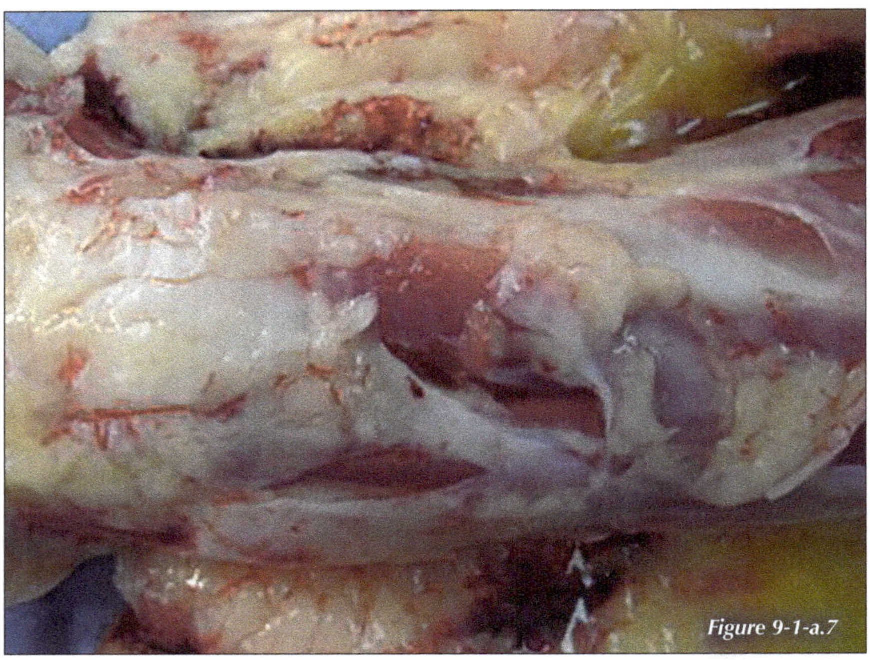

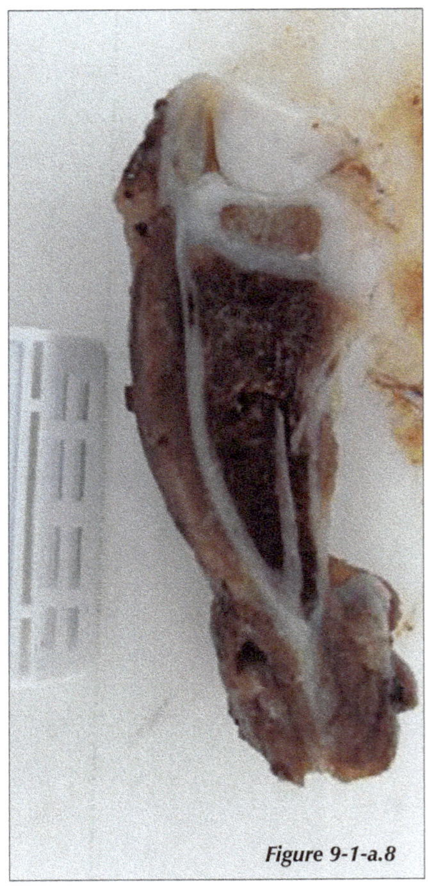

Figure 9-1-a.6. *Dissection of soft tissue of left upper extremity to show extensive soft tissue hemorrhage of dorsal proximal forearm and at wrist.*

Figure 9-1-a.7. *Dissection of soft tissue of left forearm to show hemorrhage at site of fractures of distal ulna and radius.*

Figure 9-1-a.8. *Left radius removed, fixed, and sectioned to show fracture.*

Figure 9-1-a.9. *Dura after fixation showing residual subdural hemorrhage.*

Figure 9-1-a.10. *Brain after fixation showing early brain death with disruption of right frontotemporo-parietal areas of surgical manipulation.*

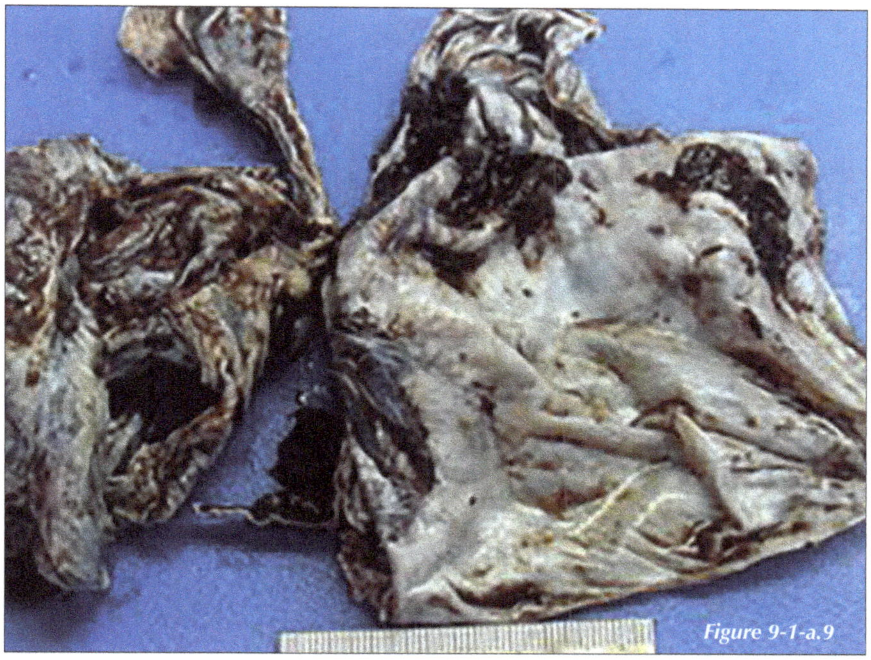

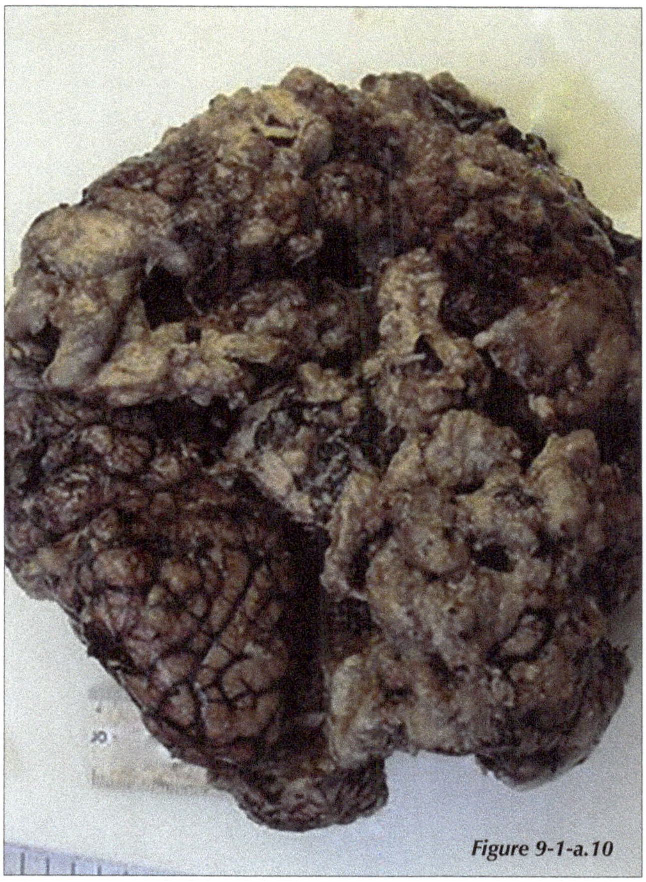

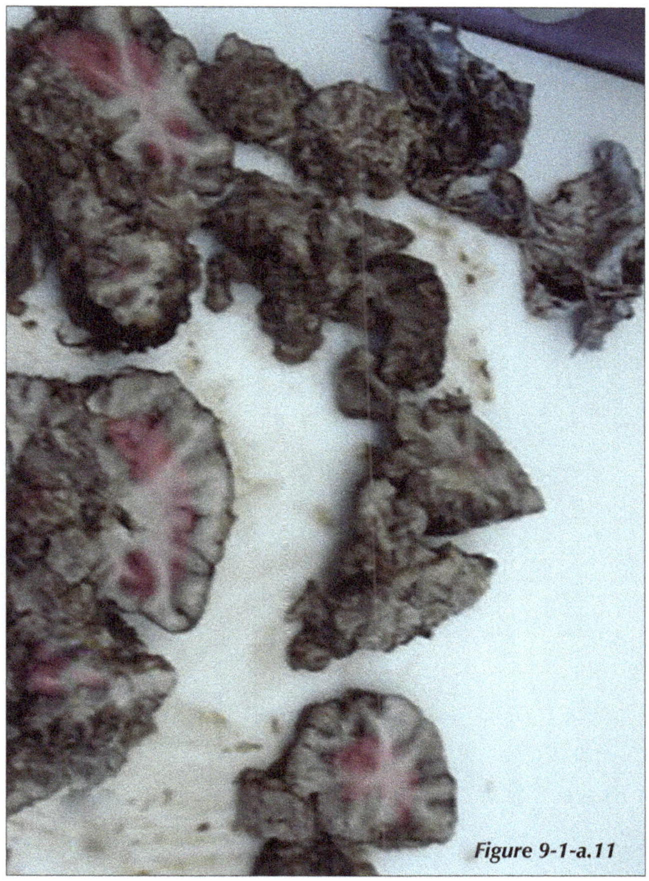

Figure 9-1-a.11. *Coronal sections of dead brain showing pink artifact of fixation.*

Figure 9-1-a.12. Eyes removed at autopsy and after fixation showing bilateral optic nerve sheath hemorrhage.

Figure 9-1-a.13. Eyes bisected to show optic nerve sheath hemorrhage and extensive retinal hemorrhages out to the ora serrata and too numerous to count.

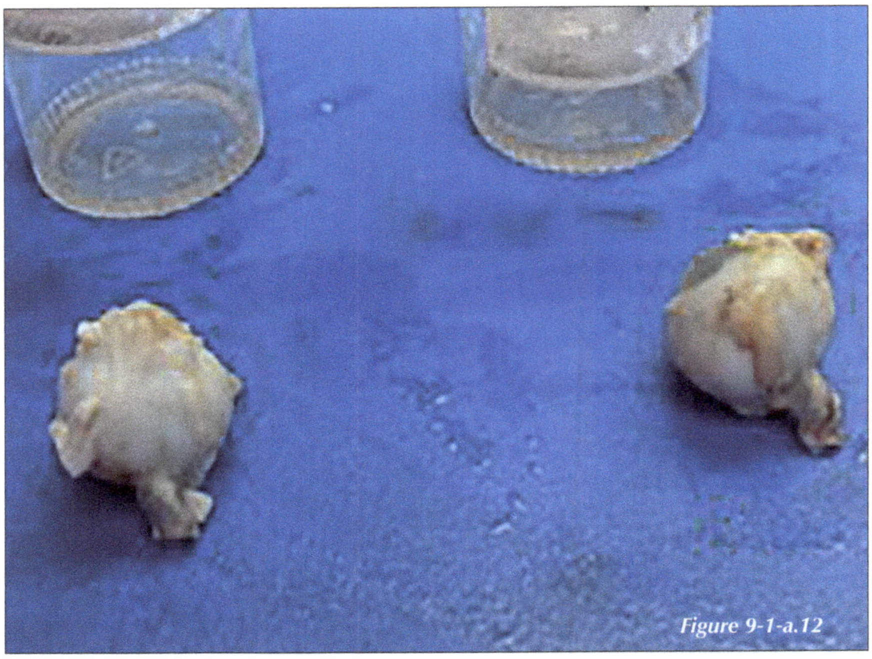

Figure 9-1-a.12

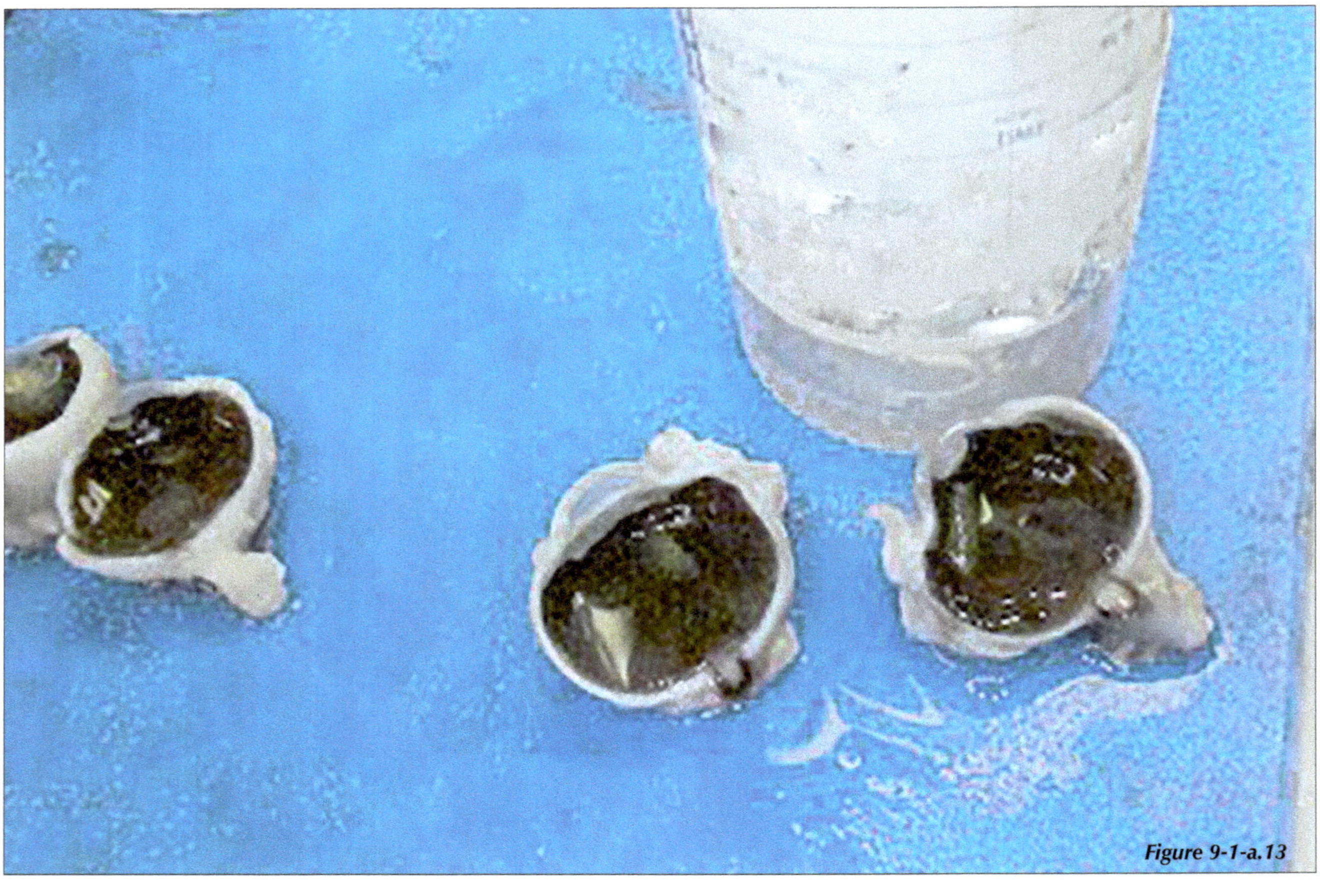

Figure 9-1-a.13

References

1. Pinckard JK, Geiselhart RJ, Moffatt E, et al. National Association of Medical Examiners position paper: medical examiner release of organs and tissues for transplantation. *Acad Forensic Pathol.* 2014;4(4):497-504.

Section IV

Test Questions

Extended Multiple Choice Questions

1. Which of these injuries are *static* head injuries? Select all that apply.
    - A. A child's head is crushed by a falling shelf while lying in their crib
    - B. A child's head is run over by the tire of a motor vehicle
    - C. A child's head is injured, and their head does not move
    - D. A child's head strikes the ground after falling from a bicycle without wearing a helmet
2. Which of these injuries are *dynamic* head injuries? Select all that apply.
    - A. A child's head strikes the chair in front of them when thrown from an unbuckled car set in a motor vehicle accident
    - B. A child's head is injured when thrown against a wall by a parent
    - C. A child's head is injured and jerks rapidly
    - D. A child's head is run over by a motor vehicle
    - E. A child's head is injured as they fall from a treehouse
3. Select all statements that are true of thoracic and chest injury.
    - A. Thoracic injuries account for 25% of all adult traumatic death
    - B. Abusive chest trauma is rarely lethal in children
    - C. Rib fractures are never caused by cardiopulmonary resuscitation (CPR)
    - D. Rib fractures account for up to 51% of all fractures in abused children
    - E. Rib fractures are commonly caused by accidents
    - F. Abusive chest trauma is frequently lethal in children
    - G. Rib fractures account for as much as 60% of fractures in infants
    - H. Rib fractures are usually caused by CPR
    - I. Rib fractures are uncommon abusive injuries, accounting for only 3% of injuries in children
    - J. Rib fractures are rarely caused by CPR
4. Select all the steps of the forensic autopsy of the chest.
    - A. Stripping the pleural membrane from the ribs
    - B. Taking radiographs of the chest
    - C. Checking for hemorrhage around the fracture site of rib injuries
    - D. Inspecting only anterior ribs for fracture
    - E. Checking for hemorrhage in intercostal muscles adjacent to site of injury

5. Select all scenarios wherein a forensic pathologist should suspect abuse.
    A. A 7-year-old child shows evidence of 1 minor fracture to the anterior ribs on radiograph after receiving CPR
    B. A 3-week-old child shows evidence of significant rib fractures on a radiograph
    C. A 2-year-old child has significant disruption of the cortex and adjacent bony trabeculae surrounding the ribs
    D. A 3-year-old child has white bulging knobs on the rib bones
    E. A 5-month-old child shows no evidence of rib fractures in radiograph
6. Select all that are potential mechanisms of death of blunt soft tissue trauma.
    A. Large volumes of bloodshed into the soft tissue
    B. Embolism released by the crushed fat of the soft tissues
    C. Profuse bloodshed though skin lesions
    D. Effects of stress associated with pain and fear
    E. Bursting of spleen
    F. Effects of stress associated with traumatic shock
7. Select all of the following that fall under the jurisdiction of the medical examiner or coroner (ME/C).
    A. Individuals who die suddenly
    B. Individuals who die unexpectedly
    C. Individuals who die of natural causes
    D. Individuals who die of possibly unnatural causes
    E. Individuals who are children
    F. Individuals who die in the custody of law enforcement
    G. Individuals who die during surgeries
    H. Individuals who die during an interaction with law enforcement
    I. Individuals who die in the workplace
    J. Individuals who die outside of medical care
8. Select all that are likely indicators of abuse.
    A. The child does not show rib fractures in radiographs
    B. The child has a deep bruise on the sternum
    C. The child has multiple rib fractures on both sides
    D. The child has large bruises on either side of the chest
    E. The child has fractures to the anterior, lateral, or posterior aspects of the ribs
    F. The child has fracture through the cortex of the inner surface of the bone
    G. The child has small fractures of the anterior ribs after CPR

9. Select all that are possible mechanisms of abdominal injury.
    - A. Direct blunt force to the abdomen
    - B. Punch or blow to the abdomen
    - C. Direct blunt force to the head
    - D. Punch or blow to the chest
    - E. Indirect forces of deceleration (eg, being thrown against a wall or object)
    - F. Motor vehicle accidents

10. What are the *requirements* for determining the cause of death as drowning in children? Select all that apply.
    - A. Some other causes of death have been ruled out
    - B. The individual was seen submerged in water or was found in water
    - C. The individual has evidence of broken ribs
    - D. All other causes of death have been ruled out
    - E. The individual was found alone in a bathtub
    - F. The individual has bruising on the neck

11. What are the responsibilities of the medicolegal system in death and crime scene investigations? Select all that apply.
    - A. Taking telephone reports of deaths
    - B. Determining the cause and manner of death
    - C. Identifying the deceased, if unknown
    - D. Arranging the transportation of bodies to the medical examiner office
    - E. Talking to other professionals in the field for their opinion
    - F. Determining the time of death
    - G. Photographing the relatives of the victim
    - H. Determining how the injuries occurred
    - I. Documenting any natural disease present
    - J. Ordering medical records and police reports
    - K. Treating the victim's injuries before death
    - L. Taking telephone reports of deaths
    - M. Documenting injuries or lack of injuries
    - N. Collecting evidence, including toxicology specimens as well as materials for DNA analysis, hair, fibers, or other types of material
    - O. Determining or excluding other contributory or causative factors of death
    - P. Responding to and investigating certain death scenes
    - Q. Responding to emergency calls with police/other responders
    - R. Providing expert testimony if the case goes to trial

Single Best Answer Multiple Choice Questions

1. Why is the need for children's tissue and organs so acute?
   - A. Because children can have adult organs transplanted
   - B. Because children need size-matched organs and tissues
   - C. Because children must have organs removed before death
   - D. Because children are all the same size
2. What is the mandate of medical examiners and coroners?
   - A. To determine cause and manner of death, remove evidence from the body, and photograph injuries
   - B. To determine cause and mechanism of death, seize evidence from the body, and document injuries and disease
   - C. To determine cause and manner of death, seize evidence from the body, and diagnose disease
   - D. To determine cause and manner of death, seize evidence from the body, and document injuries and disease
3. What is a retinal hemorrhage, specifically in relation to abusive and deadly head trauma?
   - A. Rippling of the cornea of the eye
   - B. Tearing of the iris of the eye
   - C. Bleeding of the retina of the eye
   - D. Bleeding of the iris of the eye
   - E. Denting of the retina of the eye
   - F. Bleeding of the cornea of the eye
   - G. Tearing of the cornea of the eye

Categorizing with Diagrams Questions

1. Label each image as either *static head injury* or *dynamic head injury*.

1-a. ______________________________

1-b. ______________________________

1-c. ______________________________

1-d. ______________________________

1-e. ______________________________

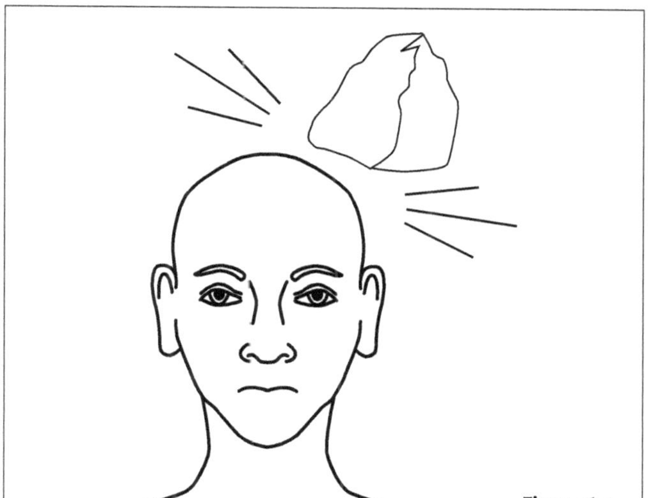

Figure 1-a

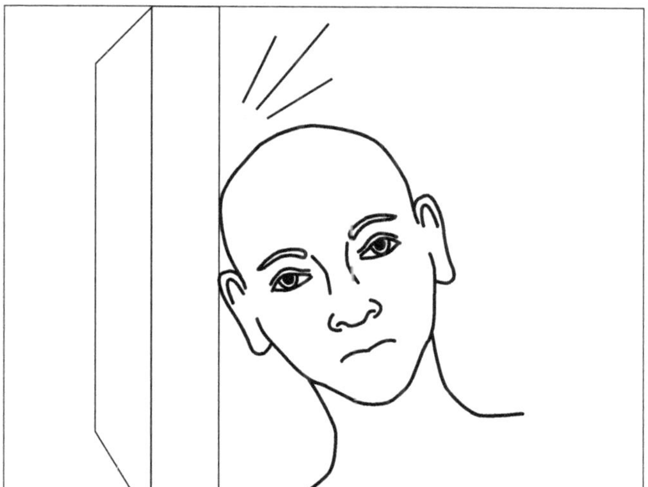

Figure 1-b

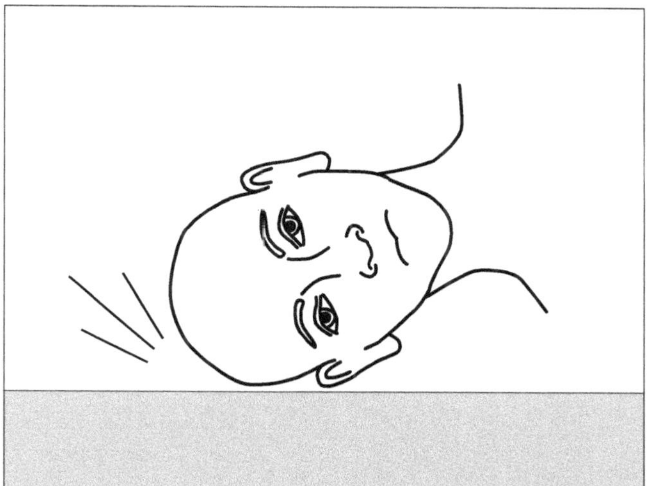

Figure 1-c

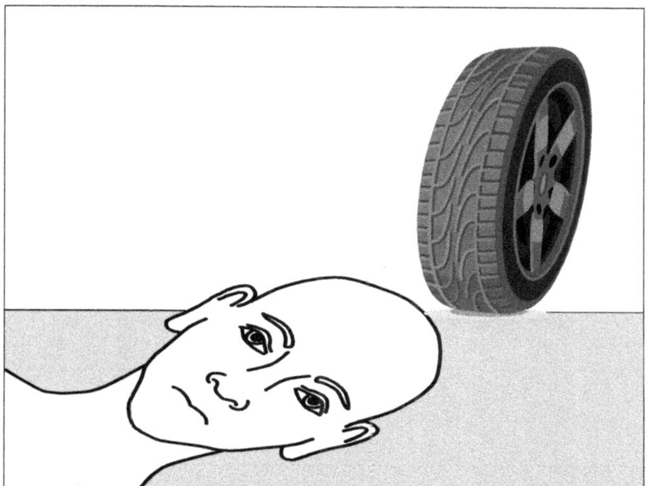

Figure 1-d

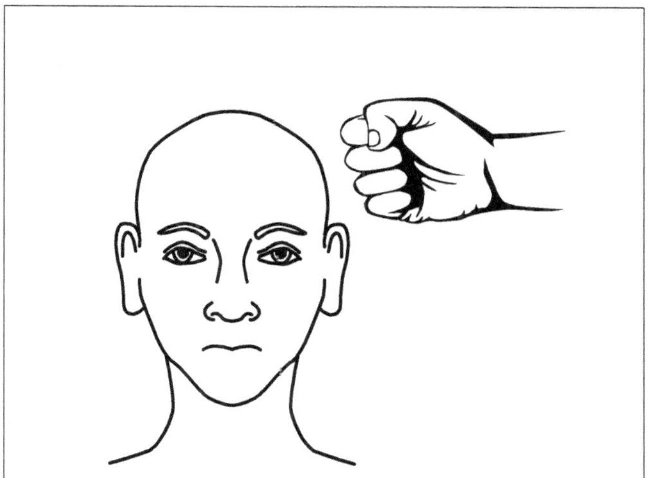

Figure 1-e

Short Answer Questions

1. How do ME/Cs determine if a child is a candidate for tissue procurement, and what steps must they take before beginning the process?

2. Define distraction injury of the cervical spine, and identify the mechanism by which it is most commonly caused.

3. How is retinal hemorrhaging related to head trauma?

4. How do the responsibilities of the medicolegal system lead to determining the cause of death?

5. What is the relationship between epidural hemorrhages of the cervical spine and abusive head trauma?

Matching Questions

Match each phrase or image to the term it defines.

Group I

1. Scalding Burns	______	A. Produced when an individual makes contact with a hot object for several seconds
2. Contact Burns	______	B. Produced when an individual is exposed to an open fire
3. Chemical Burns	______	C. Produced when an individual comes into contact with a corrosive substance
4. Flame Burns	______	D. Produced when an individual or part of an individual is held under or submerged in hot water

Group II

1. Intentional Scalding Burns	______	A. Large area of solid burn with a tide mark "a sharp line of distinction between the burned and unburned areas with no tapering off or lessening"
2. Accidental Scalding Burns	______	B. Tapering and lessening of the degree of burning in areas, no distinct line where the burn ends
3. Intentional Contact Burns	______	C. Not a full thickness burns, typically no recognizable pattern to the marks
4. Accidental Contact Burns	______	D. Usually cause a full thickness burn in a specific area and are often in a recognizable shape such as a curling iron, heat grid, cigarette, iron, or heater grate

Group III

1. Cervical Cord Contusion	______	A. Injury to the upper part of the spine, typically caused by crushing or blunt force to the spine
2. Distraction Injury	______	B. A very rare abusive injury of the cervical cord, typically caused by severe shaking while grasping the head

Clinical Vignette Questions

1. During an autopsy, a child has large amounts of blood in the subdural region of the brain. What type of injury should be suspected? How are these injuries induced?

____

____

____

____

____

____

2. During an autopsy, a child is seen to have an acute head injury. Further investigation shows a traumatically induced tear of the arachnoid and cerebrospinal fluid in the subdural space. What type of injury should be suspected? How are these injuries induced?

____

____

____

____

____

____

3. During an autopsy, a child has extensive contusions, abrasions, and pattern injuries to their chest and back. Internal examination shows large amounts of soft tissue hemorrhaging, but no organs seem to have specific damage. Analysis of vitreous fluid shows the child was not dehydrated. What is the likely cause of death? What piece of evidence supports your determination?

____

____

____

____

____

____

Ordering Parts Questions

For each group, number the steps in the order that they should be performed.

Group I: External Examination

1. ________	A. Describe each injury by size, color, and shape
2. ________	B. Examine the body's condition at arrival to the morgue
3. ________	C. Document the state of nutrition, hygiene, hair growth, unusual soiling, or congenital abnormalities as well as any evidence of dehydration
4. ________	D. Examine clothing for evidence and document
5. ________	E. Examine genitalia for evidence of injury, and, if assault is suspected, oral, vaginal, rectal, or penile swabs for DNA should be performed
6. ________	F. Examine and photograph the face, scalp, neck, chest, abdomen, back, genitalia, buttocks, and extremities, noting any identifying marks, scars, and/or fresh, healing, or healed injuries
7. ________	G. Inspect the mouth, including teeth, lips, gums, and frenula, and distinguish injuries from those that may have been caused by resuscitation or intubation
8. ________	H. Measure height, weight, and dimensions of the head, chest, and abdomen
9. ________	I. Take microscopic tissues samples of any injuries to determine the age

Group II: Internal Examination

1. ________
2. ________
3. ________
4. ________
5. ________
6. ________
7. ________
8. ________
9. ________
10. ________
11. ________
12. ________
13. ________

A. Open the head for internal examination by reflecting the scalp forwards and backwards to expose the underlying calvarium

B. Remove the brain and spinal cord, especially in cases of suspected head trauma

C. Expose the rib cage and peritoneal cavity by reflecting the skin and soft tissue of the anterior body

D. Note and photograph all presence of blood or other fluids in the pleural cavity, pericardial sac, or abdominal cavity

E. Document and photograph any injuries to the soft tissues of the rib cage and peritoneal cavity, and take sections for microscopic examination

F. Examine the head cavity for any hemorrhage or injury and describe, photograph, and document all findings as well as take microscopic sections for examination

G. Manually remove the parietal pleura from the rib cage to view each rib and note any fractures, as they may not appear in radiographs

H. Closely examine the scalp, shaving hair to expose any wounds

I. If blood is present in the periosteum of the calvarium, check for underlying skull fracture and remove the periosteum to view the underlying bone; document and photograph any findings

J. Lift off the calvarium and look for subdural or epidural blood; document and photograph any findings

K. Make incisions down the line of the back to dissect the underlying soft tissues of the back, buttocks, and extremities; look for hemorrhages

L. Strip the dura from the inner surface of the calvarium and cranial fossae, and inspect for bone fracture

M. If blood is present in the pleural cavity, pericardial sac, or abdominal cavity, attempt to measure the amount

Using Case Studies

Carefully read the following case studies and examine the provided images. Using the information found, concisely answer the questions that follow.

Case Study 1

This 4-year-old boy was sleeping in a camper with a faulty generator with the rest of his family. All family members died.

Table 1. Autopsy Results
— A few drops of blood under the nose — CO 82%

1. Using Case Study 1, identify the cause of death and manner of death and give evidence from the case study to support your determinations.

   Cause of Death:

   ____

   Evidence:

   ____

   ____

   ____

   ____

   ____

   Manner of Death:

   ____

   Evidence:

   ____

   ____

   ____

   ____

   ____

Case Study 2

This 3-year-old girl was found near a creek bed, nude, with her clothing scattered around her. The child was unresponsive with a body temperature of approximately 75°F. She was last seen playing in the neighborhood with other children. The father came home from work around 5:00 PM to find the mother passed out on the couch drunk. The mother did not know where the 3-year-old child was. The father went looking for his daughter and called police to report her missing. Three hours later, she was found by a police officer a quarter of a mile away from the residence.

Table 2. Autopsy Results

EXTERNAL EXAMINATION

— There was extensive caking of dried mud covering the entire body, including the hair and face

INJURIES

TYPE	*MEASUREMENT*
Multiple contusions and abrasions were present	
Nose was reddened and contused with an abrasion on the right nasal ala	1 mm
Abrasion on bridge of nose	2 mm
Contusion on right upper lid and outer canthus	2.5 cm x 1.2 cm
2 parallel contusions, left forehead	
Left upper lid contusions	10 mm x 1 mm, 8 mm x 2 mm
Left upper lid abrasion	2 mm
Scattered abrasions on preauricular area of right cheek and chin	
Left upper lip contusion	7 mm
Reflected scalp showed the parietal and occipital areas to have subscapular contusions on each side	5 to 6 cm
Trunk and extremities had numerous linear abrasions randomly distributed	2 mm to 2.5 cm in length
Similar scattered abrasions on abdomen	
Left lower chest contusion	8 mm area
Linear abrasions on lower extremities	2 to 25 mm
2 abrasions on right lower leg	
Scattered abrasions on back overlying scapulae and upper portion of buttocks	
Right hand, scattered linear abrasions	
Laceration on left hand index finger	3 mm
Right thigh near genitalia, multiple circular contusions	5 to 10 mm

2. Based on Case Study 2, what is your determination of the manner of death? Would your determination of the manner of death change without the details of the individual's history?

Case Study 3

The mother reported she was holding this 3-month-old girl when she went to get Pepcid, which the infant was supposed to take twice a day. When the mother looked down at the infant, she noticed the child looked blue in the face and was bleeding from her nose. The grandmother began CPR. The infant had a history of breathing problems. The mother admitted to consuming Comet cleanser periodically while pregnant with this infant. The infant was in the ED about a week before death for vomiting blood. The infant was hospitalized at that time to determine the cause of the bleeding, but after 2 days the mother discharged her against medical advice. The infant had also been hospitalized 2 other times since birth, once for apnea that wasn't demonstrated during the hospitalization and once for pneumonia. At the time of the infant's death, the mother was 3 weeks pregnant. The mother was 15 years old. There were 3 other teenagers who lived in the residence.

Table 3. Autopsy Results

INJURIES

Lungs

— Anterior petechial hemorrhages with edema fluid exuding from the cut surfaces

Thymus

— Several small petechial hemorrhages on the anterior surface

MICROSCOPIC EXAMINATION

— ***Lungs:*** Congestion, and the alveoli contained macrophages with apparent hemosiderin

— ***Kidney:*** Demonstrated several areas that showed focal segmental glomerulosclerosis and several areas of mononuclear cell accumulation adjacent to the glomeruli

3. Based on Case Study 3, what is your determination of the manner of death? Would your determination of the manner of death change without the details of the individual's history?

Case Study 4

This 2-year-old boy was at home with his father when he was said to have had an unwitnessed fall from a chair. The father had placed the child in a chair with a make-shift booster seat made of 2 telephone books. The father then left the room, and after a few minutes, he heard a thud. He returned and found the child obviously injured and called 911. EMS arrived and found the child wearing only a diaper and with a decreased level of consciousness and difficult respirations. He was transported to a hospital, where he was noted to have bruising of the chest, back, and right hip. The child arrested in the emergency department (ED) and could not be resuscitated. The father subsequently admitted to striking the child in the chest and stomach area.

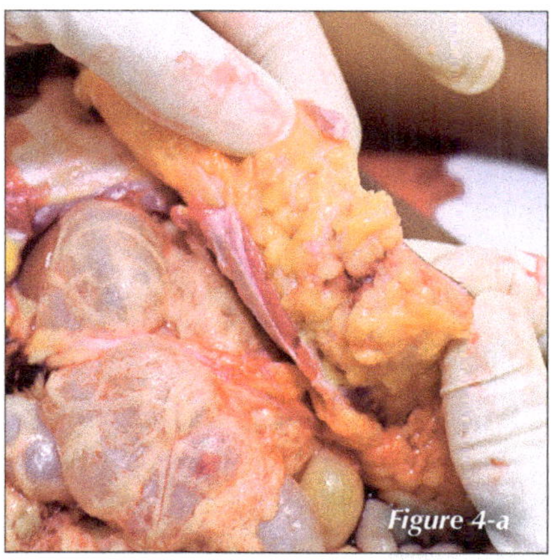

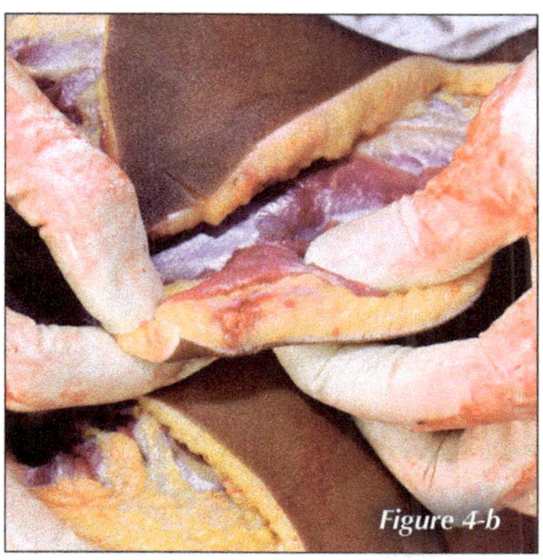

Figure 4-a and b. *Abdominal wall showing hemorrhage beneath contusions.*

Table 4-a. Autopsy Results

External Examination	
Type	***Measurement***
Left forearm scar	25 mm x 5 mm
Left elbow scar	15 mm x 10 mm
Right knee scar	8 mm
Right thigh, vertical scar	120 mm x 4 mm
Injuries	
Head	
Right cheek contusion	5 mm
Right chin contusion	10 mm
Left ear contusion	15 mm
Left cheek contusions	20 mm x 10 mm, 30 mm x 15 mm
Reflected scalp, 3 focal subgaleal hemorrhages over left parietal	3 mm, 5 mm, 8 mm
Healing abrasions on nose	1 to 2 mm
Chest/Abdomen	
Contusions over midline	110 mm x 90 mm area, 5 to 3 mm each
Right lower chest contusion	10 mm
Left lower chest contusion	10 mm
Left mid-chest contusions	5 to 15 mm
Right chest, axillary region, abrasions	1 to 20 mm
Left upper chest, healing abrasions	1 to 5 mm
Blood in right side of chest	50 mL
Blood in left side of chest	80 mL
2 contusions, right abdominal wall	30 mm x 15 mm, 20 mm x 10 mm
Left abdominal wall contusion	40 mm x 20 mm
Lower abdomen contusion	110 mm x 15 mm
Lacerations of right and left lobes of liver	
— the largest in the parenchyma of the right lobe	60 mm x 40 mm x 30 mm
Hemoperitoneum	300 mL
Soft tissue hemorrhage in the mesentery of the large and small bowel	
Severe soft tissue hemorrhage in peripancreatic fat, periadrenal fat, and perirenal fat	
Hemorrhage in all lobes of both lungs	
Soft tissue hemorrhages corresponding to contusions on chest	
Severe soft tissue hemorrhage in the chest cavity involving the mediastinum extending to the upper chest and lower neck regions	
Left parietal pleural hemorrhage	
Right anterolateral fractures of ribs 2 through 6 and ribs 8 through 11	
Left lateral fractures of ribs 2 through 11	
Hemorrhage present in tissue surrounding the fractures	

(continued)

Table 4-a. Autopsy Results *(continued)*

INJURIES *(CONTINUED)*

Back

TYPE	MEASUREMENT
Right upper back, contusion resembling a bite mark	40 mm x 35 mm
Midline back contusion	20 mm
Right mid-back contusion	15 mm
Right lateral back contusions	15 mm, 5 mm
Left mid-back, contusion resembling a bite mark	45 mm x 35 mm
Contusion, just below mid-back	20 mm x 10 mm
— with healing abrasions	1 to 5 mm
Right hip contusion	20 mm x 5 mm
Right buttock contusions	10 to 120 mm
Left buttock and left upper thigh contusion	160 mm x 120 mm area
Healing abrasions on right and left buttocks	1 to 4 mm

Extremities

Right forearm and right hand contusions (4)	5 to 20 mm
Left forearm contusions (3)	5 to 10 mm
Right thigh contusion	40 mm x 20 mm
Left inguinal region contusion	60 mm x 30 mm
Left thigh contusion	30 mm x 15 mm
Left calf contusion	15 mm

Body Cavities

— ***Mediastinum:*** Right-shifted; thymus with hemorrhage; extensive mediastinal soft tissue hemorrhage

— ***Lungs:*** Contusions in all 5 lobes with hemorrhage

— ***Liver:*** Lacerations

— ***Pancreas:*** Mild focal hemorrhage

— ***Peripancreatic:*** Soft tissue, extensive hemorrhage

GI Tract

— Extensive hemorrhage with areas of lacerations of mesentery of the large and small bowel

— Large intestinal serosa, areas of hemorrhage

— ***Adrenals:*** Extensive periadrenal hemorrhage bilaterally in surrounding fat

MICROSCOPIC EXAMINATION

— ***Lungs:*** Patchy areas of interstitial and alveolar hemorrhage present; multi-focal interstitial pneumonia

— ***Liver:*** Acute hemorrhage

— ***Pancreas:*** Patchy acute hemorrhage

— ***Thymus:*** Patchy acute hemorrhage

— ***GI tract:*** Small and large bowel mesentery, acute hemorrhage

— ***Endocrine system:*** Periadrenal acute hemorrhage

— ***Skin:*** Acute hemorrhage in contusions

— ***Rib fractures:*** Acute soft tissue

Figure 4-c. *Chest opened showing hemorrhage in mediastinum and pulmonary contusions.*

Figure 4-d. *Abdomen opened to expose liver laceration.*

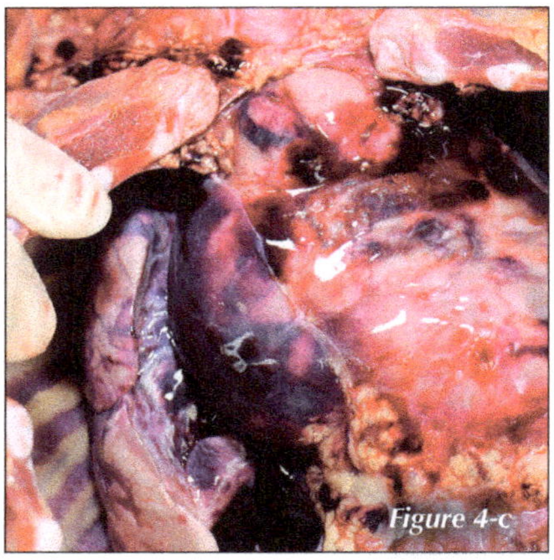

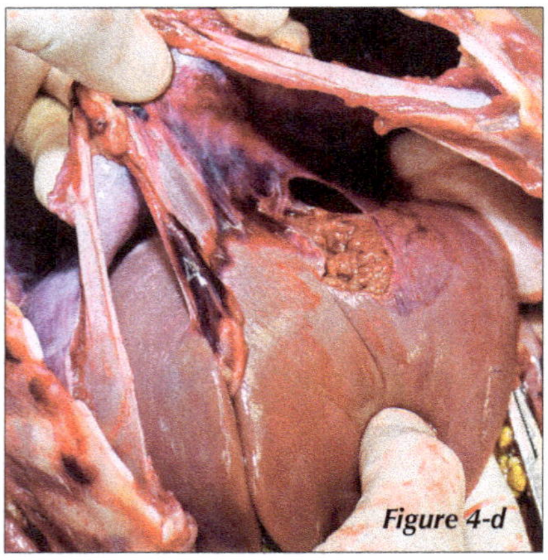

Table 4-b. Diagnoses

Blunt Chest Trauma

- Ribs, bilateral fractures
- Extensive mediastinal soft tissue hemorrhage
- Lungs, bilateral contusions
- Hemothorax, bilateral

Blunt Abdominal Trauma

- Liver, right and left lobe, lacerations
- Small and large bowel mesentery, lacerations
- Peripancreatic, perirenal and periadrenal fat, hemorrhage
- Hemoperitoneum

Integument and Soft Tissue

- Head, chest, abdomen, back, and upper and lower extremities, contusions and hemorrhage

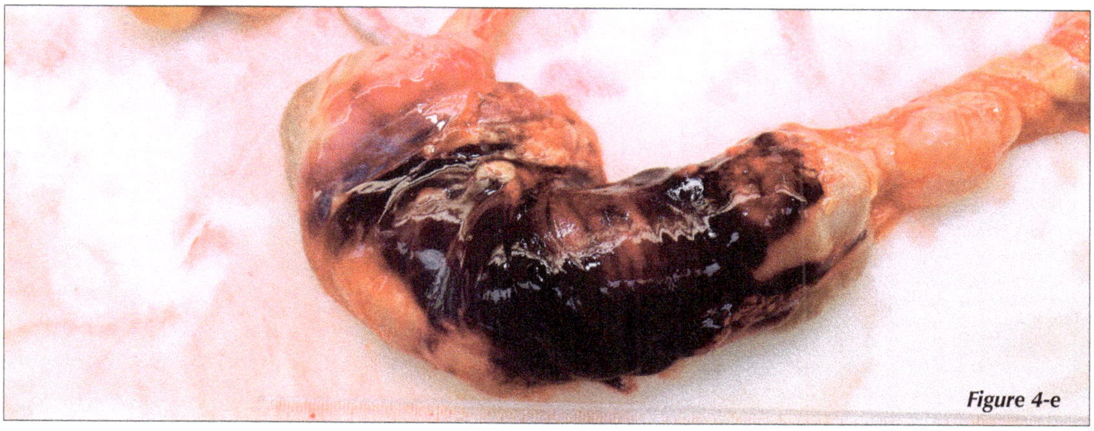

Figure 4-e

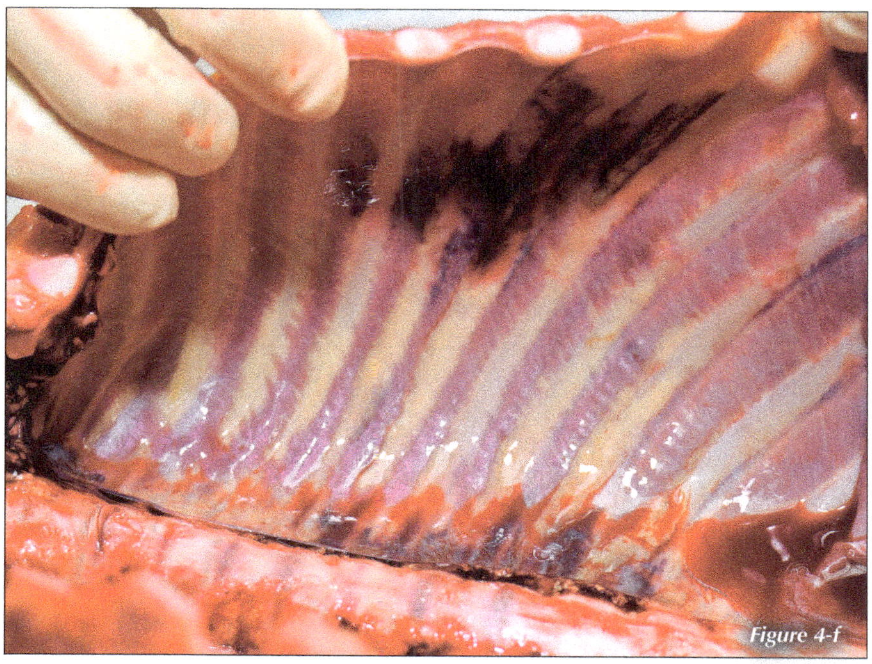

Figure 4-f

Figure 4-e. *Hemorrhage over serosal surface of cecum.*

Figure 4-f. *Left chest showing subpleural hemorrhage over rib fractures.*

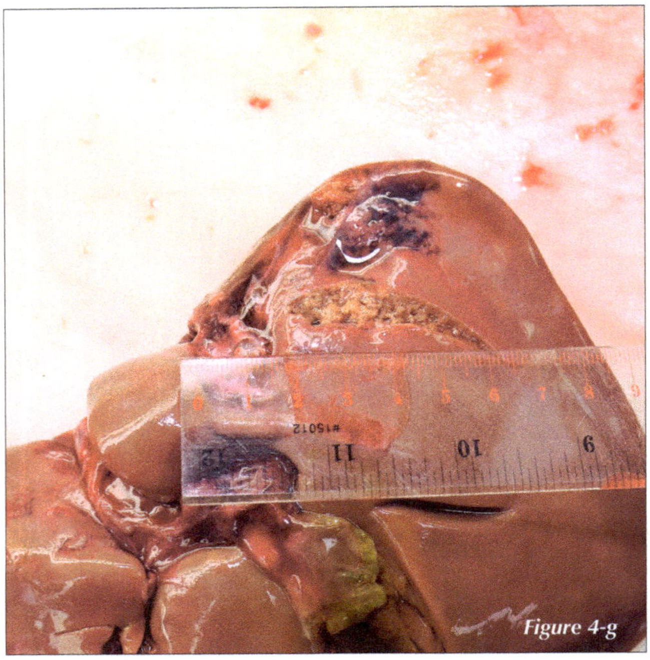

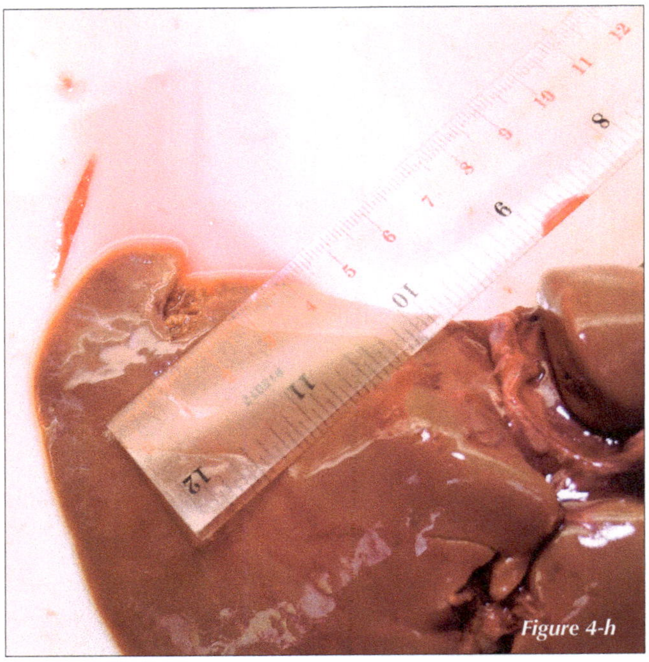

Figure 4-g and h. *Inferior surface of liver showing laceration.*

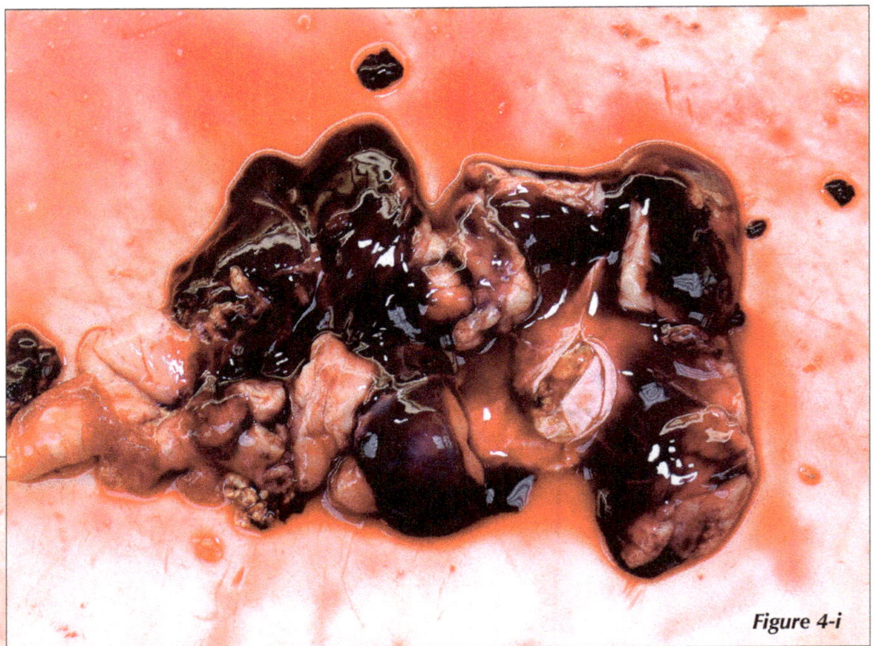

Figure 4-i. *Pancreas removed and showing hemorrhage.*

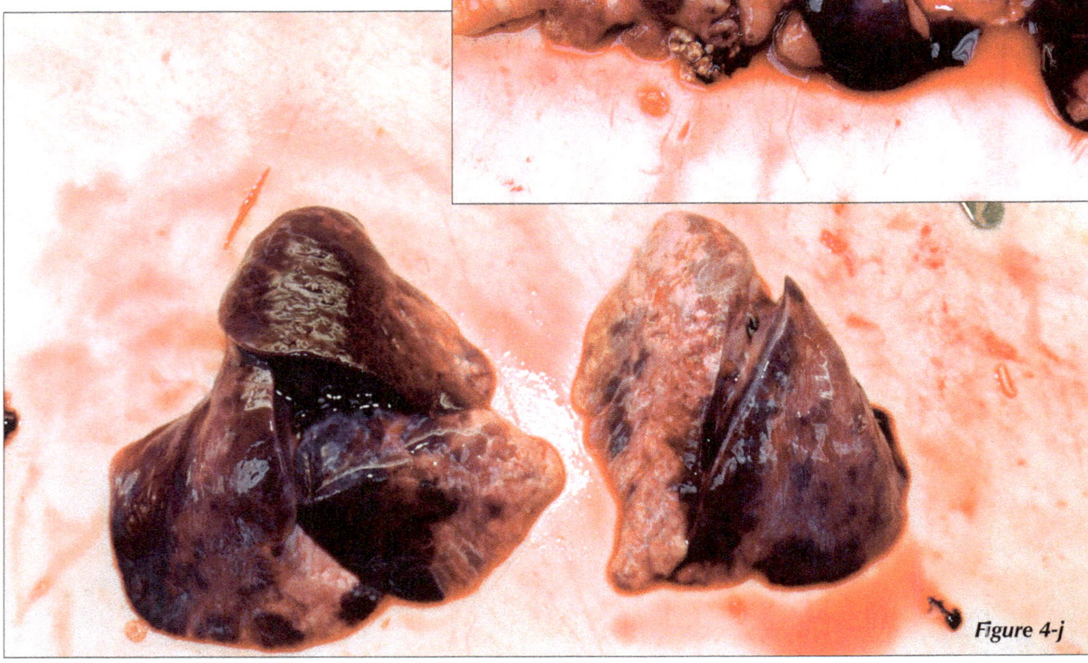

Figure 4-j. *Lungs showing contusions in all lobes.*

4. Using Case Study 4, interpret the correlation between abdominal organs/structures and the types of injuries inflicted. What type of injury was inflicted (intentional/abusive or accidental), and which organs should be looked at closely to best understand the injury inflicted?

Case Study 5

According to the history, this 2-year-old boy fell into a pot of hot water. The grandmother went to the store and left a 12-year-old child in charge. There was a 14-quart pot of boiling water on a hotplate on the floor. The water was being heated to the wash the kitchen floor. The 12-year-old said she accidentally kicked the child into the pot while she was getting something out of the deep freezer. She had been severely depressed since the incidence and was threatening to kill herself. The child was unresponsive at the scene and in the ED. He died after being admitted to the hospital with burns covering 70% of his total body surface area.

Table 5-a. Autopsy Results

Injuries

— Extensive full-thickness burns, including 90 mm × 50 mm irregular area of scalding burns on right face and upper neck
— Similar burn on base of neck and right shoulder
— Burning on anterior deltoid areas and proximal medial arms
— Anterior chest and abdomen diffusely burned
— Burning on the dorsum of the penis
— Anterior, medial, lateral, and posterior surfaces of right thigh burned
— Left thigh diffusely burned
— 10 mm excoriated area at the right corner of the mouth
— Blisters, 3 to 30 mm, with clear fluid on the dorsal surface of the right foot
— ***Body cavities:*** 1000 mL fluid in peritoneal cavity

Neck Organs

— Upper airway contained frothy material

Lungs

— Increased firmness, edema; air passages contained frothy fluid

Liver

— Somewhat soft in consistency

Microscopic Examination

— ***Lungs:*** Diffuse alveolar damage
— ***Kidneys:*** Tubules dilated and lined by flattened epithelium with focal tubular epithelial necrosis present
— ***Skin:*** Resolving scald burns

Table 5-b. Diagnoses

— ***Thermal injuries:*** Skin, extensive resolving scald burns
— Diffuse alveolar damage syndrome (ARDS)
— Liver centrilobular necrosis
— Kidneys, focal tubular epithelial necrosis
— Ascites

5. Based on Case Study 5, what is your determination of the manner of death? Would your determination of the manner of death change without the details of the individual's history?

Case Study 6

The mother put this 14-month-old girl to bed at 8:30 PM, and when she woke up at 7:30 AM, the child was missing. The father worked night shifts and would usually get home at 7:30 AM. Police were notified, and the child was found in the woods near a cemetery. The child was covered by leaves and had a jump rope around the neck. The father confessed to causing the death of the child for the purpose of obtaining the benefits of a Gerber life insurance policy.

Table 6. Autopsy Results

INJURIES

— Ligature around the neck from a jump rope to which a portion of pink ribbon had been tied; the ribbon was tied tightly around the neck

— Ligature was 3 mm wide and produced a ligature furrow, which was flesh-colored and slightly indented; ligature was 4 mm wide at the level of the middle of the thyroid cartilage and extended entirely around the neck

— Knot was on the left side, and there were 4 red dots that measured 2 mm on the adjacent skin

— Three crescent abrasions on the right undersurface of the jaw suggested fingernail marks and measured 8 mm x 2 mm, 7 mm x 2 mm, and 7 mm x 1 mm

— Ant bites were found all over the body, with active ants on the body

— Healing abrasion on the left knee, 2 cm x 0.7 cm

INTERNAL EXAMINATION

— Neck showed hemorrhage on the anterior wall of the left carotid artery, 3 mm x 2 mm

Cranial Cavity

— Inner surface of scalp had 3 areas of fresh subgaleal hemorrhage, 2.5 cm x 1.5 cm, 3 cm x 1 cm, and 0.5 cm in diameter

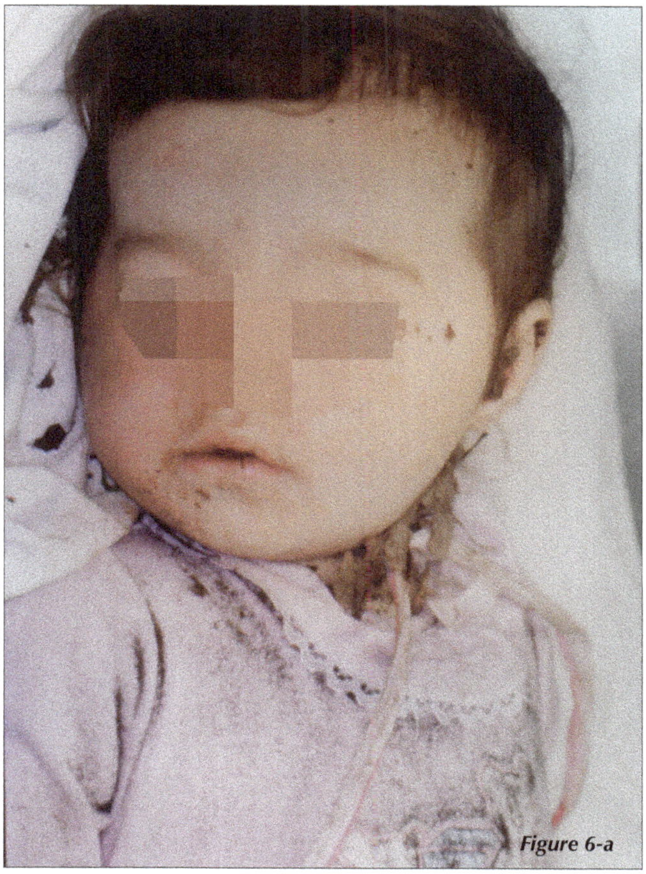

Figure 6-a

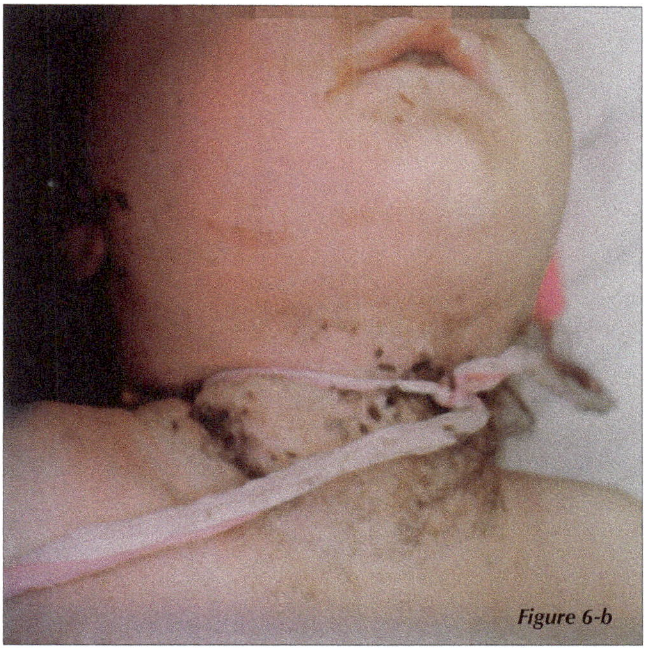

Figure 6-b

Figure 6-a. *Jump rope ligature around neck with a portion of pink ribbon tied tightly around the neck.*

Figure 6-b. *Head extended backward to demonstrate ligature across front of neck.*

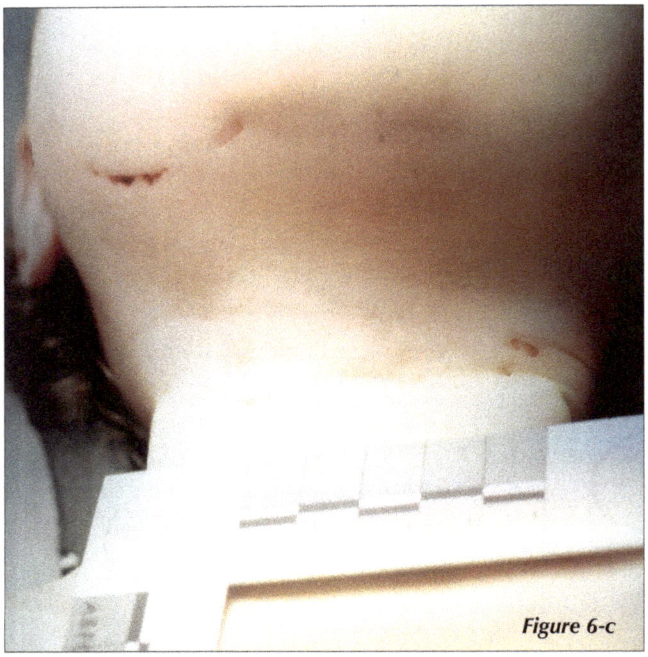

Figure 6-c

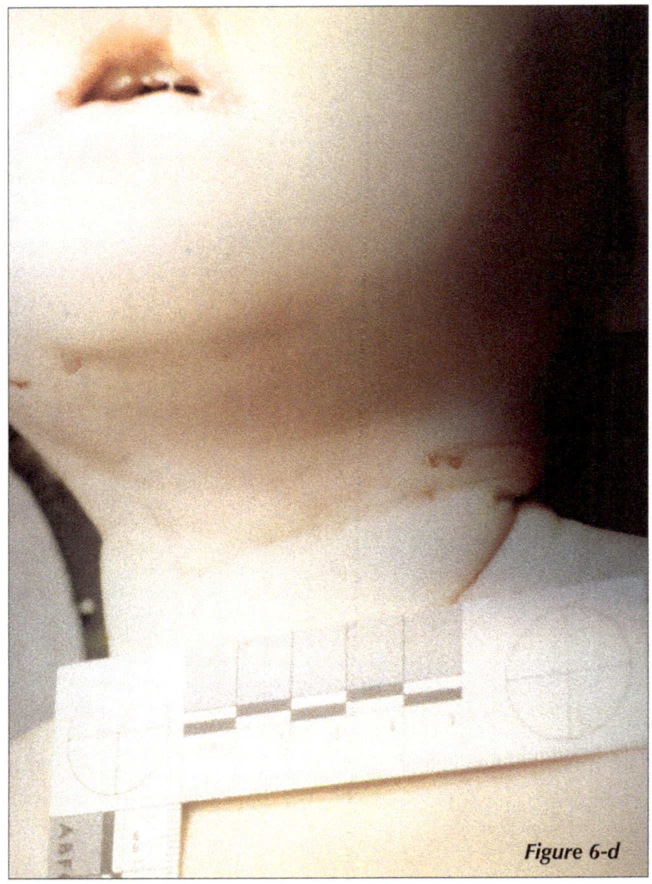

Figure 6-d

Figure 6-c. *Close-up view of 3 crescent-shaped abrasions on right underside of jaw.*

Figure 6-d. *Head extended backward to show ligature furrow across front of neck at middle of thyroid cartilage and 4 red dots on left side of neck at site of knot.*

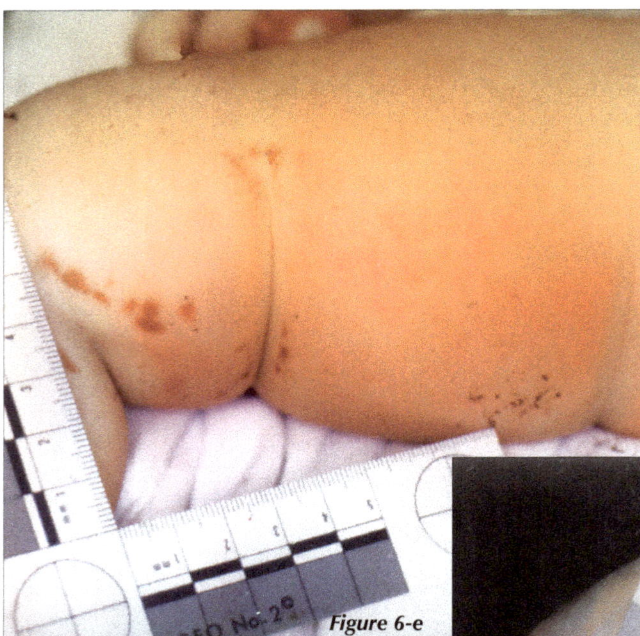

Figure 6-e

Figure 6-e. *Postmortem ant bites on right thigh.*

Figure 6-f. *Undersurface of scalp showing 3 areas of subgaleal hemorrhage.*

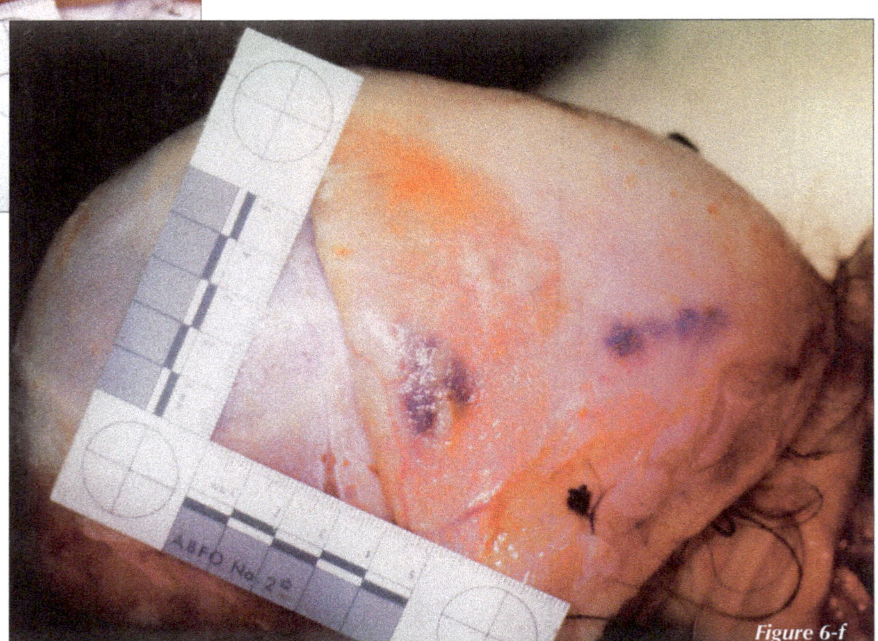

Figure 6-f

6. Using Case Study 6, identify the cause of death and manner of death and give evidence from the case study to support your determinations.

   Cause of Death:

   ____

   Evidence:

   ____

   ____

   ____

   ____

   ____

   Manner of Death:

   ____

   Evidence:

   ____

   ____

   ____

   ____

   ____

Case Study 7

This 3-month-old child was in the sole care of her father when she became unresponsive. 911 was called, and she was transported to a children's hospital. She remained unconscious and required ventilator support for 3 days because of a traumatic head injury before she was pronounced dead. A skeletal survey demonstrated that there were multiple bilateral rib fractures in various stages of healing. Permission was given for a live organ donation of the heart, lungs, and liver; the heart was taken for donation. A 3-year-old sibling of the child was born at 37 weeks and was noted to have a distended abdomen and palpable abdominal mass following birth, as well as a multicystic kidney with cystic renal dysplasia and an atrial septal defect. The child underwent a renal transplant at age 2 years and then had subsequent cellular and antibody mediated rejection. The sibling and family were well-known to the children's hospital where the child was treated.

Table 7. Autopsy Results

Injuries

Type	*Measurement*
3 blue contusions in the left upper forehead	4 mm, 3 mm (2)
Blue contusion, midforehead	10 mm x 5 mm
Right medial forehead, blue contusion	3 mm
Blue contusion, right forehead	3 mm
Subgaleal hemorrhages underlying each of the forehead contusions	
Thin layer of subdural blood over the posterior cerebral convexities and over the right and left middle and posterior cranial fossae	
Optic nerve sheath hemorrhage in both eyes	
Yellow ascetic fluid in peritoneal cavity with deep gold staining of the mesentery of the cecum and duodenum	
Entire rib cage removed, demonstrating old healing fractures of posterior left ribs 1 through 9 and right posterior ribs 1 and 4 through 9	

Microscopic Examination

- ***Mesentery of cecum:*** Numerous mononuclear cells, including macrophages; contusions of forehead all show hemorrhage of deep subcutaneous tissue with small numbers of associated neutrophils and mononuclear cells
- ***Right first rib:*** Fracture at costochondral junction with soft callus
- ***Right fourth rib:*** Fracture with abundant soft callus
- ***Right fifth rib:*** Abundant soft callus with new woven bone and formation of trabeculae
- ***Right sixth rib:*** Abundant soft callus with new woven bone and much necrotic bone being removed
- ***Right seventh rib:*** Abundant soft callus
- ***Right eighth rib:*** Soft callus
- ***Right ninth rib:*** Early soft callus
- ***Left first rib:*** Granulation tissue and dead bone at fracture site
- ***Left second rib:*** Granulation tissue and dead bone at fracture site
- ***Left third rib:*** Soft callus with woven bone at fracture site
- ***Left fourth, fifth, and sixth ribs:*** Soft callus with woven bone at fracture site
- ***Left seventh rib:*** Fracture at costochondral junction with granulation tissue
- ***Left eighth rib:*** Small fracture at costochondral junction with granulation tissue

Neuropathology

- Acute subdural blood over cerebral convexities of dura
- Small patches of subarachnoid hemorrhage on parasagittal regions of occipital lobes
- Thrombosed veins over occipital poles bilaterally
- Both eyes had prominent optic nerve sheath hemorrhage; neither eye showed any retinal hemorrhages

Microscopic Neuropathology

- Diffuse traumatic axonal injury, extensive
- Subarachnoid hemorrhage
- Acute subdural hemorrhage
- Early hypoxic encephalopathy
- Recent thrombus in cortical veins of bilateral occipital lobes

7. Based on Case Study 7, what is your determination of the manner of death? Would your determination of the manner of death change without the details of the individual's history?

Case Study 8

The father, who was caring for this 9-month-old boy, said he found the child unresponsive in a crib located in the living room. There was white froth exuding from the child's nose. The father said he fed the child and put him in the crib and then went into his room to sleep. When he woke up 3 hours later, he found the child not breathing. The child was dead at the scene. The crib had many blankets, toys, and clothes in it. At the scene recreation, the father stated that when he found the child, a heavy comforter was wrapped several times around the child's body, covering the head as well as all portions of the body, as if the child had lain on the comforter and rolled himself up from one end to the other. The arms were alongside the body, and the child was face down. The parents of the child were teenagers and often fought about the child's care. The mother worked days while the father watched the child, and the father worked nights while the mother cared for him. Two weeks before the child's death, the father was angry and threw all of the child's clothing out the door, stating he "hated the little SOB" and was "going to kill him."

Table 8. Autopsy Results

External Examination

— Blanching lividity from the mid to left side of forehead, over the nose, and over the right cheek

Injuries

— Both buttocks were heavily bruised, and on incision into the subcutaneous tissues, there was extensive fresh hemorrhage throughout all areas

Microscopic Examination

— Buttocks showed areas of older injury with iron staining and extensive acute hemorrhage

Figure 8-a. *Child at the scene where he was found face down inside a comforter that was wrapped around him several times.*

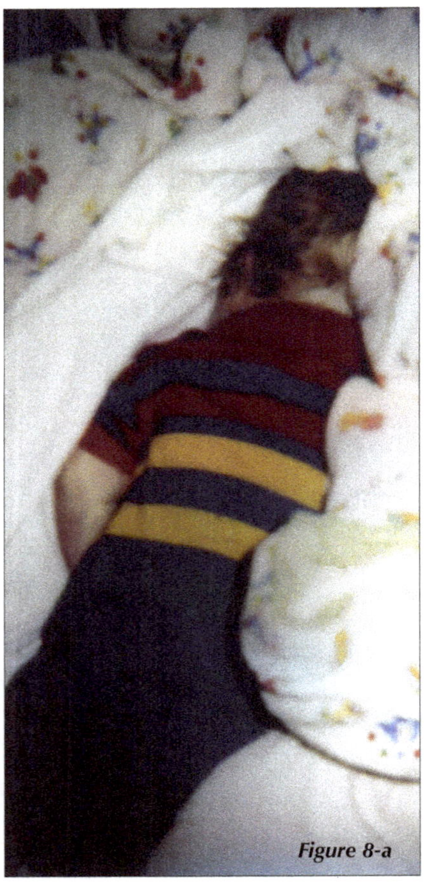

Figure 8-b. *Child turned supine at the scene after the comforter was removed, showing lividity blanched over mid-forehead, nose, and right cheek from face down position.*

Figure 8-c. *Posterior surface of lower back and buttocks with bruising of buttocks.*

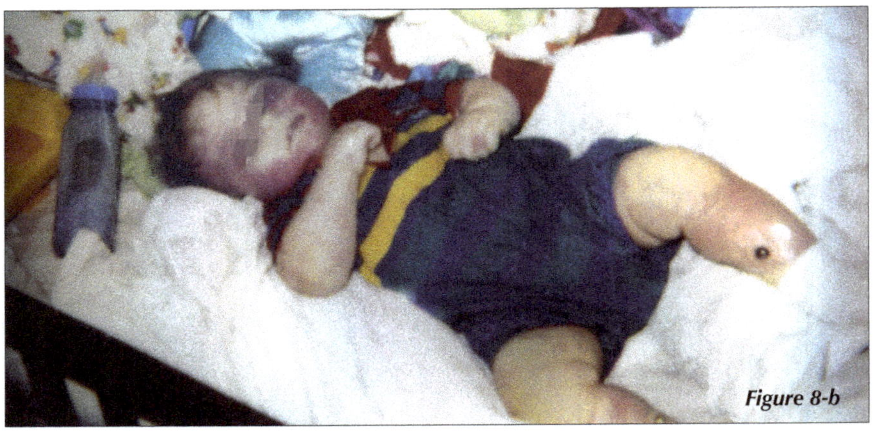

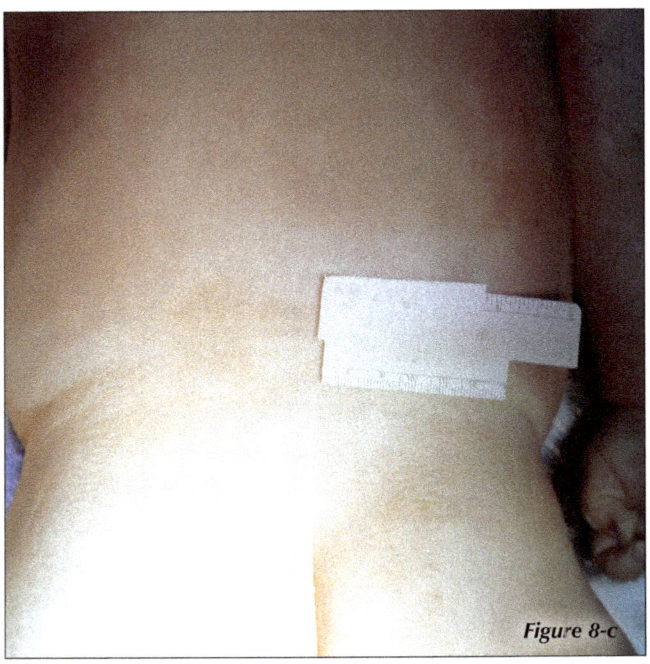

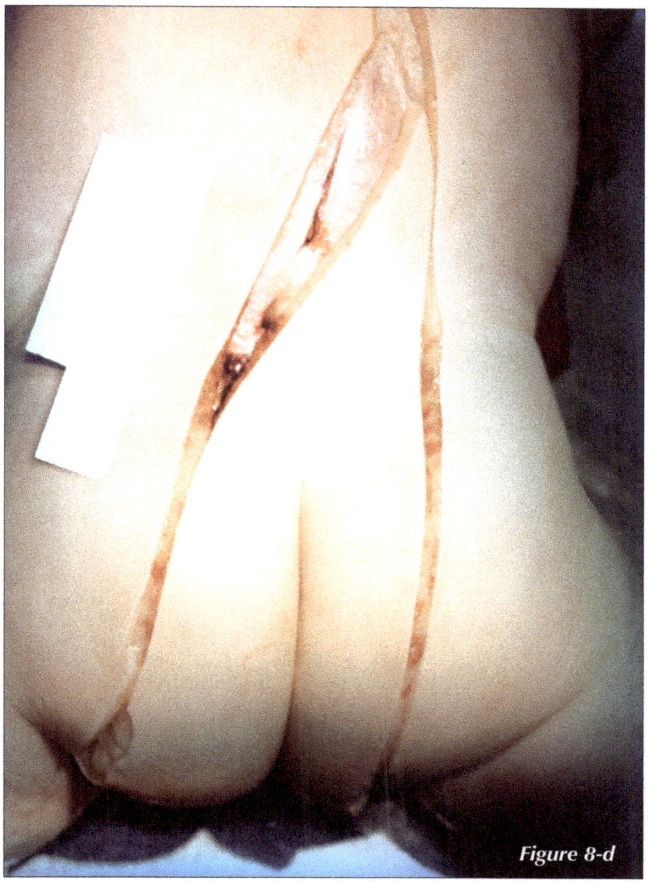

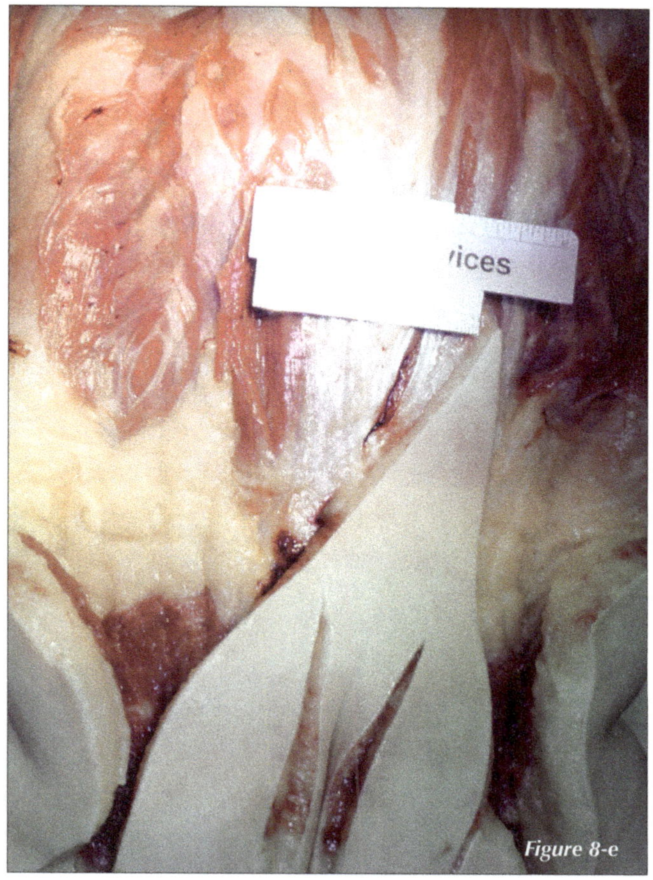

8. Using Case Study 8, identify the cause of death and manner of death and give evidence from the case study to support your determinations.

   Cause of Death:

   ____

   Evidence:

   ____

   ____

   ____

   ____

   Manner of Death:

   ____

   Evidence:

   ____

   ____

   ____

   ____

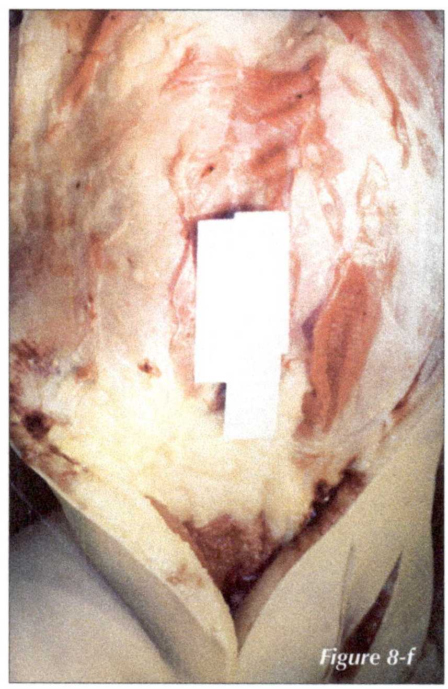

Figure 8-d. *Buttocks incised to show extensive fresh hemorrhage into subcutaneous areas.*

Figure 8-e and f. *Posterior surface of body with dissection of soft tissue of back showing hemorrhage into subcutaneous tissues of buttocks.*

Section V

Answer Key

Extended Multiple Choice Answers

1. A, B, C
2. A, B, C, E
3. A, B, D, G, J
4. A, B, C, E
5. B, C, D
6. A, B, D, F
7. A, B, D, E, F, H, I, J
8. B, C, D, E, F
9. A, B, E, F
10. B, D
11. A, B, C, D, F, H, I, J, L, M, N, O, P, R

Single Best Answer Multiple Choice Answers

1. B
2. D
3. C

Categorizing with Diagrams Answers

1-a. Static Injury

1-b. Dynamic Injury

1-c. Dynamic Injury

1-d. Static Injury

1-e. Dynamic Injury

Short Answer Answers

1. Most of the candidates for tissue and organ procurement involve cases that fall into the jurisdiction of the ME/Cs. Before a case is released for donation, permission must be obtained from the ME/C after a review of the case details. In these cases, most injuries have been documented, and at the time of death, the pathologist can review the medical records and determine whether tissues and organs can be recovered in cases where the injuries are elsewhere in the body. Infants and young children who are found dead outside hospital care will often be eligible for donation of certain tissues or organs without the fear that evidence will be lost.

2. A very rare abusive injury of the cervical cord is a distraction injury. It is most commonly caused by grasping the head and shaking the body. Distraction injury itself is the lengthening of the gap between bones, often coupled with immediate impaction, causing damage to tissue between bones or even fractures.

3. Retinal hemorrhages occur in about 85% of head trauma cases and are more common in those who die by head trauma than those who survive. They are also more common in causes of intentional or abusive head trauma than in accidental head trauma.

4. Through a separate, medicolegal death investigation and in conjunction with police investigation, the medicolegal team generates information needed by the forensic pathologist in order to fully evaluate a case. Without such extensive research into various injuries and possible causes of death, the cause and manner of death could not be determined with certainty.

5. Not all epidural hemorrhages are traumatic, and the presence of blood in the spinal region is not necessarily damaging to the spine or spinal cord. Epidural hemorrhages should always lead to an investigation into possible head trauma, but head trauma is not always the cause of such injuries. Hemodynamic forces can also be responsible for blood found around the spinal cord.

Clinical Vignette Answers

1. Subdural hemorrhages are caused by focal injuries, direct impact, or diffuse injuries (inertial loading). During the injury, the weak dural cell border or bridging veins around the brain are torn and blood floods the newly made cavity.

2. Subdural hygroma is present when cerebrospinal fluid enters the subdural space. The space is created by a traumatic tear of the arachnoid. If blood accompanies this fluid into the subdural space, the hygroma may become a subdural hematoma.

3. The cause of death in this case is blunt soft tissue trauma as there is extensive soft tissue damage but no evident injury to organs or dehydration present.

Matching Answers

Group I

1. D
2. A
3. C
4. B

Group II

1. A
2. B
3. D
4. C

Group III

1. A
2. B

Ordering Parts Answers

Group I: External Examination

1. B
2. D
3. H
4. F
5. A
6. C
7. G
8. E
9. I

Group II: Internal Examination

1. C
2. E
3. D
4. M
5. G
6. H
7. A
8. F
9. I
10. J
11. L
12. B
13. K

Text-Based Essay Questions

1. Case Study 1

   — Cause of Death: Acute carbon monoxide (CO) intoxication
   Evidence: CO level was 82%

   — Manner of Death: Accident
   Evidence: No history of maltreatment, entire family died

2. Case Study 2

   — Homicide. Given the historical details outlined in the case study, further historical evidence would not necessarily change the determination of this death as a homicide as the mother's actions in the scenario directly led to the child's death.

3. Case Study 3

   — Homicide. Given the historical details outlined in the case study, further historical evidence would not necessarily change the determination of this death as a homicide as the mother's actions in the scenario directly led to the child's death.

4. Case Study 4

— This injury is an intentional/abusive injury for several reasons. The child had obvious bruising to the chest, back, and right hip that were inconsistent with the mechanism of injury initially described by the father. In addition, the father's confession to striking the child confirms that the injuries to the child were abusive in nature. The small bowel and mesentery should both be examined extensively as they are rarely injured in accidents but commonly injured by intentional/abusive injury.

5. Case Study 5

— Accident. While this case was ruled an accident, some medical examiners or coroners may have ruled it a homicide due to negligence on the part of the caregiver. If there were previous CPS calls, other previous injuries to the child or siblings, or other suspicious activity, the manner of death may have been determined differently.

6. Case Study 6

— Cause of Death: Ligature strangulation
Evidence: Ligature from jump rope, jump rope still around neck, hemorrhage in neck

— Manner of Death: Homicide
Evidence: Inflicted injury with jump rope, confession by father

7. Case Study 7

— Homicide. Given the type of injuries, the family history of injury, and the accompanying injury of a sibling, additional historical details would likely further strengthen the determination of homicide as the cause of death.

8. Case Study 8

— Cause of Death: Suffocation
Evidence: Child found face down and had blanching lividity from the mid to left side of forehead, over the nose, and over the right cheek

— Manner of Death: Homicide
Evidence: Bruising to buttocks, areas of older injury, inconsistent history and developmental stage

STM Learning, Inc.

Leading Publisher of Scientific, Technical, and Medical Educational Resources

www.stmlearning.com

Helping professionals and students identify fatal cases of abuse and neglect

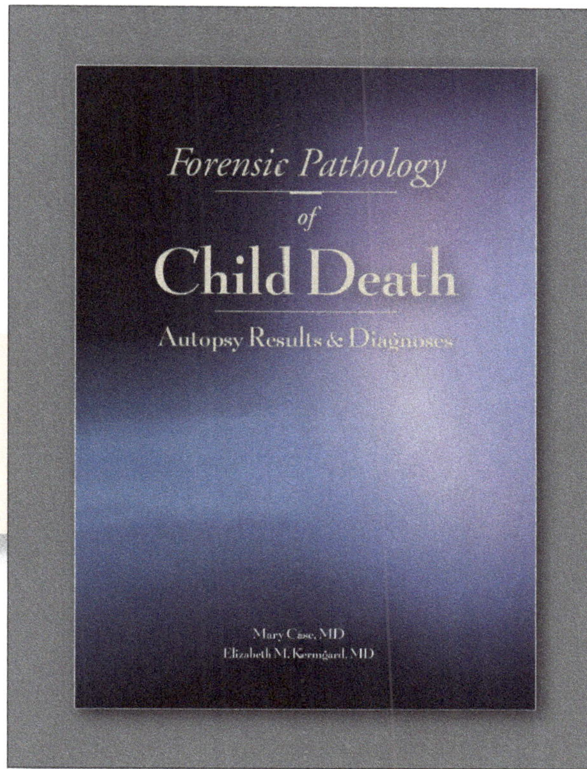

Table of Contents

Forensic Pathology of Child Death

Autopsy Results and Diagnoses

Mary E. Case, MD; Elizabeth M. Kermgard, MD

466 pages, 221 case studies, 783 images

Forensic Pathology of Child Death	*ISBN 978-1-936590-42-1 . . . . . $135.00 Print*
	ISBN 978-1-936590-81-0 . . . . . $110.00 eBook

With more than 200 case studies and 750 photographs, *Forensic Pathology of Child Death* is an exhaustive reference for professionals and students in the fields of forensic pathology, pediatrics, law enforcement, social work, juvenile court, and child advocacy. This new atlas is a comprehensive resource on child maltreatment, with high-quality images illustrating the injuries sustained and causes of death common among victims, as well as examples of accidental deaths for comparison. Each case study includes historical and circumstantial information, as well as family history and autopsy findings that medical and legal professionals might encounter in the field.

The author, award-winning forensic pathologist Dr. Mary Case, has practiced in the Saint Louis metropolitan area since 1975. For over 20 years, Dr. Case has served as Chief Medical Examiner to Saint Louis County and the neighboring counties of Saint Charles, Jefferson, and Franklin. Over the course of her career, Dr. Case has been an invited lecturer at over 400 professional conferences, seminars, and symposia, sharing her expertise with colleagues the world over. Now, with this new atlas, Dr. Case lends the full benefit of her experience to current and future practitioners in their efforts to investigate and prevent unnatural child death.

Representing a wealth of knowledge refined over the course of 4 decades in the field and in research, *Forensic Pathology of Child Death* is the definitive reference on forensic examination in cases of child fatality. This truly invaluable work will benefit forensic pathologists, their professional collaborators, and the communities they serve for years to come. It is a must-have for any in need of a more sophisticated understanding of unnatural child death and the circumstances under which it occurs.

Orders are billed for postage, handling, and state sales tax, where appropriate. Prices subject to change without notice.

1220 Paddock Drive, Florissant, MO 63033
www.stmlearning.com Tel (314) 434-2424
orders@stmlearning.com Fax (314) 434-2425